AMERICAN ELDERCIDE

AMERICAN ELDERCIDE

HOW IT HAPPENED, HOW TO PREVENT IT

Margaret Morganroth Gullette

THE UNIVERSITY OF CHICAGO PRESS

Chicago and London

The University of Chicago Press, Chicago 60637
The University of Chicago Press, Ltd., London
© 2024 by The University of Chicago
Published 2024
Printed in the United States of America

33 32 31 30 29 28 27 26 25 24   1 2 3 4 5

ISBN-13: 978-0-226-82776-6 (cloth)
ISBN-13: 978-0-226-82777-3 (e-book)
DOI: https://doi.org/10.7208/chicago/9780226827773.001.0001

Library of Congress Cataloging-in-Publication Data

Names: Gullette, Margaret Morganroth, author.
Title: American eldercide : how it happened, how to prevent it /
Margaret Morganroth Gullette.
Description: Chicago : The University of Chicago Press, 2024. |
Includes bibliographical references and index.
Identifiers: LCCN 2024013168 | ISBN 9780226827766 (cloth) |
ISBN 9780226827773 (ebook)
Subjects: LCSH: Older people—Institutional care—United
States. | Discrimination in medical care—United States. | Age
discrimination—United States. | Older people—Health and
hygiene—United States. | COVID-19 Pandemic, 2020– | Aging—Social
aspects—United States.
Classification: LCC RA997 .G85 2024 | DDC 362.1084/6—dc23/
eng/20240410
LC record available at https://lccn.loc.gov/2024013168

♾ This paper meets the requirements of ANSI/ NISO Z39.48-1992
(Permanence of Paper).

CONTENTS

PART 1

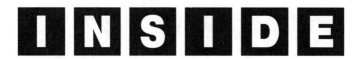

DEDICATION

American Eldercide is dedicated first of all to the people in the nursing facilities who died of COVID. Those we lost should have been better protected before the pandemic, and then, when it struck, immediately made safe by those state powers that had the utmost responsibility to protect them: the president, the Department of Health and Human Services, the Centers for Medicaid and Medicare, Congress, and the fifty states. Instead . . .

Where the residents were concerned, *instead* is the keyword of the new COVID Era. Instead, they were often forgotten and exposed. Discarded as if they were expendable. Dependent on authorities who seemed distant or witless. Unable to get away to greater safety. Often dying alone. All across the country, if an aide held an older person's hand and spoke words of love from family members or friends whom the dying person could not be with or even see, that was the best death available.

Tens of thousands of older adults and disabled people died in miserable circumstances, unnecessarily. More of them could have been saved—and in some places they *were* saved, to survive the pandemic, savor longed-for reunions, and await the next normal. Now is the time to show that the humiliating and lethal governmental abandonment of these people amounted to eldercide, and to explain how this unimaginable outcome could ever have happened, in a rich democracy, to the most vulnerable among us.

This book is fueled by anger at the injustice done to people living in nursing facilities, abandoned by our government in the hour of their greatest need. Indignation, when describing grievances and calls for a fairer world, feels useful.

"Useful" was my mother's favorite word of praise for ideas and actions. I want everyone to have what they themselves would consider a comfortable old age, as my mother did. After having worked for decades as a unionized teacher, in her early nineties she was able to move near us, into an assisted-living place she chose herself. In 2010, thankfully before the epidemic, she was able to die in her own bed, accompanied by people who adored her. I needed to call on the memory of her lifelong strength to face the suffering revealed by COVID and to uncover the full disgrace of systemic ageism.

When compassion is a passion, it may lead to social justice. Emmanuel Levinas, the philosopher, writes, "The face [we see] is the other who asks me not to let him die alone, as if to do so were to become an accomplice in his death." The story I tell aims to make readers feel as if the nation had neglected their own mothers and fathers . . . as if their own hearts would be squeezed in pain until they reach out to make amends and make sure that we never lose such precious ones prematurely again. Never again.

THOSE WE LOST

To those who grieve for loved ones lost in such unbearable conditions, the pain goes beyond words. Chris Kocher, who started a weekly support group for the bereaved, must be right when he says, "I guarantee you they are thinking about this every single day." To all of us lucky enough to still have older people in our lives, they comfort us by their presence. Repositories of family lore and legend, they dole out secrets and, for better or for worse, guide us by their experiences. We so much need our elders to be kind that we imagine they must be. "Sweet" (often paired with "incompetent") is one of the common epithets for older adults. Often, sometimes, rarely, never—younger people judge—elders manage to meet their judges' complex needs. Psychically, whatever their individual characters, those older than we are stand between us and our own mortality. With so many elders gone, however, we have lost that thick blanket of shelter. Perhaps when we complain of anxiety or isolation, as so many now do, those feelings arise because we feel more naked against the tornado winds of futurity. "Having an elder die is like watching an entire library burn down," lamented a young tribal American woman, Virginia Hedrick.

By 2023, over one million Americans had died of COVID. Several groups suffered disproportionately, especially minoritized and otherwise marginalized groups. But one particular group gained a historic significance that no one would wish on their enemies. In 2019, the

US government had provided congregate homes to 1.4 million people who needed care. These people should have been "the object not just of governance, but of *good governance*, a symbol . . . and indicator of a caring society and of national coherence and inclusiveness." Residents of those facilities were the first to die, and they began to die in alarmingly high, then seemingly unstoppable, numbers.

As of May 28, 2020, twenty-six states found that 50 percent or more of their COVID-19 deaths had occurred among these residents, who had been locked down in government-supervised care facilities. In what follows, the term *residents* refers to this group.

It is well known that the condition of convicted people in state and federal prisons was atrocious. Before the end of the first year, out of 1,215,800 prisoners, 1,700 had died. The residents' plight was far worse. The death total for nursing-home residents (as of the week ending on January 17, 2021), out of around 1,400,000, was at least 112,300, many times more. And that number is known to be a severe undercount. The government stopped counting during the first deadly months and thus made all true counts of the 2020 COVID toll uncertain.

The residents had constituted only 0.42 percent of all US inhabitants, a number small enough and localized enough for them to have been properly protected. A director of geriatrics in a resource-rich NYC hospital challenged experts "to cite another pandemic in which a majority of cases are so profoundly concentrated to one patient population and place." Nursing-facility reformers had anticipated that whenever this segment of public health was confronted by a new biological threat, the disaster would be due not to the residents' physical vulnerability but to the well-known, ongoing failures of the system. No one wants to be right about such dreadful prognostications. Reformers were distraught, frustrated, and helpless.

To say that it was just severe acute respiratory syndrome coronavirus 2 (SARS-CoV-2), a.k.a. COVID-19, that killed tens of thousands of residents and left their families bereft is to miss an important sociopolitical and ethical point. The US government was responsible for these people—for their housing, food, and health and welfare, and for their *lives*. Indeed, they are the only group that is in a position to make a strong claim on the government, as long as the US continues to have no universal national health care system. Protecting these residents is—*was*, has long been, and will remain—a legal and a moral responsibility.

When a highly contagious and potentially deadly disease strikes so special a group, the only sensible, humane response is to rush resources to them. Saving them would have been doable: There were *only* 1.4 million of them. They could have been wholly separated from contagion, like those privileged enough to afford to hunker down at home. Indeed, some facilities were fully protected. Even in 2020, a small percentage of nursing homes suffered no deaths.

Instead, the system at top government levels catastrophically failed most of them. In *The Value We Place on Life*, Howard Steven Friedman stated a sad truth: "Undervalued lives are left underprotected and more exposed to risks than more highly valued lives. . . . the young more than the old, the rich more than the poor, whites more than blacks, Americans more than foreigners, and relatives more than strangers." The residents—undervalued lives—were under-protected.

Among the millions of grieving families and friends, some suspect the truth this book will show. It was Eldercide. Indifference, rooted in preexisting ageism, killed the victims before their time. They all had more life to live, more love to give. The government's failure to protect them should strike fear in the hearts of everyone who hopes to grow old. Many of us already worry about finding ourselves, with some bodily weakness and too few resources, captive to a market-driven system that traps some older, disabled, and sick people in inadequate institutions.

For reasons that will become clear, the Eldercide in the nursing facilities did not cause outrage. The public should also have been amazed, as well as grieved, that so high a proportion of the million-plus COVID dead were older adults. My hope is that we can understand how and why this Eldercide happened and finally forge policies to prevent the next such public health catastrophe. With knowledge and goodwill, the US can achieve a profound alteration in consciousness: restoring the image of all older adults as human beings who have precious lifetimes ahead of us and an equal right to live. To emphasize why all old lives matter, I focus first on the residents.

ACROSS THE THRESHOLD, 2019

Across more than 15,400 nursing facilities in 2019, the residents "looked like America."

They represented all genders and sexualities, races and ethnicities, national and cultural backgrounds, religions, political persuasions, physical and intellectual abilities, temperaments, tastes in music, vocal tones, and life narratives. No two baby photos were alike! Only, among other Americans, by this time of their lives, they had experienced more hardships. Simone Weil, the French philosopher and activist, was viscerally attuned to how the maligned suffer from being maligned. She turned to the tragic characters of Aeschylus and Sophocles in order to find portrayals in which "a shamed spirit . . . is neither disguised, nor enveloped in facile pity, nor held up to scorn; here more than one spirit bruised and degraded by misfortune is offered for our admiration."

The residents accrued diverse experiences over the decades and became more individual as they grew older, as one does. They had witnessed firsthand and endured a long span of national history. A few had lived through the pandemic of 1918–1919. More had suffered the Great Depression. World War II. The internment camps. McCarthyism. 1968. Vietnam. The civil rights movements. 9/11. The Long Recession of 2008. In one week early in 2021, Elliot Kukla, a rabbi in San Francisco, "said goodbye to five clients who died of Covid-19 in nursing homes: one Holocaust survivor, two who survived the repressions of the former Soviet Union, one who always greeted me with a clipping about transgender rights issues (because she knew I was trans and might be interested) and one whom no one really knew."

The residents belied most common stereotypes. To start with, they were not all women. Almost a third were men, according to the National Center for Health Statistics. Immigrants held parts of two or more cultures in their heads, and two or more languages. They were diverse racially and ethnically, although most were white. At this stage of impoverishment, whiteness confers no exemption. Six percent were Latinx, 12 percent were Black. (In 2016, 12 percent of the centenarians were African American.)

Once you are inside, you see faces that recall noble artworks. (Like my father in his sixties, who had the fine profile of Giovanni Bellini's Doge Loredan.) One of Käthe Kollwitz's later self-portraits, with chiseled nose and fierce determination. A dapper mustachioed man straight out of Gordon Parks's portfolio. A man who is the spit of Lucian Freud in later life, looking stern. A head bowed by osteoporosis lifts to look you in the eye and turns into a friend of Alice Neel's as she relays gossip about the woman at the next table.

Age is not the only thing to know about them. It's not even the first. Residents covered a multi-decade spectrum of ages. Some were over one hundred. Around 16 percent of residents were *younger* than sixty-five, the so-called retirement age. ALS, Parkinson's, multiple sclerosis, Alzheimer's, diabetes, and heart disease—such maladies can all strike young.

Because of the stigmas of weakness, dependency, and dementia, and because walkers and wheelchairs are prominent in the public's visual imaginary, it is good to remember the photographer Ponch Hawkes's words: "The best thing about [having] an older body is you're still here; it's got you through so much." Hawkes photographs people over fifty and thinks we'd mollify our hard age gaze by seeing more older people in images. "All aging is 'successful'—not just the sporty version," anti-ageist writer Ashton Applewhite declares in one of her enlightening epigrams. "Otherwise you're dead."

There is no single "first" identity among residents. Not even ill health. A good number as usual were recuperating—from surgeries or strokes. Some who needed assistance with Activities of Daily Life (ADLs) like "toileting" and bathing otherwise enjoyed sturdy health. In general, older adults tend to think their health is "good" or "excellent," whatever their doctors' charts say. Either they emphasize the positive—"what I can still do"—or they have a more holistic view of health. Some were bed-bound. Some required around-the-clock med-

ical care, including replacing oxygen tubes, catheterization, and turning, because of physical limitations or paralysis. There were survivors
of polio, environmental racism, stroke, amputation, cancers. For various reasons, many more residents now are multiply impaired.

Some had mental illnesses; their number, due in part to legally required deinstitutionalization, had been going down. About half were
living within a broad spectrum of cognitive abilities, memory loss,
or loss of some executive abilities. Only 4 percent suffered from delusions. People with partial losses still have a lot of selfhood left—
telling stories, laughing at jokes, voting. At least a fifth of us—call us
the outsiders—have some impairment. A full half of us have some cardiac disease, according to the American Heart Association, so this is
the main illness residents arrive with. No ableist superiority is justified. In 2019 most residents rightly expected to live many years longer.

They remake their personal spaces on that assumption. Even if each
person has only 90 feet square (the minimum that owners must provide in my state), the presence of a few precious possessions makes
their area inside the building a bit more like "a room of one's own." On
the wall of one ward-like room hang eleven photos of family members
and a framed piece of ecru crocheting, laboriously tatted. In framed
photos taken of *them*, most occupants are smiling, looking at people
they like who took the image. Every object in a room—except the TV
for watching "the shows"—enfolds a precious fragment of the occupants' personality and history. Most prized pieces had to be left behind for lack of space. But here is a small flag. A crucifix. An open book
and tortoiseshell bifocals. A Raggedy Anne in a patchwork dress. An
award with a name in spidery calligraphy.

In the top drawer of a small bedside chest, securely wrapped: his
Swiss Army knife, the expensive one with multiple functions, the
last of his tools to go. Inside a grandmother's woven bamboo sew-
ing basket (Guangdong Province, 1880–1930), ornamented with red
silk: small snipping scissors shaped like a crane. In a bottom drawer:
a packet of the thinnest airmail letters, from Korea, via Army Post Office 246—with the one on top marked "Return to Sender."

Before the lockdowns, some residents found ways to do what was important to them. Despite age and impairment, "we don't stop wanting pleasure of whatever sort." They played Scrabble, pinochle, fivecard stud. Most bigger places had a space that could serve as a beauty parlor; people like to be as well-groomed as they were before. Some enjoyed the energetic shouting and groans on bingo days. (Don't smile. A small win can make a desired purchase affordable.) A grandparent gave a child an exhilarating ride on her wheelchair.

Food was notoriously bad, but in some places aides spoke their language and kitchens made familiar food. Residents extolled and disputed the virtues of rösti, kugel, samosas, dumplings. Some married couples could live together in a room. People met and fell in love. Parties were held when couples retook their vows, sometimes after fifty or sixty years of marriage. If staff organized a dance, there was music, cake, and crowns for king and queen.

Most residents were single: divorced or widowed, never married or, if they were LGBTQI, long forbidden to marry. LGBTQI people over sixty-five have a higher rate of chronic illnesses. They are half as likely to have life partners or significant others, half as likely to have close relatives to call for help, and four times less likely to have children — they are thus more likely to find themselves in a facility if they need care. The PBS documentary *Senior Prom* gives that term fresh, woke meaning. The film celebrates the legacies of LGBTQI people, once cruelly excluded from their own proms, who went on to become trailblazers. At the prom showcased in the movie, held in Hollywood, California, an older man, smiling proudly, is crowned Queen. "We're visible now, and we're going to keep on being visible," an activist firmly proclaims. In an enlightened culture, these words could become the proud motto of the entire world of residents.

Federal regulations mandate that appropriate activities be offered. Like much else that is "mandated," including physical care, activities don't occur if the operators skimp on hiring staff and don't get caught. In better-run places, residents choose from a range of programs — just as my mother did. Art, music, or woodworking were offered to those in the better memory units. People with such impairments retain their personhood longer if they are not sent to Coventry — if others include them. In an insightful Chilean documentary called *The Mole Agent*, eighty-three-year-old Sergio is hired to pose as an inmate in order to monitor the treatment of an isolated woman. Over those few months, Sonia, who had been sleeping during the day and shunning physical contact, becomes talkative as she responds to Sergio's attentiveness. Memory loss can produce or reveal extraordinary thoughts. Poets find them quotable. Some people write books about living with their cognitive losses.

Michael Bérubé, the father of a child with Down's syndrome, "suspect[s] that cognitive disability is the slowest-moving of the stigmas and will remain a subject of horror and avoidance for decades to come." "Treat us with patience, not hostility," one patient woman with Alzheimer's explained to a researcher who had asked what she most wanted from others.

Some new residents—maybe for the first time in their lives—sang in choruses, showed artwork, grew plants in raised beds. During lives of hard work, some had not had the leisure for such activities. Some had been movers and shakers when it counted in the movements of the fifties, sixties, and seventies. Many had been "essential workers," which we now know means people no one sees, doing valuable work for less pay than they deserve. They had been teachers, stoop labor, firemen, house cleaners—you name it, like all those articulate people in *Hard Times* and *Working* whom Studs Terkel loved to interview.

The residents were loved. Being there, in those crowded rooms, often in a hospital-like setting, did not mean they had been abandoned. Being mistreated might simply signal that their loved ones outside were also helpless to alter the system. Before the lockdowns, many residents went out regularly with family or friends, who also came to visit. In the dining rooms, people sat at tables for four or six, with their vehicles—their walkers and wheelchairs—parked nearby. Some entertained the staff. Some volunteered, using skills and talents.

Margaret Ditto, a fine-featured young certified nursing assistant (I) working in Seattle, who wears a single long dark braid down to her waist, said "I like talking to [residents] about their past, and what their marriages were like, and what their kids are up to as adults. I find a lot of comfort in that." (CNAs do 90 percent of the daily hands-on work that residents need, often work part-time in several jobs, and earn only a median annual income of under $30,000. Many, hired part-time, don't qualify for paid time off or health insurance. Some are also providing unpaid care for family members. A disproportionate number are female, people of color, and immigrants.) Younger people who get close to congenial elders must be calmed by seeing so many versions of later life, rich with jokes, songs, anecdotes, griping, and opinion—the poetry and factuality of otherness. They must admire those elders' ability to endure situations that cannot be avoided or made to come right.

Many permanent residents were well enough that they could have lived at home had they been able to afford to pay for help. In-home care is cheaper than residential care, but there's long been a counterproductive paucity of government money for it. Running out of money is the curse.

Even if they had worked all their lives, 63 percent of residents were on Medicaid, a program for low-income people and people with disabilities. It is funded mainly by the federal government, which guarantees part of the states' costs. But not all recipients started out as hardworking poor, long stuck in low-paying jobs. The well-enough-off can need skilled care—like Thomas, a minister whom we will come to know in the next chapter. Nor is it improvidence that drives people onto Medicaid. After about 1980, the US population grew steadily more unequal. Corporations chiseled employees out of their pensions. Middle ageism and outsourcing threw them out of work in their prime. Millions lost earnings that would have gone toward plumping up their Social Security benefits or laying down savings. Medical expenses pauperize many.

The economic slide has slammed many middle-class people. Having outspent their savings and assets and the short-term hospital stays paid by Medicare, they can find themselves in a facility they abhor. My mother's dear friend Vera, whose painful story I tell later, was one of them. If any of the residents had been less able to work all their lives or to save despite working hard, all the more reason to cherish and protect them from powerlessness. If the 1.4 million people in nursing facilities shared any single commonality, it was powerlessness.

Although in this book I call all of them "residents," about a third of this group at any time come for rehab, temporarily. Transients may arrive in casts or in recovery—from a stroke, joint replacements, or a prostate or cancer operation. They come for skilled nursing care, training in symptom management, or physiotherapy. They expect skilled, respectful care. In a home with adequate staffing they would get it, but adequate staffing is rare. In one small New Hampshire non-profit, however, Ms. M. moved in thinking it would be for life. She left forty-six days later, having lost more than twenty pounds with the help of a dietitian, her diabetes kept in check with oral medications. Her leg wounds were fully healed.

Most residents come permanently. Moving into congregate housing—nursing and veteran's homes, rest homes, assisted living, or continuing-care retirement communities (CCRCs)—is not a sign of being near the end of life. It's a new domestic setting in which to lead one's life. Assisted living is expensive; few such businesses accept Medicaid. People whose families adore them but cannot manage their intensive care, and people who cannot afford to hire aides, may qualify for nursing facilities. People with preexisting conditions or cognitive or physical disabilities are not ipso facto suffering. They may enjoy—one chooses the word "enjoy" deliberately—long lives. Most of the COVID dead would have. They were looking forward to visits, weddings, births, the sun rising.

Louise Aronson, author of the widely read book *Elderhood,* a geriatrician who loves to visit with her clients and give hugs, calls greater contentment a widespread fact, one of the psychosocial joys of growing older. Even when it doesn't follow a shocking disruption, however, making one "Big Move" in later life is heroic. The exchange is bound up with loss of community, status, and familiar objects. Discarding "the stuff!"—as gerontologist David Ekerdt calls it—is part of the ordeal: deciding what furniture and clothes and photo albums to leave behind, never to be seen again. The gathered possessions are a public sign of one's continuous identity. Most facilities require people to leave their pets, an added trauma. Instead, the sad newcomer may find "pet therapy," visits from pets, or robotic toys.

In any life, the Big Move may mark a grave loss of mobility, health, friends, a community, independence, or all of these at once. Moving into a feared place can feel like a wound. Doing so requires whatever people have accrued of ingenuity, patience, charm, resilience. Adjusting may take as much heroism as arriving in a foreign country with $16 in your pocket, as my immigrant grandfather did at age twenty in 1901.

After enduring such shocks, many try to recreate their normal, non-pathologized identities. It can take great effort to overcome the grief, anger, or depression at their own bodies or minds or incomes, or, sometimes, indeed, family, for failing them. Back of mind can be the possibility of losing more. People with moderate cognitive impairment may fear being seen to "wander" and then having to remove from their familiar room, however cramped, to a "secure" ward. Anxiety about this strange place can be exponentially greater than in any earlier move. Therapy, a plausible solution for anxiety or depression, is often unavailable.

But admission to a nursing facility can also be greeted with a long-pent-up sigh of relief. Some must be glad they are not homeless, as too many people over fifty find themselves. People whose rent was too high to buy medications, or who were subject to eviction, may find themselves grateful that the rent is paid. Some facilities, however, force those they consider "problems" to leave. John Oliver, in an outraged diatribe on *Last Week Tonight*, calls this practice "resident dumping." People who need specialty care—for cognitive impairments, AIDS, dialysis, head trauma, Huntington's, a ventilator, or hospice—may find a nursing facility essential. People abused by family members— beaten, raped, cheated out of their Social Security checks—are that much safer. It's a tremendous luxury—for women with huge family responsibilities, especially women of color, or widowers who never learned to do for themselves—to receive regular meals they don't have to cook, and to have someone else drag the vacuum under the bed.

Residents of nursing facilities often need to undo an aversion un-comfortably common among outsiders: their own, to being the self locked into that diminished situation. Having lived so long as community dwellers, they have imbibed the same remorseless stereotypes circulating about inhabitants of nursing homes—as soiled, degraded, abjected, and close to death. Inside, the carefully constructed social gradients and stigmas of outside still inhere. Residents may feel inferior and shamed instead of understanding "inferiorization," the *infliction* of a lower, demeaning status. Audre Lorde saw that "in a society where the good is defined in terms of profit rather than in terms of human need," a group of people, "through systematized oppression, can be made to feel surplus, to occupy the place of the dehumanized inferior." It's common enough to seem like mere common sense.

In one rare study of the desires of hospitalized older adults, 26 percent said they were either "very willing" or "somewhat willing" to move to a nursing home; but 30 percent said they would "rather die." (This wording was the only option provided for disagreement.) If they find themselves in an "institution" they believed despicable in advance, the stigma doesn't necessarily weaken. They may have trouble making friends because ageist slurs make the doors of clear perception as opaque as clouded glass.

Others find genuine, humane ways to surmount the constraints— like Lou and Joe, quoted in a lively book by Tracy Kidder about two accidental nursing-home roommates, *Old Friends*. John Leland, a journalist who interviewed people over eighty-five, sums up their achievement. "Everyone has had to find satisfactions that were still accessible—to make lives of what they had, not what was taken away. The elders have been living in this terrain for a long time." We outsiders, having lived through the deprivations of the COVID Era, not always in good humor, may now admire such abilities more than we used to. 2019 was the *Before Time*.

INSTEAD

Everyone, once inside, should be able to rely on a basic level of courteous attention: living nicely, with pleasant assistance if assistance is needed, nourishing and edible meals, exercise classes, access to the outdoors, clean rooms, and common spaces to entertain guests. Two advocates of reform say, rightly, that "the provision of care and service to residents, who are arguably the key constituents of the institution, is the entire *raison d'être* of LTC [long-term care] facilities."

However, the fact is that the government had entrusted residents' lives and comfort to a private money-making industry valued at over $141 billion. If government-monitored housing were guaranteed to be comfortable as well as safe and permanent, these locations could be desirable locations to age in place. Some are. The rest must now be made good enough so that the public officials responsible for elevating standards of care and imposing stiffer penalties on the industry for its COVID Era failures, could imagine their own parents or siblings—*or themselves*—living there.

Instead, the risk of dying was greatest precisely for those who needed assistance and chose or required congregate living in which to get it. After January 2020, most of those diverse individuals found themselves living in dangerously understaffed and under-equipped lodgings, often thought of, as we'll see in detail later, as "tinderboxes" at the start of a "perfect storm" or "wildfire." When the virus precautions ended all communal meals and activities, many were imprisoned in a room with another occupant or two or more. Pre-COVID, the worst case might have been that another occupant snored, screamed, or supported an odious political candidate. After March 2020, a roommate or an employee could pass you the deadly virus. The residents who had had little in common in 2019 except powerlessness were suddenly united by their risk of infection and a justified new fear of dying.

A DEEPER ASSERTION OF LIFE

Harold Furness, a World War II veteran called "the Colonel," is one of six survivors who turned one hundred at a home in Pennsylvania in 2021. "You think, 'Oh, I wouldn't want to live that long,' but every day is precious," he said. Before COVID, the residents had certainly expected to go on living. It's human to have such expectations—however old one is. Absent a life-threatening illness, older people do not think about death more than younger ones, and they seem more calm about it.

(Living long had certainly been my expectation in 2019: I was only in my late seventies, healthy and of strong stock. My grandfather, like my mother, had died at ninety-six. But COVID's global lethality undermined any complacency. After flying back from a huge conference where people had been too eager to hug the main speaker [me], I started sheltering at home. My husband and I wore rubber gloves to open the mail, paid a neighbor's son to shop, washed the food packaging. We kept sanitizer in the car, inside the hall, in the kitchen. We wore carpenter's masks—all we had at first—in public. Those were the known guidelines. We followed them strictly.)

Many residents felt they had a lot to live for. Ginny Dockweiler, living in LaCrosse, Wisconsin, said, after getting her first vaccine shot, "I figured I may be 86 but I have a few more years to live, and I want them to be healthy." When her granddaughter Tia was finally able to visit after a year's absence, they exchanged a long-awaited close hug, and at the same time, both said, "I love you." Ginny said wonderingly, "O, tears in the eyes?"

Billie Jean, an eighty-three-year-old in Charlotte, North Carolina, knew what she wanted: cooking, visiting grandchildren. "I definitely don't want the virus. You have the potential to die and nobody wants to do that." Pre-COVID, the idea that older adults living in facilities held assertively to life, like younger people, was blotted out of social consciousness by hearing so much about dependency, sickness, loss of abilities. In 2022, Dr. Jasmine Travers, a professor testifying to a Select Subcommittee on the Coronavirus Crisis, felt she had to rebut the alienating stereotype. "I urge the subcommittee to recognize that older adults do not want to stop living, although they may need help living."

People aging-toward-old-age need to hear that now—after the storms of mortality data and horrifying narratives of abandonment and abuse behind those locked doors. Although the whole life course from childhood on, Milan Kundera once wrote, is a "planet of inexperience," in the earlier parts we develop expectations by learning in advance about parenting or adultery or being an astronaut, through the storytelling of others. Among the true unknowns—*Whom will I find to love me? Can I get a better job?*—people seem unable to estimate in advance how long they will want to live in old age.

For some, that changed as the pandemic was prolonged, surge after surge. People learned they could die prematurely. Some discovered that they themselves, flush with life, might be considered expendable. They could hear spirit-crippling opinions. A callous Texas lieutenant governor, Dan Patrick, gained enormous attention when he said on right-wing Fox News on March 23, 2020, at the height of the spring panic, that adults "70-plus" should be willing to "take a chance on our survival" (risk our lives) for the sake of our children's economy. There was pushback to this calculated ageism: 90 percent of one Twitter sample retorted in different ways that *old lives matter*. But rebuttals are typically weaker than attacks. Not everyone who needed to hear this critique heard it. In the crisis, ageism swelled into fiendish expression and formerly unimaginable speech and behavior.

Outsiders might remain unaware of the daily threat, but residents could not remain ignorant of it. Most lived inside the cacophony. They heard the sirens of ambulances arriving and watched the gurneys depart. Hearses came and went. Phones kept ringing at the nurses' station.

For some, becoming conscious of their strong will to live in the face of danger profoundly changed their feelings about growing old. Jane Miller, an English writer who was eighty-seven and living at home, had formerly felt ashamed of being old, and had signed an advance decision to refuse resuscitation should she "lose my wits." "*What was I thinking?*" she berated herself in the midst of the pandemic. About her abrupt change of heart: "It's not just fear. It's also something better than that. It's wanting to live, wanting to come out of all this alive and changed, even ready for an altered world."

In February 2021, when the vaccine rollout had hit snags and many were refusing the jab (Twitter users, Fox viewers, "macho" men, and nurses' aides who had heard the vaccine was contaminated, among others), reporter Ginger Christ underlined "what we've seen across the country, which is that residents are overwhelmingly willing to get the vaccine." *They* were the leaders, undeterred by conspiracy theories. To them it was no hoax. Their urgency should tell us—if we need proof—that despite how hard it could be in those government asylums, however mean the aides, bad the food, or uncaring the hierarchy— that among the residents this deeper assertion of life is widely shared.

THE EDUCATION OF THE HEART

Who were they? Unless we knew someone "inside," we too may have been ignorant or indifferent. We may have unconsciously averted our eyes until the news of their dying or suffering appeared remorselessly day after day.

Ageism takes many forms. It is almost always braided into other stigmatizing social mechanisms—sexism and sizeism, ableism, racism and ethnic prejudice, homophobia. It crawls out in the hard-eyed age gaze of visual culture, with its far-fetched standard of youthful perfection, and of course in dementism, or dread of Alzheimer's-like memory loss. In our hypercognitive world, many people fear such loss more than they fear cancer. It hasn't helped that the "war" on Alzheimer's disease (AD)—an approach some critics consider to be overly "militaristic"—often engenders "emotions of fear, disgust, and anguish towards persons affected by memory loss, rather than fostering compassions, solidarity, and social inclusion."

At bottom is classism, the ingrained fear of poverty and the trained bias against the pauperized. Downward mobility afflicts a statistical majority of Americans as they retire, or if they cannot afford to retire. Residents are no longer "working," which has the modest cachet of a labor-market position. Most are indigent. Barely consumers, they are open to being considered doubly unproductive. They are the no-class poor. Compared to other groups with rights, who protest, they don't fight back. Being no-class-but-old through impoverishment has become a (silent) attribute of old age. Becoming more dependent, which can occur at any age, is also treated as synonymous with growing old. Ableism—looking down on people with impairments—is connected to fear of pain or dependency. These are the mountains of our own compound ageisms.

What does my term *compound ageism* do for us? First, it invites readers to discover whether they have been a target, since compound ageism developed long before COVID. Only a minority of our population lives long enough to be considered "old." I am one of the 16.5 percent of people over 65. We're not thought of as a minority. But skin and hair make us another of the visible minorities. We can't hide. The term *minority* helps us understand bias against our entire age group. Before the pandemic, the three things that most younger people associated with "the Old" were: Alzheimer's, celebrities (a ninety-year-old presidential skydiver), and Medicare. Almost nothing at all.

It may be useful to think of compound ageism as a Venn diagram of multiple overlapping ovals, in which the one new element, common to all, is age. Your own personal location will be there, possibly attracting banal stereotypes and life-distorting discriminations. Next, compound ageism invites readers to discover whether they are a part of the problem. A person not yet old, possessing the volatile age gaze, thinks they will never grow old. As I see it freshly now, from deep within the COVID Era, a neoliberal capitalist society deluded by meritocracy drives many people who are old enough to know better, but privileged, to feel a dumb sense of superiority. *Becoming one of* them *will never happen to me. I'd rather die.*

The societal weight of such a Himalayan range of prejudice crushed the residents into a single category, both hypervisible and invisible. Former certified nurse assistant Tracey Pompey saw how tepid public reactions were to the ghastly deaths. "People get desensitized to things like this," said Pompey. "If it happens to a child or a dog, people won't shut up." Among our minority of "the Old," nursing-facility residents—already estranged from society by America's cult of youth and by physical segregation—are possibly (with the exception of older prisoners, or unhoused older people) the most ostracized, misunderstood, stigmatized, stereotyped, and, alas, easily forgotten.

Compound ageism makes strangers out of people we formerly met as neighbors, creating condescension even toward erstwhile colleagues.

George Orwell once argued that such prejudices—his example was xenophobia—cause brutality. The loves and hatreds worm their way into a society's feelings and mental habits:

> [They] are part of the make-up of most of us, whether we like it or not. Whether it is possible to get rid of them I do not know, but I do believe that it is possible to struggle against them, and that this is essentially a *moral* effort.

Activist author David Swanson writes, impatiently, "We don't have time . . . to go on 'humanizing' away every little prejudice one at a time." Struggling against our feelings and misperceptions toward nursing facility residents is not a discipline. It comes purely from recognizing merit in *other* stories about them.

Stories bring about *Herzensbildung,* a beautiful German word that means the *education of the heart.* I started my own reeducation in early 2020, when I began wondering why the people sheltered in government facilities were the ones dying. I had to learn about them to write these pages. Coming to know them as best I could in a time when personal introductions were not forthcoming lifted some heavy stones off my heart. It replaced alienation with a kinship that proved to go far deeper than I can easily explain.

MISSED

A group portrait guides us as we cross the alienating threshold. It sweeps away stereotypes. It is fascinating and eerie to learn some of these truths. After all, we outsiders are each only one accident or acute event away from spending time in one of those 15,400 facilities, good or lethal. Or ending our lives in one of them—depending on our income and on government reluctance to expand long-term care programs into private homes and communities, as most people would prefer. Some fine people work in eldercare institutions. The rest of us need information about how the US structures its late-life options for poor folks in need.

It is also part of our human makeup that there is pleasure in discovering that we have been wrong—greater than the satisfaction of mouthing the conventional wisdom that we formerly thought correct. The residents are poignant and ordinary, like any other group innocently unaware they may soon be stricken, as if by the merciless hatred of some capricious deity.

A portrait like this one, however varied, uncovers only part of their whole human canvas. The rest has long been obscured by everyday compound ageism—casual, inhibited or openly nasty, dismissed as jokey—jacked up by our not-irrational dread of winding up in their state. Put another way, the 1.4 million—4.5 percent of Americans over sixty-five—are a special, precious group. Conscious that they had unique firsthand experiences of enduring this historic, terrifying time, I asked, *What must the people inside be feeling?* I wanted to hear their different voices. In the next chapter some of them paint a bigger part of the canvas. Many are eloquent. Absorbing truths about them, the heart opens a little wider.

Those who died, in their tens of thousands, are irreplaceable. People don't have to be perfect to be achingly missed. Millions—their relatives, friends, community members, caregivers—feel impoverished in myriad ways. It makes it worse that their deaths were premature. Not only their families but all of us should know as fact that they died before their time.

CHAPTER 1

"SWEEPING UP THE HEART, THE MORNING AFTER DEATH"

Lost. Tragically lost—because they could have been saved and because of who they were. They were the matriarchs and patriarchs; our parents, spouses, aunts, and uncles; the grandparents and great-grandparents of the children; our mentors and coaches, neighbors, colleagues, and friends; the children of our ancestors, co-builders of the nation.

In 2020, when the sudden COVID dying began, the United States became divided into two distinct and unequal groups: those who lived inside the nursing facilities—the 1.4 million—and the rest of us, outside, 330,000,000. Even amid the obfuscations of official recounts and a shifting mess of recriminations, one disproportion should never lose its grim historical power. By May 2022, at least 179,000 of those "insiders" had died. Almost 8 percent. In the same time frame, a million outsiders died: 0.33 percent of the 330 million. People who happened to be living in government facilities were *twenty-six times more likely to die* than the rest of us.

The Eldercide, viewed as a natural experiment in how a distinct, segregated group would be treated in the COVID Era, was the first prominent historic development of the new epoch. It posed a fierce challenge to the public health system's status quo. The disproportionate dying of these elders and disabled people was not only tragic but scandalous since it brought to light a new social fact: that every resident *could have* been protected. By sins of omission and furtherance of foreseeable harms, the government enabled an eldercide. Like so many other brutal sociopolitical tragedies stamped "United States bias," it could have been avoided.

LIVES CUT SHORT

Perhaps everyone we love dies too soon. That is our ego crying out, grieving, from Gilgamesh and Enkidu until today. But the harsh fact is that in 2020, in US sociopolitical circumstances, most residents of nursing and veterans' facilities who died of COVID did die prematurely. Some family members are sure of it. Marla Krohn's mother, Helen Center, died at the William Breman Jewish Home in Atlanta. In an interview, Ms. Krohn says, "My mother was only 88. I mean she lived a long life, but in our opinion, in our heart felt, her life was cut short. Because she wasn't an ailing woman." Family members who believe "it was cut short" are probably correct. The rest of us need to hear three untold facts.

The first unrecognized truth is that these residents would have lived longer than they did. Harvard Medical School professor Stephen J. Elledge explains why we didn't know it. "When people talk about deaths from COVID-19, they say, 'Well, they were old. They were going to die anyway.' . . . But people don't appreciate the fact that even if you're 70 or 75, you may still have 10 to 15 years of life left." Considering "years of life lost" brings us closer to appreciating the residents' feelings in March 2020, when they were locked in but the virus was not locked out. If they became confused or depressed, those feelings were not "natural" to being "old" but a result of their objectively frightening new circumstances. Whatever outsiders felt, the residents must have felt some mixture of longing for life, rightful expectations of receiving basic protections and care, and fresh dread.

NO ONE EVEN GOT SICK

The second truth is that no resident, however poor, feeble, or impaired, had to get infected with the new plague. We don't need to look far for proof that protection worked. In a small, nonprofit, Baptist-run facility in Baltimore, Maryland, whose low-income residents were predominantly African American, many with chronic conditions, not one person became infected during the frightening surge of March, April, and May, and none had done so as late as January 2021. Nursing homes remain highly segregated, and racial- and ethnic-minority residents tend to be cared for in a small number of larger facilities, located in communities of color, with the poorest quality of care and highly restricted resources. But in the Baptist Aged Home, everyone was protected by best practices, instituted early and with the greatest goodwill.

The director, the Reverend Dr. Derrick DeWitt Sr., instantly locked down. "When did you realize the threat was real?" he was asked. It was the day he heard then-president Donald Trump confidently proclaim that the United States "had 15 cases and it would soon be down to zero." Reverend DeWitt chose to stand solidly athwart the door that Trump left open to viral death. The place in his charge was small—only forty people—but he had already hired a full-time infection-control specialist. *Prevention* is what works best in public health; it's a tenet of the field. The readiness was all.

Quickly Reverend DeWitt brought in more personal protective equipment (the robes, gloves and masks soon known as PPE), and more TVs. He hired an extra activities coordinator. He had food brought to residents in their rooms—just as was done in fancy assisted-living facilities. He provided food for employees so that they wouldn't leave for lunch and heighten everyone's risk. His own aunt lived there. As soon as possible, staff instituted porch visits to counter fear, isolation, boredom, and failure to thrive.

Derrick DeWitt Sr., a hero of our time, was not alone. Nursing facilities should be havens, safe defensible spaces. Thankfully, some were. By one expert count, 1,950 nursing homes (out of 15,477) had no deaths at all through November 2020, the worst of times, before vaccination.

Nonprofits, often run by religious groups (Jewish, Catholic, Quaker), had lower death rates than the facilities run by for-profits.

In the three hundred Green House facilities, groups of small houses offering single rooms and baths, the median death rate per hundred residents was so low that mathematically it was statistically zero. (For facilities with fifty or more beds, the rate was 12.5 percent). In unionized workplaces, the mortality rate was 30 percent lower than in those without unions. "Unions generally demand high staff-to-patient ratios, paid sick leave, and higher wage and benefit levels that reduce staff turnover." (Turnover elsewhere could run to 100 percent a year.) The nonprofits were also "three times as likely as for-profit facilities" to satisfy the minimum staffing standard, which Joe Biden was the first president to require. During 2020, nonprofits in general were in fact able to *increase* nursing-care time per patient.

Any facility could have prepared beforehand, stocking gloves, gowns, and masks. Deciding hours per person of care should not be a profit-based business decision. Even after billions of federal dollars had been allocated for improving safety, after testing was available, and when providing PPE and enforcing safety protocols could have saved residents' lives, some facilities never acted. In law, ignoring safer options can raise the charge of "neglect" to criminal "reckless conduct."

The Baptist Aged Home, the "zero" deaths in 1,950 facilities, the Green Houses that operate in thirty-two states, the unionized places, the successful nonprofits—these are all important models. Every facility regulated by the Centers for Medicare and Medicaid (CMS) should be a model. The best-case scenario for a country like ours? Respect those who have no place else to go. Those who took direct care of the residents, mostly women of color, many of them immigrants, now honored as "essential workers," could also have been protected better, at least inside their work sites. Protect them all, starting with thoughtful, caring, prevention. It's as simple as that.

OLD AGE IS NOT A DEATH SENTENCE

The deep misery, the posthumous regrets, were avoidable. Some residents protected from COVID certainly died in 2020, as many do in normal years—but the others need not have died *then*. Everyone dies eventually, but not during a panic, from air hunger, in a terrible breathless death; not alone, not in an atmosphere of chaos and crisis, not in squalor, nor feeling disdained.

Ageist ableism blinds observers to biological facts. Here is the third truth, after "They would have lived longer" and "More could have been protected": Becoming infected with COVID was not always a death sentence. Although 28 percent of residents in some Connecticut homes tested positive (601 people), only 11.7 percent of an asymptomatic group went on to get symptoms. An early study from Italy, from the worst period, shows that even among people hospitalized with COVID, frailty and multi-morbidity, not age alone, predicted death.

In the US, we became so transfixed by the horror that the *survival* of residents was never discussed. Here is the startling data. Of the 1.4 million residents alive in 2019, subtract those who were exposed to COVID and became infected—by 2022, at most a million cases. That means at a cautious estimate, four hundred thousand went unscathed—either so well protected they never got infected or asymptomatic and then resilient. Among the infected million, how many survived? A question never asked. The welcome news I bring is that *hundreds of thousands* of this group survived—ultimately, perhaps as many as 80 to 90 percent of the people considered most frail and vulnerable.

One was Emogene Stamper, ninety-one, a Black woman who lives in Co-Op City in the Bronx. She had worked helping ex-offenders find jobs. The first nursing home "was like a dungeon, and they didn't lift a finger to do a thing for me," she told veteran columnist Judith Graham emphatically. In her rehab hospital, her new doctor acted surprised she was ninety and still alive. Ms. Stamper's comment: "That lets you know how disposable they feel you are once you become a certain age."

Geneva Wood, age ninety-one, even survived the Life Care Center in Kirkland, Washington. Ms. Wood was to be discharged, but she broke her hip in late February, just as that Life Care Center, advertised as a "five-star" facility, became a code word for elder death. Ms. Wood told AARP, "My roommate was coughing. Everybody was saying bronchitis. Then I got a cough and could hardly breathe. Thought it was pneumonia. I remember them saying I had a 102 fever. I guess I didn't know enough to be scared."

As they died, the residents of care facilities were being counted, however incompletely. The media reported that they constituted an astounding percentage—"30 percent" or "40" and then "55"—of the deceased in a given state.

The data blizzard, blinding as a sirocco, hid the fact that in unimaginable circumstances, surprising numbers of residents who caught COVID were tough and lucky. Surviving, many had an amazing story to tell. *Survival* comes as a surprising perspective. By offering it, I don't intend the fact to be used unscrupulously, to lessen our pity for the dead or concern for the living—many of whom still contend with long COVID or PTSD—or to discount the need for nursing-facility reform. My point is that the fact of survival wasn't noticed because it was scarcely conceivable. Survival did not confirm the implacable COVID Era assumption: "the Old were gonna die anyway." It was wrong to take this belief for granted. Had the survival numbers been known, however, they still might not have challenged our erroneous beliefs or feelings.

CALL IT ELDERCIDE

With clearer vision, the COVID Era Eldercide can be recognized as an avoidable governmental failure. If that story is not yet known, the reasons are complexly historical, political, and psychological. Hannah Arendt explained a certain American obliviousness as a national characteristic. Soon after she arrived as a Jewish refugee from Nazi Germany, stateless, she described the US as a country that has

> the passion to straighten things out, not to tolerate unnecessary misery—all this has a flip side, however, which is that nobody worries about what cannot be changed. . . . The basic response when

someone dies or when something goes irrevocably wrong is: Forget about it.

The Eldercide was an "irrevocable wrong" being hastily transformed
into a *necessary* misery. During the pandemic, few assertions about the
splintered collective called "Americans" were possible. But the belief
that "the Old die" helped create a sweeping sense of futility. *American
Eldercide* tracks and disputes that culture of feeling.

Fighting futility, we now have the three facts about the residents to
keep in mind; almost everything that seemed "irrevocable" could have
been different. We have a concept we formerly lacked that allows us
to account for our collective blindness as social bias: *eldercide*. Eldercide had previously been narrowly understood as private intrafamilial
or parricidal violence: Lizzie Borden with her axe, giving her mother
forty whacks. Now this Eldercide must be redefined, as the abandonment of this concentrated and confined group of older adults to exposure and death, on a mass scale, by those responsible for their welfare.

Eldercides have occurred in the US before. In Hurricane Katrina
in New Orleans in 2005, no one under five died, but 64 percent of
identified victims were over sixty-one, clustered in poorer, low-lying,
mostly Black neighborhoods. Those responsible called the events "a
natural disaster," but there is no such thing for people who are old
and poor.

The *American* Eldercide is specific to the US, distinguishable from
the COVID eldercides in other Americas, such as Canada or Brazil.
The term is sometimes *geronticide* or *senicide*, from the Latin words
geron or *senex*, old man. *Eldercide* is a more powerful keyword—
immediately understandable and weighted by the inclusion of women
and by respect for old age. The term urges us to resist stereotypes,
prejudice, and discriminations and to seek causes.

The first responses to COVID—inside the lockdowns of March
2020—made this Eldercide undeniable. The residents were captured
in a public health system that promised decent help, starting with
"safety," the protection of life. Reformers had long known, however,

as proved by the forthright six-hundred-page 2022 report from the National Academies of Science, Engineering, and Medicine (NASEM), that "U.S. nursing home care is ineffective, inefficient, inequitable, fragmented, and unsustainable." "Care" could also be cruel and lethal.

In many facilities, a silent eldercide had been going on for decades; indeed, it continues. Researchers suspected that many owners' pattern of understaffing for profit led to abuse or neglect and thus extra deaths. But evidence was sparse; there were the crime scenes, but the crime was typically undetectable. Residents died one by one. The bodies were buried decorously, one by one; mourned quietly, family by family. The public believed that residents died *naturally*. And we lacked a name for the phenomenon. A named concept reifies, clarifies, leads to further questions. Then came the Coronavirus pandemic, and the deaths came fast, from everywhere, all at once—too many to be ignored.

Within the limits of their powers of love, every bereaved family in the US loved their lost relatives and friends. Some now sorrowfully or bitterly believe they did wrong by "putting" their relative into an institution. But that blame is misplaced. It was the system that made the disproportionate deaths predictable. The Eldercide of the COVID Era could not be hidden. It demanded a forensic exam. Proof was there for the digging.

THE GREATEST HUMAN FORCE A POPULATION KNOWS

The new facts about these COVID deaths—that they were avoidable and premature, that protection was doable and survival possible for many—ask us to point an objective accusatory finger at first causes. In the steep pyramid of government, state power is the greatest human force a population knows. It is most beneficial when it works for the benefit of the vulnerable, the most potentially deadly when adverse. One property of state power, I submit, following Simone Weil, who wrote forcefully about vulnerability in her notable essay on the *Iliad*, is its ability to suddenly turn any creature in its charge—whether a migrant, a prisoner, an enemy, or a nursing-facility resident—"into a thing while he is still alive. . . . He is alive; he has a soul; and yet—he is a thing." Abandonment by a government that holds your life in its hands is a harsh fact that the Greeks in their tragedies recognized as the gravest injustice. They worshipped capricious deities, but they were clear-eyed about the difference between what the gods decreed and an overlord's cruelty.

When the pandemic began in early 2020, the government failed us *all*, as political philosopher Danielle Allen shows in *Democracy in the Time of Coronavirus*. But residents are a special responsibility of the public health system, and they were the first to die. The abdication of duty—nonfeasance—started with then president Trump's dismissive lies, uttered in his trademark brisk offhanded tone: *It's a hoax; it will end like a miracle; it will be over by Easter*. The indictment includes Congress and the part of Health and Human Services (HHS) with prime responsibility for the residents, the Centers for Medicare and Medicaid Services. This is the agency I focus on in the next chapter. Seema Verma, its director, followed Trump's lead—unconscionably slow to mask up or serve the special people in the agency's care. Verma abandoned the residents to the oversight of the facility owners, a fatal step.

Congress's shaping of the institution had almost guaranteed irresponsibility and lack of coordination. Congress invented a joint state and federal program in which Medicaid—which covers long-term care for eligible people—is constrained by hybrid public financing. The residents are considered "indigent" even though they pay monthly for often stingy care with every possible private resource that the facilities can garnish: pensions and Social Security checks, received after years of work and paying taxes. Once inside, residents control only a "personal needs allowance"—set at rate that is both infantilizing and low. (In Massachusetts the allowance was $18.20 per week, a sum that had not been raised despite decades of inflation.) Bureaucrats who never read Dickens's *Oliver Twist* must have seriously debated whether granny needs more. In some states, residents can't afford a doll for a grandchild or disposable adult underwear. Toward board and keep and care, Medicaid pays "about two-thirds of what Medicare pays for the same services, framing Medicaid recipients as worth about two-thirds of other people." It's a harsh discrepancy.

When Senator Ron Wyden's Finance Committee held a hearing headlined "A National Tragedy" in 2021, Professor Tamara R. Konetzka, who had looked at data on 13,312 facilities, testified that those "serving more (>40%) non-white residents experienced more than three times as many COVID-19 cases and deaths as those serving primarily white residents." Racism harmed and killed people of color disproportionately. Yet the great majority of residents were white. One counterintuitive conclusion is inescapable: in this Eldercide, the elite white establishment left even its white elders unprotected when they were old and poor and dependent on others for care.

The neglects of 2020 were heinous. Congress, as the first branch, should have immediately imposed a national face-mask mandate for nursing-home employees. Such a mandate would have saved lives and established a national anti-ageist standard hard to oppose. (The Centers for Disease Control recommended *cloth* masks only in July 2020.) Trump used the Defense Production Act to produce some equipment; late as it was, that equipment could have been sent directly to nursing facilities. Executive responsibility by law was handed off to the states that regulate, partly fund, and are supposed to monitor nursing facilities. Their departments of public health are the next line of defense. By April 8, 2020, when the CDC had developed a good test, Trump had stopped testing. But states could have tested residents and staff, as West Virginia's governor was first to do.

The situation was chaotic, but many good feasible steps were neglected. Lacking CMS leadership, *states* could have initiated immediate surveys and required facilities to reduce their part-time employees, who were more likely to be carrying the disease between facilities. None did. An AARP vice president, Elaine Ryan, reported that some facilities offered staff on-site housing to contain community spread. Some separated patients on COVID-only floors or buildings, a practice called cohorting. "These actions could have been mandated by all states or the federal government, but were not." In December 2020, a post-holiday surge was hitting nursing homes hard, *again*. An

AARP spokesperson in Florida said failure was ubiquitous: "No state is protecting frail elders well."

Congress had handed responsibility for part of the Medicaid budget to the states. Some states begrudge the expense. State budgets swing wildly depending on the business cycle. Some legislators siphon off money or set rates low. States individually license owners of facilities and monitor them, but harm to residents had long gone on, largely undetected and unpunished. Bureaucracies defeat the people who are trying to do right, one of 3,500 county health officers fiercely explained. "Sins of commission got you fired. Sins of omission you could get away with, but they left people dead."

RESPONSIBLE

What happened to the main institutions that should have galloped to the rescue? The fact is that the jobs of top officials and operator/owners entailed a duty to act to "promote and protect the rights of each resident." The definition of *neglect* in the Elder Justice Act, reauthorized in 2017, is "the failure of a caregiver or fiduciary to provide the goods or services that are necessary to maintain health and safety of an elder." CMS "is responsible for ensuring that nursing homes nationwide meet federal quality standards." Laypeople may correctly assume that responsibility for the residents' rights and lives depends at bottom on the Constitution: the respect for "life" which alone makes possible liberty and the pursuit of happiness. The Eldercide—past and present—can be seen as a widespread violation of law and statute, residents' rights, citizen rights, and human rights. The residents were not "vulnerable" as much as endangered.

The most endangered fell out of their nation's formalized social embrace. Their tragedy was our disgrace. The word "embrace" comes from the word for *arms*. The arms of the nation did not uphold our elders, long almost invisible in their tiny multi-occupancy rooms. COVID was the most dangerous pandemic illness since the global influenza epidemic one hundred years before. As before and again now, people directly responsible for their welfare did not treat the residents as precious, in need of special consideration. A negligent system exposed them.

Once COVID-related decisions were made—or, more typically, omitted, within this country's fragmented public health system for older and disabled and indigent adults—the local consequences were fated. The people at the bottom struggled in circumstances not of their own making and out of their control.

INSIDE THE LOCKDOWNS, TRAPPED AND WAITING

There is a time "that will be forever burned into our minds as the month everything changed—March 2020." The COVID Era began as a series of delays with dire consequences. China announced a virus in Wuhan in December 2019. The US lost precious weeks for prevention. The World Health Organization announced a pandemic on March 11. Only in mid-March (too late) did nursing-home lockdowns begin. The Seattle outbreak had occurred in February, when Geneva Wood fell sick.

Many people remember the exact day when they stopped shaking hands and started buying Purell sanitizer, putting the mail in the oven on low heat, and wearing a scarf before the N95 mask became available. People who could, stopped going out. If they met friends, no hugs were exchanged. People bumped elbows instead. You may recall how endangered you felt and what precautions you took or neglected. Mid-March 2020 has become like 9/11: Some of us will be telling stories about it to our grandchildren.

(For me, the memorable date was March 11, 2020, when I flew back from that huge friendly conference. COVID was believed to be a death sentence. At home, my husband and I self-quarantined for fourteen days—then considered incubation time. I was one of billions of people startled to notice they had just been in contact with others, at a mall, in a movie, a place where someone was spewing a medieval mace with devilish rusty spikes—the mesmerizing emblem of the Era, a fuzzy color-enhanced drawing from an electron microscope. I wondered what to do if these were my last days. No activity seemed serious enough, while calling people to say goodbye would have been absurd. But in that torpid condition I read triage guidelines that permitted hospitals to exclude older patients from access to lifesaving ventilators. The revelation was appalling: Unashamed, undisguised medical discrimination was signed by apparently honorable, even distinguished physicians. The critique I wrote in haste—published March 21—was the first impetus for this book.)

Even before the end of that month it was clear danger was shared unequally. The residents of nursing facilities were dying in heavy clusters, isolated from family and friends. A tired woman hospitalist in Coventry, England, said, "No one should have to die alone and in pain. Yet that was happening every day. That is not dignified . . . It's cruel."

Overnight, most "homes" were transformed into perilous units. An AARP state director from Arizona testified to a Senate judiciary committee that, unlike others on the outside, "LTC residents don't [choose their level of risk]. They were not even allowed to leave. They were locked in and families were locked out." They couldn't get out to buy masks or gloves. Residents were shut away from the very people who had supplemented staff assistance—family members or volunteers who had helped them bathe or eat, who monitored the quality of their care and the cleanliness of the surroundings; social workers, if any; the state ombudsman, who dropped in to ask if they had complaints. When it most mattered, communicating became more difficult. Not all residents had phones, tablets, or Wi-Fi. Unless they had a medical appointment, people could be confined to their small rooms or beds for twenty-four hours a day. Exiled in their room aside from the hours of care allotted to them (if performed), some said they felt helpless, as if they were "in prison." Everyone was turned into an inmate.

The lockdown dragged on. A retired professor of English, then ninety, my friend Mary Mason was living in a well-run retirement community. But "the description of the 'new normal'—confinement, unpredictability, social separation, is 'the old normal' for many with disabilities." The quarantine, she wrote for a disability journal, is "hard: relentless, inevitable, and suspenseful as I hear statistics and reports on all the media."

In those frightening circumstances, were the residents resilient, as a residue of lifetimes that included suffering? Or is that virtue attributed to elders to save us from asking them directly if they felt loneliness, panic, dread, or sorrow? No group portrait is possible of the disruptions of habits, of feeling unsafe. A million-plus people; a million-plus ways of dealing with danger, neglect, fear, or loneliness. There are no documentaries of what occurred in the crowded bedrooms and empty halls as the year wore on.

Understanding the pandemic requires listening to these survivors' stories. Unfortunately, their voices were rarely heard in news reports. It was as if yellow police tape barred the entrance to most of the 15,477 buildings: "Keep Out." About the residents' concerns, our imaginations continued to be stunted. I wanted to cross the forbidden threshold, mentally. I had done so physically years before, visiting a dear friend of my mother's. (I tell Vera's story in the epilogue.) It took extensive research to find even the fragments of their stories that I quote here. Those fragments proved vivid and expressive. Funny and touching. Informative. Endearing. Sad. Enraging. *Essential.* I want to make more of their stories indelible.

"what's important, and what's not"

In mid-March, Beverly Breitenbach Thomas, of Pittsburgh, who was eighty-one years old and needed dialysis three times weekly, worried: She had lost a grandmother to the 1918 flu pandemic. A family photo shows Ms. Thomas's curly white hair, oval silver glasses, light-pink lipstick and engaging smile. Ms. Thomas did not trust caregivers. "I've been to a lot of football games at Three Rivers Stadium and watched those women come out of those stalls and run out not washing their hands," Ms. Thomas said. "Dreadful." Her daughter, Mary Ann Thomas, a reporter, feared the facility would become "a death trap."

Some residents felt safe. Grace Barnum, seventy-six, in New London, Connecticut, said, "We were really lucky to have such precautions taken, you didn't see that everywhere, and the people really paid the price." Some residents were profoundly grateful and emotional. The aides were "angels." This fact is important to remember for the future—given that some people will always need congregate settings for assistance, and they could be made safe. Some well-run homes were cradles, not barracks.

Deprived of activities but ensconced in a single room with the door shut at the Hammond Lane Center in Baltimore, Sheila Liles watched Netflix, assembled puzzles, and kept in touch with outsiders by phone. In a news photo, Liles, a Black woman aged sixty-five, was shown outdoors enjoying winter weather, wearing sunglasses and a warm watch-cap. "When you're restricted like this, you start realizing a lot of things—what's important, and what's not," she said. "People are starting to realize how connected we really are, and how we need each other, worldwide."

Some of the exiles took charge. They kept amazing equanimity and instilled confidence in others. Charles Miller, age seventy-three, in Connecticut, told his family not to come. "Keep my family safe," he said. "That's important. . . . It's tough on the elderly, but I think it's tough on everybody," he said judiciously. In one Pennsylvania facility, a rebel sneaked into another wing to see her buddy. "They got together and laughed and had some fun." At one point, Hebrew Home in Riverdale, the Bronx, was "the leader of deaths from Covid complications." In 2023, the chief operating officer, David V. Pomeranz, recalls, "The most calm people during those times were the residents. They [had] lived through wars, diseases. They were a source of comfort for staff who were very anxious and nervous." How many of us would have done as well?

A Massachusetts psychotherapist, carefully gowned, gloved, and masked, interviewed a patient of his who had "a mixed experience" amid the pandemonium:

> On one hand, I received good care from the aides—at least in the
> early stages, and when I was sick with COVID, and I got good phys-

ical therapy, and that got me walking again. I also got a little insensitivity, at times, because the workers needed to take care of their needs rather than mine, or so it seemed.

Some complained about lapses of cleanliness and care. James Stalker was living in Pleasant Lake Villa Nursing Home in Cleveland. (It had a five-star rating.) "'There is no accountability anymore because all you have to do is say it's COVID,' Stalker said. 'How does COVID allow you to leave a [soiled] bed pan by my TV?'"

Floyd Dalseth was one of the transients in rehab who got stuck inside, recovering from a bad fall in October 2019. He was interviewed by Chris Serres of the Minneapolis *Star Tribune* in May. "Dalseth tried not to panic as he watched three of his roommates at the St. Therese of New Hope nursing home die within the past month," Serres wrote. "Now Dalseth, 85, has contracted the deadly virus and fears he may never make it home. 'I just want to get out of here,' said Dalseth. 'Death is everywhere.'" He couldn't go home before testing negative. Tests were hard to come by. "'It's a case of horrible timing. Now I feel trapped and I'm kicking myself for not acting sooner.'"

Thomas M. was also trapped, separated from his wife, Patricia. After two falls that hospitalized him, he told Patricia he was willing to go into skilled nursing to get physical therapy, alone. Alzheimer's was going at a nice slow pace. "I'm not going to let Alzheimer's ruin my life; I'll just enjoy life for as long as I can," he said. "I'm sorry I'm not the man I was." A retired Unitarian Universalist minister, a mainstay for his parishioners for seventeen years, at eighty-four Thomas stood six feet tall, with keen blue eyes and a boyish, triangular chin. Patricia wrote me about him. Thomas had said that "it was too hard for me to take care of him and he didn't want that for me."

Patricia had planned to spend every day with him. But it was that treacherous March. The new facility didn't tell her that a resident had contracted bronchitis. "Had I known . . . I never would have allowed Thomas to go there." Only by phoning constantly did she discover that he was suddenly to be transferred there out of hospital. Richard

Mollot, executive director of the Long Term Care Community Coalition, explains that transitions are often badly managed even in normal times: "You're not given a lot of time and choices when you leave the hospital." Patricia staked out the parking lot of the nursing facility. As Thomas was being wheeled rapidly inside, each called out "I love you." There was no time to say more. She could not have known that would be their last sight of each other. Thomas died of COVID soon after. At Belmont Manor, at least sixty out of 135 people died of COVID. From its five-star rating, no one could have known that its reported nursing hours had fallen 20 percent below the state average.

Everywhere, relatives were calling, frantic. Phones ringing shrilly at the nurses' station were not always answered. Some inmates heard panic in the aides; some guessed at it. Many suffered from lack of activities and loss of chosen company. "Why does no one come to visit me?" was the question from those who could not understand that visits were no longer permitted. "They used to have music, they played movies for them, played games," Dr. Michael Wasserman, a geriatrician and past president of the California Association of Long-Term Care Medicine, explained. "During the lockdown none of it was happening. So they have [had] no stimulation of the brain for at least a year. This is why they got worse in their manifestations." Many of us outsiders also got worse in our own manifestations.

In March, Melissa West's ninety-five-year-old mother-in-law was living in a nursing home. West couldn't stop mulling over her situation. "I just think of her being there by herself. Just sitting in her wheelchair all day. Being trapped and waiting." After the SARS epidemic, even though that disease had been quickly contained, scholars noted that trauma had arisen among people identified as at high risk. In the facilities in 2020, it's likely that being supremely singled out, as residents clearly were, heightened anxiety. My friend Mary Mason felt they were bombarded by bad news. PTSD is worsened when trauma is not alleviated by therapy. In Massachusetts, Dr. Asif Merchant, partner of a company that runs medical services for forty-five nursing facilities, walked the dreary, empty communal spaces.

"It's a very grim picture to have to paint it," Merchant said. "It felt like the silence of death in the hallways. And a lot of people lying there in their bed, listless."

"THEY DO NOT SPEAK THEIR BIGGEST FEAR"

Griping about the activities director, lack of visitors, and mediocre food were the bland topics that now characterized the "good old days." Isolation gave people plenty of time to think.

The new danger was death from a terrifying unknown disease with a sudden onset. Incoming COVID was a constant threat. Residents could not practice self-quarantine if they lived two or more to a cramped cell, with only plastic shields or a curtain dividing bed from bed. Aides could bring in the disease at any moment. In the next bed, sick people were coughing. Roommates died. Healthy people must have been on watch for the telltale cough, chills, loss of taste and smell. Residents could anticipate hospitalization, intubation, coma, asphyxiation. Calling an aide or nurse, a family member, or — in desperation — 911, people were crying out, "I can't breathe."

For over a year, and in many places much longer, the inmates were like soldiers in war, forced to lie low in trenches, subject to the unscheduled terror of incoming bombs. The boredom was more like wartime pauses between attacks.

In mid-March, Sara Sidner, a CNN interviewer reporting on Kirkland, wrote, "They do not speak their biggest fear, but they are acutely aware coronavirus has killed 22 people associated with this facility; 18 of them were patients." Janet Siebrecht, a New York State resident, said, "There's a lot that we don't know are dead or alive because we can't go from wing to wing." In New Haven, in a facility that was to see sixty-nine residents infected and twenty-nine die, Grace Davis caught COVID. She survived — another centenarian who did so. She and others were, Davis said, "petrified that tomorrow we're going to pass."

Ruby Walling, a ninety-four-year-old woman with some cognitive impairment, arrived at a West Texas facility in June after testing positive. Nursing facilities in Texas typically had fewer employees than they needed even before the pandemic. Walling started calling her daughter Barbara, "hysterical and sobbing." "She said she would kill herself if I didn't get her out of there," Barbara told a reporter. At a time when it was not easy to get in, she managed to take her mother out. She found her "'filthy,' as if she hadn't been bathed during her stay there."

Geraldine Garcia, admitted April 4 to a Nevada facility for nothing more than a broken ankle, was able to check out ten days later. At one point Ms. Garcia, seventy-four, had to hold herself up on a bedpan for forty minutes before help came. She heard that a man had died from the coronavirus. "I thank God that I yelled and told them I wanted out of there. I just couldn't take it no more," Garcia said. "I could have been one of those that was stuck in there and maybe died."

That fate befell Maria Alimusa, who had come to a Nevada facility to recover from a stroke. A nurse for thirty years, she knew enough to worry because the care was so poor. She left a voicemail for her son in California. You can hear her pleading. "It's really getting bad here and I just don't feel safe anymore. I need to transfer to another facility, so I need your help." Then COVID struck. In a quavering voice, a later voicemail told him, "I just want to say I've been thinking about you, and I feel like I'm going to be passing soon." Alimusa died in hospital on April 14, just as Garcia was quickly leaving.

Ms. Cowan-Hills, a resident heard live on an AARP special, took initiative. Like others, in desperation she called 911. "I want to go to the hospital and they're not letting me," she told them. On the recorded call you can hear her voice, hoarse from lack of oxygen, as she accurately answers the questions. Chills, yes. Sore throat, yes. "Yes, I can't breathe." She was transferred to a hospital and died a day later. Many were left too long untended.

Most could not have left, even without COVID. They had no place to go. If a relative had been abusive or become meaner as a woman needed more physical care, she couldn't go back: The perpetrator was still there. Some residents had sold their homes. Chuck Sedlacek, who needed rehabilitation after breaking a bone, was admitted to the Life Care Center on February 20, 2020, just before it became infamous.

Sedlacek, eighty-six, soon tested positive. "If they were so concerned about this respiratory outbreak, why were they taking new patients?" Sedlacek's daughter asked in March, in utter frustration. "No other rehab center will take him."

There were other baleful wrongs. Administrators not allowed to raise wages. Aides not being tested. Aides working inhuman amounts of overtime forced to neglect some patients, too rushed to wash their hands between visits.

Don Odom wrote to the governor of South Carolina. He was willing to risk his life to see his wife.

> These are my wife's most important days of Hospice Care and dementia. They say she is not dying but as I view her through the window daily, I see in her eyes that I'm losing her. I want so bad to be with her and hold her fetal restricted body in my lap and rock her. She just looks back at me in the window, then turns her head.

SUSPENSEFULLY, LIFE WENT ON

Some owners extended the lockdowns long after governors ended stay-at-home orders for us outsiders, possibly to avoid outside eyes on the activities. The wearisome isolation and broken communications that brought sorrow and pain, desolation and death, also heightened tenderness among those lucky enough to have family or friends. If they could, people FaceTimed or Skyped or called each other on WhatsApp more often.

Family members came in the cold months, bundled up to talk and smile through windows. In March, Carly Boyd came to her grandfather's window to say she had gotten engaged and point to her sparkling ring. She looks woebegone. "I just told him I love him, and he said, 'I love you, too, and I hope to see you soon,' like really see you.'" How many photos we saw of relatives with their hands on an icy pane of glass or holding up babies. The shadowy face of an exile could be seen waving or looking puzzled and mouthing words.

In November 2020, a traveling "hug tent" with plastic-encased sleeves, arriving for four hours in a nontraditional facility in Denver, Colorado, finally allowed Vince Shryack and his daughter Carol Braun to embrace for the first time in eight months. "That was marvelous," said the craggy vet, a ninety-seven-year-old white man who had worked as a petroleum engineer, beaming broadly on TV. "I had to hug her; the tent was in the hug as well. But that was okay."

In San Francisco, Mildred Hamada's family moved her out to keep her safe. But Ms. Hamada, aged ninety-six, missed her friends; her facility had actually been a *home*; she had lived there with her husband before he died. She cried regularly. "When she was able to go back to the facility she snapped back to being her normal jovial self." Many warm relationships were dismally severed when common rooms—dining rooms, salons, exercise and activity rooms—closed. But some togetherness, creativity, and ritual survived. In some facilities, staff organized birthday parties, bringing cake to the celebrant. Altruistic aides kept up the spirits of the living and held the hands of the dying. They wore plastic bags for lack of PPE. They cried in private and carried on.

As if they had died in a distant war, thousands of people were buried with no one attending their funeral. When we most needed communal rituals, they vanished, replaced by Zoom funerals, home altars, and solitary visits to headstones. Organizing impromptu rituals, safely, from their doorways, masked, some residents said words of comfort and remembrance. Roommates said "Goodnight, sleep well, see you in the morning." Time passed. With death either remote or all around them, somehow life went on.

The survivors were the first and closest witnesses of the mayhem and nonfeasance, of the humor and emotional support. Some enjoyed amazing recoveries; others developed long COVID and PTSD. The most humane truths and the most gruesome facts that they experienced deserve to be recovered. Only now, with legacy stories like these collected, can we properly value the exceptional qualities it took to endure their ghastly conditions so long. Hearing residents in their own words changed my relationship to this book. It had to be dedicated to the living as well as to those who had died. It had to bring into being more admiration for their fullness of life.

HELPING THE HEART GROW
CONGRESS DECIDES WHEN THE BEDPAN ARRIVES

Outsiders may feel indifference or aversion to residents unless they know someone living in a facility. If you arrive to find that your sister's room "doesn't pass the smell test," you don't walk away from her eager, embarrassed, welcoming face. You run out for an aide. You won't complain to the nursing director—wary of retaliation, a common problem—but you know whom to blame for slackness. "They don't hire enough staff here," you grumble, so your sister won't think the neglect comes from animus against her person.

Your sister rolls her eyes. "You know what happened to Raúl?" she says. "He walked up to the aides yacking but couldn't make clear that he needed to go, poor guy. Ellen actually came over and sniffed his pants front and back. Jerod wanted to help him but Ellen said to leave him be. They dicked around with him until he went away, he was so upset at being teased. Then Raúl got angry later. He made trouble." She shakes her head, exasperated. "Who can blame him?"

"We haven't had a champion in the House since Claude Pepper," says your sister, who lived in Florida until her mini-strokes. "I voted for dear Claude Pepper every time. He had such a kind face." Her eyes are more animated now, and her pink cheeks make her look like the little sister of childhood. She is wearing a vintage cross-stitched satin bed jacket from the 1930s, which you always take home to wash so it doesn't disappear.

"Congress decides when the bedpan arrives," you joke.

"Ye-e-es," she says, doubtfully. "But it's the manager who keeps Ellen on, despite the ombudsman's complaints."

Explaining our stunted feelings toward residents became more complex as the pandemic exacerbated stereotypes. In this book I return to the topic again and again. To start with, how did we *imagine* life in a facility? Most of us had stupefying blanks or stupefying assumptions. The very place of their exile estranged us. Even if you have never visited, your images of the atrocious surroundings may be vivid. The 1946 Hill-Burton Act set in cinder block the medical model of building hospital-like buildings and long wards. "The legacies of the poorhouse and the hospital persist, creating panicked views of the nursing home as a dreaded fate," Sally Chivers and Ulla Kriebernegg write in their edited collection, *Care Home Stories: Ageing, Disability, and Long-Term Residential Care.*

As members of a society that is focused, when it focuses on residents at all, on their afflictions, our fears of age, impairments, and destitution can suffice to weaken our ties to these imagined people. Mean-spirited profiling would have it that they are "unproductive" in a society that messily divides the productive, the most highly productive, and the rest. "Moochers." "A burden." If once they had been lauded as consumers or "taxpayers," on a personal needs allowance they are no longer. But it is the government that permits the owners to understaff, so that an ageist aroma leaches outside the walls. We had been taught disgust but not the sordid money-grubbing, the two-thirds frame that Congress ordained.

Location, location, location (a real estate truism) sums up how intimately status is linked to abodes as much as to bodies. Their stigmatized housing is unconsciously harmful to right thinking about them. Long before lockdowns turned the habitations into jails, Chris Gilleard and Paul Higgs, British gerontologists, sagely observed that "nursing homes"—the mere name—had "become the condensed image of . . . rejected old age. They represent a fate to be resisted, if not avoided altogether, a fate worse than death." It is as if the people and the places merged perceptually, as lepers once became indistinguishable from leprosariums.

In 2020, inmates paid dreadfully for their degraded status, at the federal and state levels and at most of the 15,477 facilities. In one fully irresponsible way, they were not considered at all. Early in the pandemic, as if anticipating that the industry's own negligent acts would result in death or harm to residents, the lobbyists asked states for

immunity from liability. The industry had spent (since 2010 alone)
$30 million lobbying lawmakers. Many states—not all—rushed to
protect the industry, not the residents. Most never restored liability. A new, activist president who led the general mourning was in-
augurated, but despite the urgent reasons for mandating new rules—
contagious variants, startling surges, the fact that unvaccinated staff
were carrying the disease inside—Joe Biden was unable to require
vaccinations for "patient-facing" personnel until September 2021.

Recognizing that many tens of thousands of residents could have
been saved and that ethical restraints were loosened or disregarded,
this book asks the elemental question, *What was wrong with the systems and with our culture, that the 2020 Eldercide could occur at all?* No
"conspiracy" is necessary to explain the deadly patterns, the worst of
which remain to be examined. My analysis shows that where care-
fulness should have guided care, a compound of ageist ableism, dementism, sexism, racism, and classism had settled deep.

THE SOCIAL HUG

The egalitarian ethics that should arise from unequally shared peril
could not be clearer now. "Everybody, whatever their level of education and whatever their level of income and whatever their level of
connections, is entitled to a certain kind of basic respect. Everybody,"
asserts philosopher Kwame Antony Appiah. He adds, "That's a very,
very radical thought." Perhaps ethical injunctions are more necessary
now, in the COVID Era. After so much national, personal, and famil-
ial turmoil, driving us inward, a generous imagination may be needed
to enable us to think collectively again.

Of the many brutal social biases exposed during the pandemic,
none needs stricter scrutiny now than compound ageism. Until so
many facilities simultaneously became dying fields, even experts could
not see how treacherously ageism had damaged public-health politics and created morbid assumptions about older adults. Almost everything that went desperately wrong inside the facilities depended
on misbegotten systems from the past, crumbling like rotten walls.

This book exposes the bitter weirdness of the assured belief that "the old die," in a nation where many acts or omissions entailed *letting* the people in those institutions die.

Alarming historical failures require an entire society to *think together about a problematic* that has long gone unseen. The Eldercide demands first that we comprehend the magnitude of our losses, as I have tried to do in part 1, "Inside." The Eldercide's roots, further explored in part 2, "Instead," could provoke anger-galvanizing resistance—in the media, in the courts, in Congress, and most of all in our minds. Trying to prove (in part 3, "Ahead") that our elders do matter could lead to changes more life-affirming than activists have previously dared call for. "Reckonings," the epilogue, considers the odds of uncovering the crimes and restoring the health of the body politic.

> Sweeping up the heart
> The morning after death
> Is solemnest of industries,
> enacted upon Earth.

These are the words of our national poet of mourning, Emily Dickinson. Industriously, the narrative arc of this book takes us from elegiac lament to exposés, from close analysis to historical understanding, from insight to consolation, from memorials to true reform. This is the order of the service.

PART 2

INSTEAD

CHAPTER 2

INSTEAD . . . THE FIRST MONTHS OF 2020

When Ageism Hardened into Eldercide

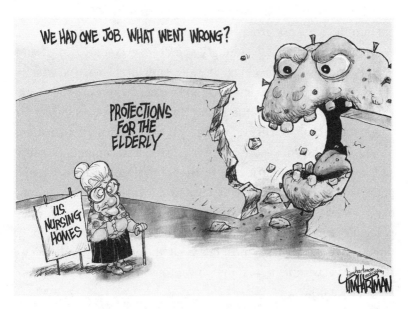

FIGURE 1 Tim Hartman, "We Had One Job. What Went Wrong?" *Philadelphia Inquirer*, May 9, 2020. Image courtesy of and updated by the artist on December 6, 2023.

THE HIDDEN TRUTHS OF A CORRUPT WORLD

The first mass of deaths in the US—the Eldercide—began in the facilities. At first it seemed the virus was felling *only* people living in nursing homes—in terrifying clusters. The media focused the country first on one nursing home in Kirkland, Washington, piously and commercially named the "Life Care Center"—the epicenter of the outbreak. By March 7, thirteen people had died (the *Guardian*). By March 23 (*Wall Street Journal*), thirty-five. Over a dozen technicians swarmed in to disinfect the place (*Washington Post*), wearing white hazmat suits with hoods and thick black snouts like WWI gas masks.

By no later than March 23, 147 nursing homes across twenty-seven states had, by the CDC's cagey count, "at least one resident" with COVID. On March 18, in what was to become a media pattern, the *Seattle Times* treated the dead as a data point. "About a fourth of the coronavirus fatalities in the U.S. have been linked to the nursing homes," it reported, and added: "[The disease is] especially dangerous for the elderly." Jumping from "linked to the nursing homes" to "the elderly" was a journalistic leap that swept *all* older community dwellers into the high-risk group. This category error was to have fateful consequences for all older adults, and indeed, everyone.

The mortality was shocking. The images of inert bodies on stretchers were shocking. The hazmat suits and gas masks were beyond shocking. The world agrees that the Trump government's delays started the whole tragic chain of US events. There have been many explanations for his original sin of apathy. Many are correct, but compound ageism adds a crucial element to his conscious political motivations. Trump's personal response was reluctant, belated, and inadequate because the mass of deaths was occurring there, in those dim places, among *those negligible people*. Society's most implicit bias is widely shared, but in those early weeks when it most mattered, the president, almost alone as head of government, had the power to *embody* obliviousness and model it for others.

Ethics starts by asking who has been harmed and who is responsible. History is about understanding "causes, effects, needs and strategies," which, one cultural historian contends, "show themselves more plainly in times of rapid emergence." For understanding what happened in the Oval Office and elsewhere in government, the first crucial time frame ran from the date of the first known US deaths in late February through March and April. These weeks shook the country.

The residents alone soon constituted over 40 percent of the US dead, a figure wildly disproportionate to their minuscule share of the population. But these staggering tolls did not seem as surprising as they should have. The mortality rate confirmed a dehumanizing stereotype of residents as fragile. Dying was the normal next state for such needy, dependent old people. Aversion exists at the intolerant end of a range of emotions toward lesser others. Aversion was evoked or heightened by fears of being old—of being *them*—in the new COVID Era.

For Trump, the chain that linked residents to old age, sickness, disability, and expendability was so taut and distasteful that he literally could not count them. At the end of August 2020, when the CDC was estimating that nearly two hundred thousand people had died, he (re)tweeted the claim that there really were only nine thousand deaths [*sic*], since "most of the deaths are very old Americans with co-morbidities." Political strategy required that he minimize the numbers, but the pejorative image in his head decided which victims he would discount.

Only months later, running against Joe Biden in that election year, Trump told Fox News, "He's mentally gone." Biden was a few years older than Trump, and the age of the candidates was briefly a main topic for the press. But Biden was Trump's opposite in obvious ways. Biden was known for energetic exercise like bike riding; Trump used a cart to get around the golf course. Trump was a germophobe, "notoriously squeamish about physical disability." On the campaign trail, he mocked a reporter with arthrogryposis, a congenital condition affecting the joints, by flapping his own arms and hands loosely and manically in the air. Trump tweeted a Photoshopped image of his Democratic rival in a wheelchair seated among elderly people in what appeared to be a nursing facility, captioned "Biden for resident."

Although then president Trump was overweight, male, and age seventy-four when he carelessly let himself become infected, the Eldercide did not fell *him*. Instead, a top hospital gave his important body bespoke care. He emerged from his unique treatments at Walter Reed shedding a mask he had long refused to wear, as arrogantly as if his individual body had personally triumphed over death. He crowed about how much younger he felt. He identified with wealth, the symbolic color gold, rich donors, his idea of lithe pulchritude, fastidious cleanliness, power. Privilege meant power to repudiate. To such a man, the residents, uniquely associated with death, were possibly the remnant of the "bag ladies" and "bums" he had seen in New York in the 1980s (when he was a wealthy young man-about-town). Indigent old people or (since women were known to live longer and become shorter and poorer, the older they get) the stereotypical "little old lady," may have been the object he associated with the epithet "nursing home." Stereotypes tend to survive facts.

Trump was often called a "narcissist"—but the charge was levied with no thought to how far spoiled vanity might carry Narcissus once he has grown older in a youth-oriented society. Aging in the body—no longer seeing a once-adored face in the mirror—can feel like a "narcissistic wound," psychoanalysts say. Psychically, this aging male at the top of the political hierarchy had to dissociate himself from the ultimate unwanted others, whom COVID would select out.

There's a touch of superstition in aversion, as if one type of ageism—warding off one's own personal decline—demanded another type of ageism: hating or shunning old people. It doesn't. Combining the two types of ageism—shunning other old people while regretting and denying one's own losses of masculinity, virility, youth—can be toxic.

A whole ideology preached by Republicans seeps into many of us, justifying any inability to empathize. When fitness is a virtue, ill health can feel like a moral failing: Residents have sinned, QED. Institutionalization can be felt as a just outcome for people who let themselves go financially—losers in the competition to get and stay in the middle class—"dependent" people in a society where interdependence is made to seem a personal weakness, not a human condition. Their segregation may make them seem socially unwanted. Their poverty can feel like a disgrace. Undermining empathy is the true violence of compound classist, racist, sexist, and ageist ableism.

Such collective failures are common but don't entirely explain the Trump administration's first policy "decision"—to do nothing effectual to rescue those living in the epicenters of the plague. It would have been possible to keep the virus out of such spatially segregated places. Trump had received coronavirus news—which then included US nursing-home mortality data—on at least twelve occasions in early January and February 2020. (Trump disputed this reporting.) The president could have ordered personal protective equipment (masks, gloves, gowns) for the depleted National Strategic Stockpile, the emergency medicine chest for the nation. PPE was urgently needed to save the lives of residents and keep the hospitals' ICUs from overflowing. For public health, having an appropriately sized national stockpile means being prepared for an emergency on the scale of the pandemic flu of 1918–1919. An adequate stockpile is a test of the basic competence of the administrative state. Despite public calls to use the Defense Production Act to produce PPE, Trump did nothing. Congress could have acted, but it was controlled by his party, and it did not.

A CEO of an eldercare association, Shawn Bloom, calling nursing homes "the neglected cousin of the health care system," knew what was missing. Bloom reported that "we were very, very much hindered in getting and prioritizing the distribution of PPEs to long-term care facilities early on." Dr. Mark S. Lachs, the director of geriatrics in the well-resourced New York-Presbyterian Healthcare System, was shocked by the disparity between what the hospitals received and what the facilities had to make do with. "Nursing homes should have the best PPE and access to testing and infection control experts. During the pandemic, they had the worst," he wrote. It wasn't until April 30, 2020, that Trump formed a special commission on nursing-home quality and safety. Publicly he called nursing homes "a little bit of a weak spot."

When that Commission on Nursing Home Quality and Safety report came out, a full four months later, in September 2020, it merely "urged" those facility owners to do right. Enforcement mechanisms—the teeth in any reform—were not added, according to a dissent from a member of the commission, Eric Carlson, a lawyer for the reliable NGO Justice in Aging. The Commission's slack report came prettied up by an overview from the Centers for Medicare and Medicaid Services (CMS), headed by Seema Verma, who praised "the robust public health actions the agency has taken to date."

"Robust" was a dishonest term to use. September 2020 was the month I felt grim despair at what seemed an unending catastrophe inflicted on those isolated people. By then, residents of long-term care facilities in my state, Massachusetts, constituted 66 percent of state COVID deaths—a worse record than that of most states. I had not yet discovered that a March 2020 "guidance" to all US facilities, promulgated by Verma through CMS, had heightened the residents' jeopardy. Verma had operationalized abandonment.

Calling out *a failure to protect the residents* is important. No one can explain an outcome properly if they misname it or are looking only at other outcomes, like the larger US disaster. Those million-plus deaths are variously attributed—with good documentation—to lack of preparation, bureaucratic incompetence and infighting, avoidance of science, confidence in American exceptionalism, and the Republican fear of disrupting the economy and losing the November 2020 presidential election. Trump may also have underplayed the menace in order to lull himself with hope that the problems posed for his presidency would magically solve themselves.

But ageism and ableism, classism and dementism, which often have fantastic, unconscious motives as well as rational and cynical ones, also help to explain the US failures. By the fall of 2020, it was obvious that the virus had long before jumped the confines of nursing homes and seemed likely to reach a toll of what then seemed a horrifying number: two hundred thousand Americans. At that moment, at a rally in Ohio, Trump again plainly revealed his age bias when he asserted that the coronavirus only "'affects elderly people, elderly people with heart problems and other problems.... But it affects virtually nobody. It's an amazing thing.'"

"Virtually nobody" to him meant nobody *young*. COVID was indeed mainly killing older people with multi-morbidities. But this statement conveyed coldhearted compound biases toward sick and dying people around his own age. Trump always intended to be widely quoted; he was. He had eighty million Twitter followers. (A study of thirty-eight million English-language publications in mainstream media showed that he was the single largest driver of COVID misinformation—mostly about "miracle cures.") His assertion that there was no danger to younger adults from the coronavirus endangered everyone.

AGEISM GOES VIRAL: THE FIRST PHASE

Age scholars believe that the disease might have gotten an instant government response if its first victims had been *children*. If ordinary, uninstitutionalized children had been asphyxiating, preventive measures would have been taken as widely as they were in the polio epidemic of the 1950s, when parents kept children out of swimming pools and other public places. Even parents sporting MAGA caps—Trump loyalists espousing his ways of Making America Great Again—would have kept their kids from cavorting in groups without masks. The Centers for Disease Control and Prevention (CDC) would have quickly received their banished funding and much more, to provide tests, masks, and contact tracing all across the country. If children had been the ones needing protection, almost everything that should have happened, would have.

Instead, rather than focusing on what had produced the life-threatening conditions in most nursing facilities, the mainstream media obsessively fastened attention on bare statistics of "the Old" dying. In a crisis, there is sometimes a pivotal period when "the real" first gets turned into a rigid story. With regard to the residents of care homes and older adults in general, spring 2020 was that major interpretive period. A Harvard professor, Cass R. Sunstein, anticipated the tenacity of whatever story gets most persuasively retold. "For a long time to come," he wrote, "people will be influenced, both politically and economically, by their understanding of the pandemic, [by] whatever narrative about it crystallizes for them."

The ageist, ableist narrative I am following crystallized fast and early, blotting out complex realities. The residents first, and then "the Old," became separated out, identified, classified, profiled as people who were doomed to die, who could not be helped. (Ian Hacking, the philosopher of the creation of kinds, called this sort of storytelling "making up people.") A society sickens morally when it assumes a subordinated group of its members is consigned to an unavoidable fate. Both the causes and the results of that careless narrative need to be thoroughly examined.

COMPOUND AGEISM WORSENED THE PANDEMIC

Data about residents dying of COVID made the danger outside the facilities seem negligible. Trump himself early on knew otherwise. In March, he blurted out what he considered "some startling facts" to journalist Bob Woodward. "It's not just old, older. Young people too, plenty of young people." But, he confessed, "I wanted to always play it down. I still like playing it down because I don't want to create a panic." He had known since January 25 that the fierce new contagion was dangerous to all ages. Publicly, he said, "Take your hat off to the young because they have a hell of an immune system." His silence about the risk to the young served his political fortunes. Woodward too kept silent.

As early as March 8, Nina A. Kohn, a professor of law at Syracuse University, wrote in the *Washington Post* that "those who wanted to persuade politicians and the public to take the virus seriously needed to emphasize that 'It isn't only the elderly who are at risk from the coronavirus.'" Nevertheless, news stories often pointedly repeated how low the risk was to younger people or children. As public health information, this claim was disastrous.

It soon became too late to correct the narrative. Trump's binary fantasy—that "the Young" went unscathed while death's scythe took "the (ignobly weak) Old"—was shared. It slackened the urgency of trying to save the residents. Tweets were filled with hate speech against the old people dying, much like the hate speech levied against Wuhan, or Chinese people, as if the residents were originating or spreading the disease. The sickness of ageism, having done its sullen work throughout the body politic, erupted in extreme forms. Twitter-hate was only one.

Many trusted that non-Old people were safe. Young and midlife adults showed this trust by engaging in risky behaviors. Surges of illness to outsiders came as a surprise in place after place, despite learned warnings. And the complementary belief, wish, or excuse, that people younger than, say, fifty would by nature remain healthy, led to many of the belated and repeated closures (and premature re-openings) of "the economy," and then to drastic unemployment; and on to the reckless, politically divisive and at times suicidal resistance of anti-vaxxers.

Saving the residents first would not only have been the right thing to do. Protecting them would also have been the *safest* thing to do in the face of the pandemic, for everyone. Had state authorities not been ageist, they would have immediately developed the resources to protect the 1.4 million residents—underscoring that they survived when protected—and they would have had valuable time, not much but some, to practice the capabilities needed for protecting 330 million others. Not as karma but as consequence, the abandonment of the nursing facilities jump-started nationwide calamities. Saving the residents first—whether out of anti-ageism or public health responsibility—should have been treated as a national security issue. Instead . . .

Simple-minded biology—the belief that "the Old" must die—left no room for the deeper history I am telling, a history of the multiple interlocking causes of all the unnatural, unnecessary losses of the COVID Era. In that context, residents' lives matter immensely. Albert Camus helps explain why. In his novel *The Plague*, Camus described that deadly disease *politically*, as "thrusting up to the surface the abscesses and pus that, up until then, had been doing their work internally," bringing to notice "the hidden truth of a corrupt world." The obvious abscess was the ferocious long-term failure of eldercare provision. The tiny nursing-care part of the vast public health system was in the charge of CMS, then under Seema Verma.

In the COVID Era, ageism became ubiquitous and yet more baffling. The narratives that got public attention about the Eldercide were contradictory. When apparently well-meaning (like the report of the

Commission on Nursing Home Quality and Safety), they could be incorrect, exaggerated, even harmful. When sentimental, they were potentially feral. When most data-driven, misleading. When disguised as rational (the lockdowns that isolated the residents from the people who most wanted to help them), lethal.

Ageism is not a universal transhistorical phenomenon. This Eldercide needs its own timeline in history: how attacks began, accumulated, became explicit or rhetorically devious, worked subconsciously, twisted discourse, denied truth, and directed conduct. Such a timeline shows how Year One of the COVID Era went wrong from the very start.

"THIS IS COMING TO YOU"

Many officials and people all around the country ignored the danger to the particular elder and disabled population that the government was responsible for. Senator Patty Murray of Washington might have had many important reasons for jumping into public action at the pandemic news coming from her state in January and February. She was the ranking Democratic member of the Committee on Health, Education, Labor, and Pensions, whose website promised to "protect against public health emergencies." That committee had received the first short briefing from Anthony Fauci, then chief medical advisor to the president, on January 24. Senator Murray had already heard about the first confirmed case of COVID, a man from Wuhan, China, who was hospitalized in her own state. Murray spoke to Lawrence Wright, the author of an exposé of early public health "mistakes" (which found little to say about nursing facilities). Murray said that she told herself at that point, "Wow, this is kinda scary. And this is in my back yard." But a back yard is not your home.

A month later, on February 29, after the first widely reported death in the country occurred in that nursing facility in Kirkland, Washington, Murray again apparently did not respond with public warnings. She knew that very facility; one of her relatives had stayed in it earlier. (Within the next four-week span, thirty-nine residents of Life Care died from complications related to COVID.) Murray said to herself, as she put it to Wright, "Wow, this contagious virus, it can't have just stayed in a nursing home." To her the idea that contagion was spreading *beyond the residents* was a reason simply to urge her friends to get tested. But her grandchildren attended schools near the afflicted facility. It was only when Murray's daughter texted her to say, "They closed the schools," that the senator said she told her colleagues, "My daughter's school closed. This is coming to you." *Now*, suddenly, it was coming. Not to residents who lacked supplies, but to "*you*."

The residents were treated as objects—like chattels or furniture, to be moved at someone else's will toward sickness or death. In mid-March 2020, researchers at the Massachusetts Institute of Technology warned the governor of Massachusetts, Charlie Baker, and his health secretary, Marylou Sudders, during an evening meeting at the home of the MIT president, that his nursing homes—where 40 percent of residents were over eighty-five—were dangerously exposed to COVID-19. "We said, 'Here are the facilities, you need to protect them,'" Retsef Levi, a management professor, later told the *Boston Globe*.

That wintry March when I was safe at home, discovering triage-by-age in the official ventilator guidelines, Governor Baker was ordering that some residents be moved out of their facilities—on such short notice that many did not know where they were going. People were wheeled out into the cold, leaving possessions behind. New York, New Jersey, and Michigan also ordered nursing homes to accept patients with active COVID infections who were being discharged from hospitals. The president of the Foundation for Research on Equal Opportunity wrote, "The most charitable interpretation of these orders is that they were designed to ensure that states would not overcrowd their ICUs." They preferred to infect residents in unprepared nursing facilities.

Eugenics—the labeling of groups considered "unfit," going back to the nineteenth century—plausibly plays a hidden role in the clear preference for trying to save community dwellers over residents. A legal scholar, Laura I. Appleman, argues that these "long-held but little discussed eugenic beliefs [are] endemic today" and underlie "our legal and medical treatment of the disabled, detained, and dependent." Such beliefs, conscious or not, explain the "State's minimal effort put forth to protect these members of our community. Specifically, the State continues to prioritize the healthy, free, and able-bodied over the medically fragile, incarcerated, and disabled." *Children's* lives matter to officials. The lives of their peers in the community matter. Older people segregated in nursing homes? Not much.

HOW TO OPERATIONALIZE ABANDONMENT

In a democratic bureaucracy like that of the United States, any top-down program authorized by Congress must be operationalized through administrative agencies' regulations, reported in public documents. Given Trump's unwillingness to rescue the 1.4 million residents via the most effective means (targeting PPE and testing to nursing facilities, investing in contact tracing, and funding direct staff at a higher level), the panic and the publicity around the residents' dying-off made damage control absolutely necessary.

On March 13, 2020, Trump and the HHS administrator, Alex Azar, had declared a public health emergency. In an emergency, executive agencies—"often overlooked despite the power they wield over the way our country is run"—are granted even greater leeway. In this desperate moment, CMS had to provide a program for the states and the facilities they monitor that would defer to Trump's inadequate cover story about the facilities ("a little bit of a weak spot") yet look fine on paper. In other words, some ideologue in the upper echelon of the executive branch had to give abandonment a friendly, authoritative public face.

As chief of CMS, Seema Verma was that face. Three years before, she had been the hatchet-woman for cutting $880 billion dollars from Medicaid—"in charge of deciding exactly how skimpy Trumpcare plans will be," said Senator Ron Wyden, then the ranking member of the finance committee, in opposing her confirmation. Medicaid is popular. But Verma was praised by politicians who aimed to curtail Medicaid funding.

In 2020, as COVID began, there was a lot at stake for Verma. She needed to provide good news about health care in advance of the boss's 2020 election. Her own job was on the line. She had spent almost $6 million of CMS funds to hire an expensive team of outside Republican contractors, rather than her communications department, to help her craft "her public profile and personal brand," in violation of federal contracting rules. In the wake of career-damaging revelations about her self-dealing, the inspector general was investigating. The White House had prepared a list of potential replacements for Verma and her HHS boss.

In March, COVID cases could double in a day. Doctor John Okrent of Tacoma, Washington, who worked in a community health clinic, wrote his first sonnet on March 17. "Everyone's eyes seemed wider / above their face masks." On March 20: "The sharp curve of new cases / like a middle finger from a fist."

CMS had to look active, proactive, and concerned with residents' safety and the quality of services. The problem for Verma was that she had to manage at least two audiences whose interests or expectations had often conflicted and now potentially clashed. On the one hand, there were the beneficiaries in nursing homes and their well-wishers, whose existential expectation would remain optimum possible care in the newly perilous conditions. On the other hand, there were the nursing-facility trade industry and its Congressional allies, whose settled expectation for a Republican government would be less regulation no matter what. The for-profit lobby had long advocated for less oversight, which translated into lower budgets, higher profits, and degraded quality-of-care standards. When market forces and good governance collide in a crisis, whose "expectations" matter most? Power decides. Influence confirms.

The injunctions in the Social Security Act as to how to "promote maintenance or enhancement of the quality of life of each resident," appearing in section 1819, had been meticulously detailed. The "authority to waive requirements during national emergencies" is known as section 1135. Declaring a public health emergency was right and proper; changing rules or regulations is legitimate. The issue was that emergencies hand agencies special powers to undo even well-conceived Congressional requirements without public comment. By fiat. With its new 1135 waivers, CMS found a way to deregulate nursing facilities beyond that industry's wildest dreams.

That spring was the critical time frame for preventing an eldercide, for keeping the new virus out of the facilities. Some 1135 waivers were welcome. Skilled facilities with dialysis equipment would be allowed to use them, sparing patients the risk of going out frequently and being exposed. California got authority to provide temporary housing for unhoused people with COVID. For the indigent, an 1135 waiver made getting accepted by Medicaid easier. Telehealth by FaceTime, Skype, or phone would enable communication between doctor and patient without travel or touch. On the other hand, it eliminated patients who lacked technology and if limited to audio made diagnoses of all kinds more difficult. A death from COVID might go unreported, lowering the numbers, as the president and his party also preferred.

On March 23, 2020, in a major press release about "Facility Inspections," Verma's speechwriters produced an apparently innocuous public document about the "national strategy." Read with care, it turns out to have been shockingly duplicitous. The states are responsible for "oversight," monitoring the residents' well-being. Inspectors, typically trained nurses, supposedly make unscheduled visits to the facilities, measuring standard indicators. In theory, the system threatened operators with retribution—fines, closures—for injuries and death, to deterrent effect. In theory, the residents enjoyed layers of protection. Inspectors were key.

In practice, oversight often worked like the opening of Nikolai Gogol's 1836 play *The Inspector General*, with the boss saying "Gentlemen, an Inspector is coming! . . . Put clean nightgowns on all the patients." When the health cops were on the way in America, suddenly there were mold-free bathrooms, supplies, rodent control, new hires. The states often delayed responding to adverse reports, thereby making information-gathering impossible. CMS's secretive appeals procedures demonstrated *strategic inefficiency*, a common way to get complainants off bureaucratic necks. At the best of times, the system for collecting damning violations was as porous as a weir in a flood. Spring 2020 was the worst of times. CMS rhetoric claimed the states would "target" inspectors by sending them only where the need for "infection control" was greatest. Making this the sole priority permitted officials to ignore other problems, like understaffing.

The press release made it look as if the pandemic, not officialdom, rendered regular rescue inspections impossible. The trick rested on Verma's ability to say that protective personnel equipment was "at a premium." It was. It was widely unavailable.

The underlying truth was that the administration had no intention of using its legal power to pressure manufacturers to produce more for the Strategic Stockpile. (Alex Azar had asked Congress for more PPE but a budget committee had cut his request 40 percent. Trump had made a trade deal in January and February that sent personal protective equipment away to, of all places, China.) Those decisions left fifty governors fighting one another to procure PPE, because—even at a desperate time—competition was the Republican way. In my state, the New England Patriots' owner sent a plane to China to pick up a million N95 masks for "our brave front-line workers." Did that honored group include aides in nursing facilities?

If CMS's inspectors had regularly gone out *then* to encounter the horrors, had they not been limited to infection control, everyone concerned might have been galvanized into doing their jobs right. Certain forms of speech, philosopher Rae Langton observes, "set norms through orders, or more subtle alterations of permissibility." "Permissibility" indeed changed.

Verma's press release anticipated as if with regret that there would be times "when a facility is experiencing Coronavirus cases and inspectors can't enter"—precisely when inspectors would be most needed. "Others will be limited in what they can carry out due to limited supply of personal protective equipment," the release continued. Facility owners in distant offices would have clearly heard: "no PPE, no inspections." The "guidance" gave them a perverse incentive not to buy more. (Trump had shown himself averse to masks. At the annual CMS Quality Conference in July 2020, held in person, no mask was visible in the audience. Verma's partisan loyalty to Trump was unmistakable, despite the danger of creating a super-spreader event that Dr. Anthony Fauci, director of the National Institute of Allergy and Infectious Diseases, was warning against.) When early on, in June 2020, Congressman Lloyd Doggett of the House Ways and Means Subcommittee held a hearing on the government's failed responses to COVID, Verma declined to appear.

CMS boasted that its "emergency declaration blanket waivers" would work well for industry "flexibility." The main objective stated was to give "relief": as immediately worded by a global firm with "a deep bench" of lawyers, "to provide the healthcare industry *relief* from various requirements under the Social Security Act." When Verma offered the owners "our innovative self-assessment tool" in lieu of inspections, the owners heard that they would be let off scot-free—free to postpone audits, free to ignore any execrable conditions of aides and elders.

The "guidance" may have provided an additional incentive to investment firms to buy up nursing facilities, unpropitious as the deadly conditions might have made them appear. Starting in April 2020, the month after CMS's ruling, the New Jersey–based Portopiccolo Group, a firm with a history of serious safety violations in its nursing facility portfolio, went on a "nursing-home buying spree," according to *Barron's*, "snapping up" twenty. By December, the *Washington Post* was reporting that at four of its new Maryland properties, Portopiccolo's operating companies failed to buy enough supplies and protective equipment and asked some employees to keep working after testing positive. Andrew Cockburn discovered that the market performance of companies involved in long-term care (Janus Long-Term Care ETF, market symbol OLD) was up 38 percent from its low by April, and by June, it had climbed almost 70 percent.

Verma did not personally need to feel aversion to the residents in her charge to operationalize Trump's careless, ageist leanings. His top-down bullying had sapped initiative at many tiers of government. But she shared the neoliberal ideological mission: avoiding "micromanagement" and "unnecessary" regulation for welfare medicine. And the neoliberal package is chockablock with ageism: shrinking Medicaid rolls, delaying the age for getting Social Security, transferring Medicare to private "Advantage" companies. Her explanation of feeling overwhelmed in February and March suggests that the 1.4 million residents did not loom large in her value system:

> We had geriatricians, surgeons, infectious disease doctors working day and night to put guidelines together. For me this was a life-and-death issue. We knew every single day could make a difference. And keep in mind, nursing homes were only one piece of it. The CMS has jurisdiction over the entire health care system.

"The main mission of CMS was to pay the bills of [*Medicare*] beneficiaries," I was told by Paul Elstein, a veteran of decades in quality control there; "otherwise . . . uproar." Residents of the facilities on stigmatized Medicaid were a small piece of Verma's trillion-dollar department. That said, she knew the deadly clusters were occurring *there*. The urgency was *there*—to keep the residents alive. The next weeks of her "jurisdiction" would determine how hard the facilities had to work to do that.

If any ordinary readers chose to peruse that two-faced speech, they might have been soothed by apparent upgrades—"innovative self-assessment," "revised Infection Control protocol"—and by correct sentiments: Kirkland was a "tragedy," nursing homes were valued as "permanent homes," filled with our "mothers and fathers, sisters and brothers." (*When sentimental, potentially feral.*) Readers could easily have missed the ill omens, hidden in that mass of warm gelatinous rhetoric. Verma succeeded in one way. Trump, admired by fans for shouting, "You're fired," on his TV show, and hasty in firing his own department heads, never fired this star subordinate.

Three days before the press release, CMS's director of Quality, Safety, and Oversight, David Wright, had already issued a letter directly to the states' survey agency directors about rules for "the prioritization period." That was code for permitting reduced or no "standard" inspections, even for "life safety" (the fire code). The 1135 waivers also removed "revisits" (for checking that corrections to deficiencies had been made) unless they were associated with "immediate jeopardy." Little immediate jeopardy had ever been found. The inspectors who were able to come would "use a streamlined review checklist *to minimize the impact on provider activities.*"

In the checklist that followed, personnel were required to "remove gloves and perform hand hygiene between each patient or dialysis station." Did they in fact do so? Did they really? *Could* they? Without enough PPE, with many aides out sick, with less training required, such rules were likely to be skimped on, although one failure could be fatal to many.

Perhaps the deadliest form of "flexibility" was that owners were not required to report any information on staffing hours per resident; rather, they were allowed to self-report whether or not the facility was experiencing staffing "shortages." Representative Richard Neal of Massachusetts, a strong advocate for improving residents' welfare, later called this metric "a significantly less comprehensive measure of staffing capacity." Candidly, CMS admitted that the "Nursing Home Compare" website—which ranks facilities from one to five stars, based on inspectors' reports on quality measures—"has been stagnant because providers didn't have to submit the data due to the passing of the waiver in April. . . . CMS believes that they can utilize the data from assessments conducted and submitted prior to January 1, 2020, to calculate quality measures." This claim made no sense. CMS promised (really, *warned*) that the very lowest-ranked facilities would have "their ratings temporarily suppressed."

The harms could have been foreseen by someone with any concern, let alone medical knowledge. Physicians and practitioners were not required to perform in-person medical assessments but could delegate them to a less well-qualified person. Federal law required nursing assistants to pass a certification exam within four months of beginning work, but the 1135 waivers removed certification requirements for new nursing assistants or lowered training rules from seventy-five hours to as few as eight. Training for "paid feeding assistants" went from sixteen hours to one hour.

For specific waivers, states had to apply. Forty-eight states asked to suspend the requirement that each resident receive an annual updated care plan. New providers were not required to undergo criminal and background checks. The document promised what it surreptitiously withdrew. In a very ecstasy of hypocritical reassurance, Verma told residents they should not "hesitate to ask staff directly: 'what are the results of your CMS self-assessment?'"

Lockdowns rendered the residents as isolated as convicts. Their families had been excluded. The ombudsman program had been suspended. Now Verma reported as simply "plain fact" that "state survey agencies" "can be pulled away by their governors" to "fulfill [other] state public health duties." The last bit of rescue that might have come from oversight was vanishing into a void. (*When disguised as rational, most lethal.*) CMS had mandated surveys of only one supremely important measure, the Focused Infection Control. In June, Quality, Safety, and Oversight reported that only a little over half of nursing homes had performed it. Inspectors started to resume regular work, slowly, only in September 2020.

Over the second quarter of 2020, observers discovered grim results of nonfeasance. Dr. Jasmine Travers of NYU attributed the stench she noticed to lack of inspections. Understaffing put aides in impossible positions, doing their own exhausted triage among people who needed changing, turning, oxygen, meds. Lee Fleisher, the top doctor at the Center for Clinical Standards and Quality in CMS after June 2020, and colleagues admitted that skilled nursing facilities saw rates of falls causing major injury increase by 17.4 percent and rates of pressure ulcers increase by 41.8 percent. "The pandemic [*sic*] degraded patient safety so quickly and severely," they declared, as if human agency—their own agency—had nothing to do with it.

THE APPEARANCE OF COMPLIANCE

The waivers were supposed to last for three weeks—ninety days at most. Two years later some waivers were still in effect; Human Rights Watch noted that some facilities continued to use lack of PPE or tests to keep inspectors out much longer.

CMS, under a new head, Chiquita Brooks-LaSure, appointed by President Biden, no longer had to fear retribution for honesty. In April 2022, CMS—in a document signed, like the first, two years earlier, by David R. Wright, as director of the Quality, Safety, and Oversight Group—plainly announced that the 1135 waivers had "removed the minimum standards for quality that help ensure residents' health and safety are protected." It didn't explicitly blame the prior administration. It wasn't a mea culpa. "The waivers" were at fault, not the former president, Congress, the secretary of HHS, or the director of CMS who had acceded to the well-known wishes of business operators.

The honest admission would have been that the March 2020 guidance made the nursing home catastrophe worse than it would have been if CMS had found a way to fight for PPE, to require frequent inspections, not fewer; if it had demanded better conditions for aides, not quiescence in what quickly turned into disastrous understaffing and consequent abuse and mortal peril. Silent people kept their jobs. Bureaucracies muffle responsibility. But there is always an option to go public. An agency head could have resigned with explanations. The Daniel Ellsbergs, the Edward Snowdens, courageous enough to blow the whistle, are few, but they make history.

The perspective presented here is informed by "state–corporate crime" theory. In *Critical Criminology*, Joseph Greener, a lecturer in sociology, social policy, and criminology at the University of Liverpool, shows how malpractice can occur in the presence of ample regulations. He writes: "The role of regulatory regimes in actively legitimizing sectors, such as the residential care industry, even in the face of routine violence [is accomplished], *by bureaucratically ensuring the appearance of compliance with formal rules*."

Ideally, the major science-based institutions of the government (such as the FTC, FDA, EPA, CDC, and CMS) are "apolitical." They govern for the public good. They attract the best minds to career public service. In practice, executive agencies are rarely free of relations with corporate bodies or the ideology of a party in power. "State capture" may mean undue, not total, influence. Under the influence, CMS quietly dropped the residents out of the social embrace.

That indefatigable journalist, I. F. Stone, discovered his bombshells about government misdeeds during the Vietnam War by seeking the deceptions hidden in plain sight in the official public record—debates, obscure committee hearings. The facts are there, he believed: just read between the lines. Performative compliance may not entirely conceal the source of injurious effects. A particular form of close reading is necessary to reveal the truth.

But who was reading the CMS documents? The media paid little attention to Medicaid. For bureaucratic rhetoric, the yawn factor is high. That makes it likely even in crisis that the public record will be ignored or be presented by journalists just as its writers intended. This phenomenon marks totalitarian states. In our country, because nothing appears to happen unless it happens in the media, we are supposed to have watchdog journalism.

Is it a surprise to learn that nursing facilities were almost never mentioned specifically in mainstream 1135 reporting, except for the blanket ban on visitors? For sage apprehensions, one had to look to the advocates' own websites, like the testimony of a lawyer from the Center for Medicare Advocacy to Representative Doggett's committee. And so it went: nothing to see here. Already, this early in my narrative, some readers may have chalked the word *forgotten* on their mental blackboard, tallying the times the residents lose. This time won't be the last.

In fact, there was little coverage of these drastic emergency waivers at all, although they would affect everyone covered by Medicare or Medicaid and the Children's Health Insurance Program (CHIP). With dry understatement, the authors of a textbook on health law note, about the agencies, that "they often work out of the public's eye." (We could find no coverage of the waivers in *Newsweek*, *USA Today*, *HuffPost*, *Vox*, or *NBC News*.) Analysis was cursory. Like government mouthpieces, the media took its role to be *announcing* the waivers.

A few mainstream articles even took a positive, explanatory tone. Waivers would allow for increased capacity in hospitals. They would permit medical professionals to cross state lines to "areas of greatest need," or, vaguely, "unlock extra powers"; they would "facilitate delivery of healthcare services." An outlet covering industry revenue, *Rev-Cycle Intelligence*, however, got it. It openly reassured investors: the waivers will protect providers "from potential financial penalties or sanctions stemming from care delivery rendered in good faith under extreme and uncontrollable circumstances." Weren't many circumstances more "controllable" than they wanted the public to believe? Was "good faith" to be taken for granted?

Some people make excuses for the facilities: the managers acted out of panic; they were just following orders from the governors; many workers went out sick or were afraid to return. But not every facility reacted in harmful ways. Some retained staff; some achieved a better staff-to-resident ratio. The long-term problem, posing the danger of future eldercides, is that while the efforts CMS made on behalf of corporate relationships had evil effects, in the emergency they were probably legal. Legal can be lethal. Many terrible forms of ageism are legal.

The evidentiary search, however, needn't end. An indefatigable journalist with an interest in aging, Lauren J. Mapp revealed in 2023 one result of the waiver in San Diego County. Before COVID, in 2019, out of 2,738 complaints, surveyors found 1,648 deficiencies. In 2020, complaints remained relatively steady, at 2,549. But predictably, surveyors managed to investigate only 393. By the time relicensing inspections resumed in April 2021, the trails were cold. Witnesses disappeared. Justice was impossible; correction, unlikely.

What would promote real reform, is an exposé from within—if some knowledgeable employees would come forward to explain the decision-making of March 2020. Most valuable would be those employed in Quality, Safety, and Oversight. Crony politics must be painful to honest civil servants. Some must have foreseen perilous consequences. Those forced to act against their conscience were exposed to moral injury. *Were any tempted to resign?* How did CMS make particular decisions? Postponing fire safety? Permitting fewer training hours for so long? Thousands of rooms were lying empty. Did they consider requiring that roommates be separated whenever possible, rather than breathing behind plastic shields or flimsy curtains less than six feet apart? The larger political question is how we protect public agencies from being waylaid by donors.

The editorial cartoonist whose succinct judgment is shown at the beginning of this chapter didn't think his upstanding woman with the cane and colorful scarf was moribund. Instead, as early as May 2020, Tim Hartman portrayed a monster chewing up the wall of her "protections." Hartman grasped the ethical situation. "We had *one* job." He was asking for investigations. "What went wrong?" Concerned people who knew the system had already guessed.

CHAPTER 3

HOW AMERICANS LEARNED TO ACCEPT THAT "THE OLD" WOULD DIE

The media taught the public how to think anew about "the Old" in the chaotic and desperate early circumstances of the pandemic. After decades of oblivion, they made the 1.4 million residents hypervisible. Some narratives about them were unavoidable. The terrifyingly quick mode of perishing in the grip of a choking illness began with them. They were also notable for dying in clusters. To the public, they could therefore hardly be visible as individuals, capable of vividly recounting their private situations—the two generations embracing in the hug tent, the woman who desperately called 911 for rescue, the man prevented from holding his dying wife. Instead, they became passively fused as a singularly vulnerable group because of the uniform ways they came to be described: as mortality statistics, through frightening, naturalizing metaphors about their susceptibility to the disease—as alien bodies emerging from "death pits."

Cultural analysts used to assert that in the US, death was a taboo topic. It may still be so, as a general rule, but the topic was not taboo when it was the residents of nursing facilities who went first. Then, tallying death's toll became obligatory. In the bald, detached form of *counting*, journalists early and frequently tallied the raw counts, as best they could in the absence of government data. The numbers they could count were alarming enough, and then, as available data did nothing but rise, they became apocalyptic. "Counting," Jacqueline Rose wrote somberly, is "a system for classifying the horror and bundling it away. . . . Counting humans, alive or dead, means you have entered a world of abstraction, the first sign that things have taken a desperate turn."

That spring, getting accurate data about residents became impossible. Until May 24, all through that winter and spring, the federal government, shamefully, did not request reports on cases and deaths. That decision, according to Danielle Ivory, an investigative reporter for the *New York Times*, "essentially missed the worst part of the outbreak in much of the country." True. In those months, sixteen thousand to forty thousand nursing-facility residents, or more, may have died uncounted. (See the appendix.) No one can ever know for sure.

Starting with Trump, some people in the administration were hoping to fool the public by minimizing danger. If they thought that not getting official numbers would stymie the media, they were partially wrong. Some journalists kept counting. Ivory's team began "a totally manual collection effort. We were going state by state, calling county officials and medical examiners' offices." People also tallied the rise of the *nation's* totals; the authors of *A Deeper Sickness*, a diary, reported nine hundred deaths by March 25 and seven thousand by April 3. By early April, Ivory had identified "more than 7,000 deaths in nursing homes" alone. It might have seemed as if *only* the residents of the facilities were likely to succumb.

The media focus on fatalities, although riveting, was unlikely to drive attention to the political failures behind the deaths. This shift in attention was the swivel that Albert Camus made, to confront the causes behind the plague. In the US, making that swivel would have meant reporting not only "tragedy" but scandal. In a crisis there is no substitute for reports given by those most affected. More early stories from survivors might have helped make the brick-and-mortar locales a cause for activism, aimed at saving the residents immured inside. From amid the horrors, we've heard some who were capable of speaking authoritatively, *validating their humanity*—sounding grateful for care or conscious of wrongs, courageous or scared, cynical or outraged, resigned or accusatory. Most stories, however, were told *about* them—often by adult offspring anxious about being unable to visit. Data without stories, a compound bias. This lacuna made it possible to profile the residents en masse and yet contradictorily. Hypervisible as dying people, thought to be uniformly old and frail, they were simultaneously invisible and inaudible. (Other marginalized groups— young Black men, "menopausal" women—are familiar with similar ornery objectifications applied to them.) Age scholars consider the term *the Old* negative and obsolete. I use it in scare quotes to emphasize the residents' imagined homogeneity and fatal vulnerability and everything that befell them as a result.

PITIABLE

One effect of these failures of representation was that in 2020, pity, indifference, or even aversion to the residents could seem warranted. Their appealing qualities (as depicted in the prologue and in chapter 1) had historically been barely visible in film, in photography, on TV, on the Web, or in newspapers. The residents had been stigmatized for the kind of inadequate attendance that left them lying in feces or wandering in hallways seeking help. The proximate cause of misery and harm was understaffing. Anguished family members, overworked aides, and indignant reformers had long suspected that many owners achieved profits by keeping staffing lean, a practice that inevitably overworks the remaining employees and leads to mistreatment of the captive audience.

Understaffing leads to neglected turning; poor skin care leads to pressure ulcers, grinding pain, sepsis, even death. Delays in responding to calls lead to falls and broken bones as people with limited mobility try to help themselves. Understaffing is correlated with more use of antipsychotics or (illegal) restraints. The practice was widespread, but Black or Latinx residents were likelier to suffer. Understaffing also leads to infections, a main source of misery, pain, and death long before COVID. CMS needed to mandate, not merely "urge," higher standards.

The walls of protection that should have kept COVID outside, had been made porous—by governors who ordered hospitals to send patients with the virus to the ill-prepared nursing facilities, and by skinflint operators, whose overworked aides had to pass in and out to similar second jobs, in risky contact with other residents. Staff attention was fragmented by heightened workloads and by anxiety about themselves and people they cared for.

In May 2020, the General Accounting Office confirmed the worst suspicions by reporting that understaffing had been a chronic issue prior to COVID and that its gravity had been neglected by CMS. In the pandemic the damages became only graver and apparently more widespread. An important symptom might be missed as just another appearance of aged frailty. A hacking cough might not get noticed by a tired aide in time. Isolated and fearful, some people who had been okay lost abilities to wash, dress, or control excretions. People who needed help eating were left alone long enough to die of dehydration. News stories recounted the conditions of those who had been neglected: their open sores, nasty sheets, cries for help, helplessness.

Such graphic accounts of abuse left the impression that the residents were merely bodies, weak, pitiable, physically disgusting. Confusing the inhabitants with their locales, a crude existing problem, became far more likely. These conditions and mortality data heightened the already repugnant image of "homes" as deadly warehouses. In April 2020, a former lieutenant governor of New York State was quoted in the *New York Times* referring to nursing facilities as "death pits." Squalor became attached to the dying inhabitants as a group. The result was, I fear, a perverse appeal to a squeamish side that many of us possess. Lacking fuller context, this side is third cousin to bullying. It is first cousin to aversion. It is the bad brother of indifference. These are ways that public emotions get constructed, almost invisibly.

It is apt to contrast the residents with another group noted early on as vulnerable: medical personnel working extra shifts. They too were endangered, but their deaths were not described as squalid or pitiable; their bodies were not portrayed as helpless. They were properly regretted. "Our Heroes," read appreciative signs that popped up everywhere. (That made the forgotten workers in nursing homes say,

"Heroes work *here* too.") The group of "the Old" was obviously un-heroic, inessential, useless, frail.

Frailty has a "rather vague definition" medically: even after age eighty it affects a minority. But in some ugly part of the social imaginary, it meant *just waiting to die, moribund.* In April 2020, Ron DeSantis, the governor of a state populated by many older adults, thought fit to say out loud what others merely thought: "Florida is ground zero for the nursing home; I mean we're God's waiting room."

In Simone Weil's remarkable essay on the *Iliad,* the French philosopher of domination and subordination analyzed how power works between unequals. It "rests principally upon that marvelous indifference that the strong feel toward the weak, an indifference so contagious that it infects the very people who are the objects of it." What is "marvelous," perhaps, is that some of the stronger don't even *see* these "objects." The mass of residents dying was just a big number changing so fast that no one could remember it.

NOT OUTRAGED

Season after season in 2020, a million family members and friends were grieving their share of those 112,000 or 128,000, or 152,000, or 178,000 losses. Millions of others, despite their own preoccupations, must have been upset by the number of deaths or the pathos of the inmates' situations or touched by the sorrow of the families. But why was there not more outrage? This question is not rhetorical.

The lack starts with the misperceptions demolished in chapter 1. Finding yourself in congregate living is not a sign of being near the end of life; it's either a short convalescent stay or a new home. People living with impairments and preexisting conditions and new troubles may enjoy long lives. Those who died would have lived longer if they had been protected. Being old is not an imminent death sentence. Getting COVID is not necessarily a death sentence.

Ignorance stifles outrage. But—this is a sad, odd, shamefaced admission—I too was slow to grasp those facts. That's why the facts are placed early in the book. My mother's long life, my grandfather's, should have removed my misperceptions. Strong people can live to be old, having survived whatever adversity throws at them. As an age critic, I didn't need to disidentify with residents, as Trump did. Yet I too started in March 2020 ignorantly assuming that many residents must have been frail enough to be close to death. Research taught me that the false assumption about "frailty" was widely shared, deeply distorting the public narrative.

In this place it is worth remembering "super-survivors" like Sylvia Goldsholl of New Jersey. She had also survived the deadly 1918 "Spanish" flu. In May 2020, on the occasion of her second return to health, Alexis Shanes quoted the 108-year-old saying, of her family and herself, "They knew that I was a wonder. . . . I met their expectations." For the interview Ms. Goldsholl wore crimson lipstick. Her blue cardigan was embroidered with flowers; her white hair beautifully coiffed. She was as vivid as a Jasper Johns' flag. "My mom was educated in Russia," Ms. Goldsholl said. "My father came from a very high-class background. I made the best of both." She had been a letter-writing activist. Goldsholl was far from the only wonder. Seeking counternarratives while watching those preventable deaths mount, I was a contrarian searching for a way out of wretchedness. It was some relief to figure out that although residents had suffered hundreds of thousands of infections, hundreds of thousands recovered.

While COVID was raging, even if fear was gripping them with no end in sight, residents who found someone to listen showed they wanted to live and were obstinately trying to do so. In our culture, truths about fortitude and the tenacity of older bodies and spirits will have to be repeated emphatically, many times, to undo just one of the common sets of blinders.

BAD APPLES?

Age is not, it never is in later life, "just a number." Ageism savages that smiley-faced adage. Many residents—turned into "inmates" by the lockdown—died from callous neglect, directed at them not only from high up but from close by.

One brutal story is of the Soldiers Home in Holyoke, Massachusetts, a "state-funded, fully accredited long-term health care facility that offers eligible veterans quality health care [and] hospice care." Union officials had long warned about inadequacies. In that harrowing situation, leadership ordered staff to merge two "dementia" units, cramming residents with COVID in with uninfected people. Suddenly, residents were jostled by rude and hasty hands, hustled or carried without warning into an unknown space, deprived of familiar objects, bewildered by lack of information. Many must have been perfectly aware of the panic, the chilling absence of caring touch; the opposite of dignity, humiliation. Being used as an "instrument" for the benefit of others obliterates our intrinsic value. An intimidated employee who helped move them said it felt like walking them "to their death." Seventy-eight residents died. An independent report found the "mistakes" "utterly baffling."

Everywhere, people with Alzheimer's or other cognitive impairments died in higher percentages than other residents. One early study found that while residents diagnosed with dementia accounted for 52 percent of COVID-19 cases in the nursing homes, they constituted 72 percent of COVID-19 deaths there. Dementism, or neuroageism, has to be considered as a contributing cause of the Eldercide—not in one spot in Holyoke, Massachusetts, but in every place with evidence of disproportionate mortality rates. Stephen Post, a philosopher, coined the term *dementism* to capture "the specificity of resentment against the deeply forgetful."

Lethal neuroageism should seem no more baffling than racism. Professor Konetzka's testimony to the Wyden Committee revealed that people of color who died of COVID had often been caught in for-profit establishments, in larger residences more reliant on stingy Medicaid, cursed with inadequate staffing. Use of the word "mistakes" avoids shame and evades assigning guilt. Deciding what is "criminal" in the Eldercide has been slow, piecemeal, rare. Nailing owners and fraudulent corporations is just. It must be done. But case-by-case arguments about punishing "bad actors" do not bring institutional transformation. The courtroom dramas, if there are any, must not distract us from unraveling government irresponsibility. The public did not know, but now can now, where blame truly lies—how systems that we ignore at our peril actually work.

UPSTREAM

"Look upstream." As I have heard, this activist saying refers to a bunch of good souls who are rescuing babies as they float down a river. Day after day, they pull babies out of the water. There's no end to it, but they are patient, dedicated. Finally, a bemused person coming by asks, "Who is up there throwing the babies into the river?"

Congress had thrown sicker and needier and less able older people mainly to the private sector, in an ill-conceived government-run system. Congress thus made their care into a commodity rather than a right. Capitalism does not work well for health care; other nations know this. Once a political system puts profit in charge, if that top goal is not continuously and staunchly resisted, the system tends to favor moneyed interests; lobbies ask for favors. Then, by dividing funding and responsibility between the federal and state governments, Congress left too much power to those states that never cared enough.

"I like to follow the money," says my friend Andrew Wengraf, a retired philosophy professor, "and the smell in my nostrils at the facilities I've visited is the whiff of the entrenched racket that 'care' of the elderly is." Year in and year out, the nursing-facility industry maximizes its assured cash flow, which is derived from Medicaid, Medicare, tax advantages, private payers, and residents' Social Security, for the upkeep of a continuous clientele of captives. About 70 percent of nursing facilities are privately owned; 58 percent are owned by corporate chains. The for-profit industry is represented by the American Health Care Association.

"The current Medicare and Medicaid system is biased toward institutional rather than home-based care, underwriting a $240 billion nursing facility industry," Meg Coffin states. Coffin is the CEO of a nonprofit center that advises cities and people with disabilities. That's the short explanation of how compound ageism became institutionalized.

The Eldercide illuminates its own past of neglect. Elizabeth Dugan, a gerontologist at the University of Massachusetts Boston, told the *Boston Globe*, "We don't [even] think of nursing homes as part of the health care system. We could have done better. We should have done better." Writing in the *Journals of Gerontology*, Edward Alan Miller and his colleagues bluntly observe that "long-term care is the ugly stepchild of health policy. It is widely understood that . . . the sector is inadequately financed and ineffectively regulated."

The entire public health care system was neglected. In 2003, SARS, the first coronavirus attack, provided a moment of sensible warnings to improve disaster preparedness to "avoid future events that might be catastrophic for the global system." As Arthur Kleinman and James L. Watson once declared, "SARS scared the hell out of everyone." It did not scare us enough. The funding petered out. In at least ten government reports from 2003 to 2015, federal officials predicted a shortage of ventilators, masks, and other supplies if faced by a large-scale infectious disease outbreak. Administration after administration had not adequately replenished the stockpile.

That said, it turns out that preparedness for nursing homes and home-health agencies has typically not been included at all in disaster planning efforts. Hurricane Katrina's abandoned nursing facilities proved as much, in 2005. The safest course in a pandemic is for government to have done everything necessary the day before, including demanding a high minimum number of hours per resident day and providing funding for face-to-face staffing.

UGLY STEPCHILD

By 2020, a run of CMS failures had put residents at notable risk. Some facilities had been cited repeatedly for years over serious deficiencies that CMS never forced them to fix, as the General Accounting Office finally reported in the midst of the crisis. CMS had the power to levy fines, but the Trump administration had reduced the amounts of those fines even when harm resulted in a resident's death, reversing guidelines put in place under President Obama. Under Seema Verma, the CMS lowered fines from hundreds of thousands of dollars to a maximum of $22,000. This amount was a gnat to the nursing facilities owned by private companies. Was reducing fines also a "mistake"?

Medical reforms made in the Obama era were also stymied: "In July 2019, the Trump administration proposed new rules relaxing the requirements [so that] there was no longer a requirement for a full-time, hands-on expert in infection contamination on-site." Many operators then reduced the hours of those essential experts. An analysis from *American Progress* contains a damning summary: "This lack of additional oversight—combined with the prior regulatory rollbacks on staffing ratios, fines levied for injuries, and requirements for arbitration—served to undermine safety for nursing home patients and staff."

THE LONG, SILENT ELDERCIDE

In fact, as said earlier, an eldercide had been occurring all along, but one that lacked documentation because people suffered or died prematurely, one by one. The system let many operators go slack; negligence and crimes were rarely caught. Responsibility was hard to pin down. Facile excuses, muddied financial records, and, from the government side, vast user-unfriendly official data sets and careless auditing easily concealed perpetrators.

In 2021, finally, came "shattering and bulletproof" statistics showing that private-equity ownership (PE) tended to be fatal. "Going into a PE-owned nursing home increase[d] the short-term probability of death by about 10%, implying over 20,000 lives lost" over twelve years—and these losses were occurring *before* the pandemic. In the first year of COVID, for-profit facilities made up a disproportionate percentage of those with extremely high infection rates. More than 1,300 for-profits had an average overall mortality rate close to 20 percent, according to the Office of the Inspector General, the watchdog.

Seventy percent of owners were for-profit companies. Fifty-eight percent were operated by corporate chains; some chains are owned by hedge funds. Investors get rich. No doubt some facilities are "struggling businesses barely avoiding bankruptcy." But Dave E. Kingsley, in his blog, *Tallgrass Economics: Economics, Finance, and Politics of Aging*, overturns this "false impression." He writes:

> Industry media such as *Skilled Nursing News* and *McKnight's Senior Living* reinforce this narrative, which is based on the pervasively faulty and misleading cost reports—not consolidated financial statements.

Sophisticated owners and their CPAs devise ways to hide profits. They shunt Medicare and Medicaid dollars from their "struggling" facility to "related-party" companies that they also own: a real estate entity, a management company, or a staffing agency that then charges them an arm and a leg for management, food, or rent—"costs." More than eleven thousand nursing homes—almost three-quarters—had such business dealings, according to an analysis of financial records by Kaiser Health News. Some owners are rightly called "slumlords." Gretchen Morgenson devotes pages to these "privateers" in her co-written 2023 book, *These Are the Plunderers*. Owners who hide profits beg for more funding, and they continually lobby legislators for less oversight. We've seen how that turned out with CMS. It is hard to believe that anyone who had ever worked in CMS was surprised by the scale of COVID deaths or the causes.

Bill Pascrell, chairman of the House Ways and Means Subcommittee on Oversight, complained, "Understanding the web of transactions, it's like a Russian nesting doll. A lack of transparency in private equity ownership makes proper oversight by regulators nearly impossible." Investigative journalist Moe Tkacik uncovered a way in which some firms nest the dolls. As landlords, real estate investment trusts (REITs) collect rent from nursing facilities. In 2020, some US companies stopped paying rent or negotiated lower terms. One nursing chain whose landlord was a private equity firm, however, paid out "millions in administrative fees, and most infuriatingly, more [than] a million dollars in annual rent. . . . Unlike the bailouts for airlines and small businesses created by the Coronavirus Aid, Relief, and Economic Security (CARES) Act, the nursing home bailout program did not require recipients to use funds primarily for payroll," Tkacik discovered. Some facilities paid steep rents while cutting aides and food budgets. In one place residents were going hungry.

But how hard had regulators been working to restrain the owners of the nesting dolls? *Oversight* has two antithetical meanings. One is "supervision," which CMS was responsible for maintaining, to prevent harms and deaths. Failure points to the other meaning of *oversight*: *We missed it and didn't even notice. Just an oversight.*

In 2020, disgraceful failures to treat the residents as if they were as equally worthy of living as anyone else had been preceded by decades of federal negligence. Inspectors managed to report serious violations—including dirty medical equipment—at about 3,500 homes. CMS continued to "clear" most violations. Roughly two-thirds of all COVID fatalities linked to nursing homes from March through August 2020 occurred in facilities that had previously received "a clean bill of health." Most facilities avoided paying any fines.

"I can't think of one decision that CMS made properly," Professor Charlene Harrington told the *Washington Post*. Harrington, a sociology and nursing professor at the University of California at San Francisco, had scrutinized the industry for more than thirty years. "They just rolled over, whatever the nursing homes wanted. CMS made it so much worse than it could have been if they had just kept their oversight in place."

The Centers for Disease Control and Prevention (CDC) also made a fatal decision. Testing was an absolute prerequisite for diagnosis, isolation, and treatment. When the CDC finally produced an accurate test, they then failed to identify long-term care residents as the highest priority for getting it. The 15,400 residences could have been treated as sentinel surveillance sites. Such sites test everyone, including those who are apparently well, in order to discover unseen transmission. Protecting the asymptomatic protects others. Keeping residents well should have made sense even to those who prioritized community dwellers, so the residents would not flood the ICUs. Instead, CDC gave testing priority to hospitals. PPE went to hospitals; other supplies went to hospitals. By May one critic called the failures in nursing homes "senicide." Cindy Sanders of Austin, Texas, who saw her mother lose a dozen peers by the end of July 2020, had a more vivid name for it. "It didn't have to be this way. If rapid, robust ongoing testing had been in place, we would not have this carnage."

LIABLE

Liability suits for harm to residents not only restrain an industry, as genuine timely and frequent inspections also do. Legal discovery is a vehicle to learn exactly what happened to cause residents to die. Many families don't know and will never know. The racial disparities in death tolls strongly suggest that immunity laws hide and perpetuate racist disparities, while the high overall death rates also suggest ageism, sexism, ableism, and dementism.

The nursing-home lobby had long sought immunity for substandard care. Now "the industry has seized on this public health crisis to pursue that objective," the American Bar Association tersely commented. In May, Alex Azar told the governors this shield was "imperative." Two hundred and fifty national, state, and local advocacy organizations objected. On May 28, 2020, they penned a letter urging Congress to reserve the right to sue, which they sent to Republican majority leader Mitch McConnell and minority leader Charles Schumer. The letter refrained from using the concept of *corporate state capture*—"where private industry uses its political influence to take control of the decision-making apparatus of the state, such as regulatory agencies, law enforcement entities, and legislatures." Some legislators receive donations from the for-profit lobby. It can be hard to discover which ones do.

The authors sent a beggars' letter, forceful but anticipating its futility. They wrote:

> Stripping residents of their right to hold nursing homes accountable for substandard care will put more residents at risk and inevitably result in increased resident deaths. We implore you to keep

this fundamental right in place . . . It would be perverse to ask facility residents to pay with their lives for the woefully insufficient emergency preparedness and substandard care of nursing homes, while allowing nursing homes themselves to face no repercussions for their egregious behavior . . . years of cost cutting and profit maximizing, by relieving them of responsibility.

Some states behaved with astounding perversity well into the catastrophe. The *Journal of Aging and Social Policy* noted that "lawmakers have often looked to cutting Medicaid eligibility and services for savings." In 2020, the state of New York first passed a budget with $1.6 billion in Medicaid *cuts*. Ohio made similar cuts. Eventually, thirty-eight states eliminated the residents' right to sue. Nina A. Kohn, a Yale law professor, concluded that "operators could be increasingly confident that they would never be held accountable for decisions that harmed their residents." Did their being given sudden freedom from legal liability as well as from inspections and fines explain managers who made little attempt to separate a sick person living in a double or triple room, or the owners who refused to give paid sick leave to aides?

Conferring immunity was deeply perverse. From the end of May, when official counting began, to late October 2020, resident deaths per week more than doubled. The industry protested that staff could not be found. But the willing invented solutions. Owners raised wages and paid sick leave so aides could stay home to recover. Several administrators brought in mobile homes and paid frontline staff to live in them, rather than returning home to their families.

The deadly fact is that a full fifth of facilities that had reported severe shortages of PPE and staff in May—those with infection outbreaks, low ratings, and more Medicaid patients—did not meaningfully improve those conditions by July. (Some people had bedsores neglected so long they sustained gruesome injuries. In June, one wound "went down to the bone with exposed tendon." This place, in Pennsylvania, had not lost staff, it had *cut* staff.) Protective gear was finally procurable and billions of federal dollars had been sent to eligible owners. An early 2020 federal program offered to train facilities in infection prevention; some facilities failed to take advantage of the offer. Some operators acted responsibly. Others could have. Instead, callous decisions were made.

Many more residents could have survived. From 571,410 to a million people became infected; many might have been saved. Healthy people who had signed Do Not Resuscitate orders, "just in case," might never have needed them. The residents were betrayed by the very government institutions that should have driven resources not to the owners but toward them.

THOSE WHO TEND TO DIE

The image of older people as those-who-are-always-about-to-die, no-matter-what, was created by the overlapping early–COVID Era reasons already noted: the obsessive media counting, the belief that younger people were safe, the media assertion that they were safer, and the lack of individualized resident voices.

In addition, "doomed to die" was becoming part of a rapidly forming, apparently scientific narrative. Writing in the *Hill* (the largest independent political news site in the US at that time) in April 2020, three colleagues at Northwestern University's Feinberg School of Medicine claimed that "because of the communal nature of these domiciles and the fragile physiologic state and attendant comorbidities of these residents, the odds of survival is low." We know they were wrong. The authors, two MDs and a geriatrician, did not speculate on whether some "communal domiciles" might be kept free of infection (as we know some were), or wonder what percentage of hospitalized or non-hospitalized residents were surviving. Their aim was kindly: they wanted to convince Beltway insiders of the urgency of universal testing, hoping not to lose "this terrifying war." Their prognostication of slim odds of survival matched what people already believed about how "fragile" residents were. That was the ableist part of age profiling.

Language, forceful, poetic, or shocking, makes particular narratives stick in our imaginations. "Coronavirus outbreaks like 'wildfire' at US nursing homes under lockdowns," read a *Guardian* headline of

April 2, 2020. In the same month, when New York City was the epicenter, Governor Andrew Cuomo, at the time often quoted as a reassuring guru, even more powerfully visualized the same destructive simile. "This is like watching a fire going through dry grass with a strong wind," he said. "And it's blowing the fire, and a couple embers wind up on one side of the field and embers start to catch fire and that's a cluster. . . ." Two medical authorities, Joseph G. Ouslander and David C. Grabowski, hoped to "calm the perfect storm" that started the "wildfire" by urging that nursing facilities be prioritized for PPE and testing. They called the homes "a tinderbox."

The language that accompanied the data storm supported the narrative of futility that was becoming dominant. This language, of fire, embers, wind, storm—forces considered "natural"—made it seem that humans had no control, even though, as usual, in every phase of a disaster—"causes, vulnerability, preparedness, results and response . . . and the difference between who lives and who dies"—fateful decisions were being made or avoided. (*When apparently well-meaning, ineffective or even harmful.*) As hyperbole swept through the media like wildfire, older people and residents alike became "dry grass"—ready to flame up quickly and helplessly die out to ash. In that frightening, panic-filled time, the most hysterical public projections about hecatombs in "tinderboxes" did not seem preposterous. Since no one had yet wondered if many, or any, residents were surviving, the rhetoric of natural forces overpowering weak bodies may well have left the impression that few of the 1.4 million original residents remained alive. All, all doomed. Fire and ash—funereal, Biblical, apocalyptic—became the national atmosphere that observers breathed in with the data.

Before COVID it was possible, sometimes, to imagine that at the approach of death our older folks might say calmly, "Well, I've lived long enough!" People want to hear classical serenity. If this book's alternative explanation had taken hold—that the residents wanted to live, and that the government was neglecting helpless people, harming them, even sacrificing them—that reality might at the time have been too painful to contemplate. The likelihood that their loved ones were being abandoned rendered the families of the residents desperate but helpless. Advocates who knew exactly what should be done have told me they were driven by impotent wisdom into outrage.

ALIENATION

Forecasting the futility of rescue was to be the most dangerous effect of these discourses. As long as the entire group was represented as doomed, that portrayal created lasting doubt that anyone was to blame, or, for the suspicious, uncertainty about what or whom to blame. Alienation from the residents thus became emotionally easier. The British psychoanalyst Adam Phillips wrote decades ago about personal psychic retreats from "unpleasant thoughts," which to him included generational otherness, aging, and dying. A positive desire to escape encapsulated misery justifies turning away. Psychologists say that *justifications* "facilitate the release of genuine prejudice in a way that does not severely compromise one's egalitarian self-concept and does not induce guilt or shame." Adam Phillips concluded, as if in a footnote to Hannah Arendt, "Common-sense equals, get rid of what you cannot effectually succour."

Phillips's universalizing "common sense" about how alienation or expulsion work in theory needs a specific US history and a cultural dimension. Inchoate public emotions about pitiful, aged otherness surely varied across a staggering spectrum. Experts and some in the government hierarchies must have observed the blatant obstacles to rescuing the residents (the feral interstate war over PPE; the flabby inspection regulations; the abominable apathy of some facility owners). For distressed publics it was easier to believe that *biology* explained the death toll. Detailed media narratives that represented the residents as helpless bodies—wheezing, crumpled, smelly—may have alienated squeamish temperaments. Imagery becomes torture porn if readers believe only that rescue is destined to fail. Some will feel hatred, aversion, or simply indifference to the abjected.

In the "Before Time," Americans had already been exposed to relentless discourses about the burden of having to provide intimate long-term personal care to their elders or spouses. Responsible individuals want to provide good care. Alzheimer's disease, represented as a demographic catastrophe, added to those painful anticipations. In fact, its prevalence is relatively low. Dread could arise from ignorance about the breadth of the dementia spectrum (even severe losses do not always end in mutism or inability to recognize the caregiver). Resentment about needing to care for people in the late stages of the disease is expressed in some recordings (found on TikTok under the #Dementia tag), mocking people with Alzheimer's or escalating arguments with them.

At worst, dementism means, *It doesn't matter so much if "they" die. They may want to. Who would care to live that way?* Alleging that people lumped together in this man-made category prefer suicide to living has no equivalent in racism or sexism. As we'll see, the wish that old people might want to die prematurely was promoted publicly, with the justifications that their doing so would save taxpayers' money and relieve adult children of trouble and guilt. It was a fantasy of euthanasia.

Nursing homes had served, back of mind, as a last resort—sobering and unwanted perhaps, but possible. Then a global disease turned the facilities into charnel houses and made something like the fantasy of euthanasia a fact. Along with the mortality data, images of ambulances in front of signs with euphemistic names like Villa or Happy Valley rendered facilities as akin to morgues, antechambers to death. Some part of the adult population was forced to imagine caring for a helpless adult, a spouse or parent, on their own, with COVID lurking, without that default option. Others, already giving unremitting care to needy loved ones, found themselves unable to reach a doctor or recruit anyone for respite care.

WERE ALL THEIR DEATHS EXTRA DEATHS?

Although the ghostly disappearance of residents did draw constant attention to the cumulative death toll, the rapidly rising numbers were badly misunderstood. In any epidemic, deaths exceed normal mortality rates. Public health officials call these "excess deaths." In 2020, deaths of people in nursing facilities were up 32 percent over the normal rate in 2019, according to the indispensable Office of the Inspector General. Dr. David Grabowski of Harvard Medical School, a learned researcher, was taken aback. "I don't think even those of us who work in this area thought it was going to be this bad. This was not individuals who were going to die anyway. We are talking about a really big number of excess deaths."

Remember the 1,950 facilities that protected their residents and suffered *no* COVID deaths in the first ten desperate months? Knowing that many other deaths could also have been prevented, we need a stronger explanatory concept than the gross statistical label of "excess" deaths. When the economist Amartya Sen, who would go on to be awarded a Nobel Prize, discovered all the female babies, girls, and women who were missing in misogynistic societies, he decided societies needed the term *extra deaths*. Simply, no one had noticed the lost females before, or asked why and how they went "lost." Sen noticed, counted, asked, and answered. *Extra* deaths are unnecessary, avoidable. Even if they are uncountable, they are enormously significant.

The deepest question now becomes, "Was every unexpected COVID death in nursing facilities in that year a premature, extra death?" Compound ageism and ignorance may have prevented us from noticing them as such. The concept of *social determinants of death* moves us surefootedly past biomedical explanations of futility to the search for overlapping discriminations on the part of those with most power. Except in cases like the Holyoke Soldiers Home, the media left the fog of ignorance intact, often noting individual abuses or early concentrations of deaths but not emphasizing *patterns* of potential wrongfulness. When deaths were represented as the result of individual despair at the isolation, this assumption (like that of biological frailty) obliterated the possibility of neglect—with its known connection to understaffing. This oblivion reminds observers of the way police malfeasance used to go unnoticed, until brave videographers connected the depraved-heart killings to often unpunished acts of violent racism.

In possibly the first criminal case in the US brought against a nursing facility caretaker who "Wantonly or Recklessly Commits *or Permits*" bodily injury or abuse, neglect, or mistreatment to "an Elder or Disabled Person," the Massachusetts attorney general indicted two administrators of the Holyoke Soldiers Home. An amicus brief to the court supports the argument that a "caretaker" is a person responsible for "primary and substantial assistance for care." Can an agency head, or a business owner, who "permits" understaffing, be determined to be a "caretaker"? Can researchers show further that CMS's 1135 waivers of inspection were responsible for exposing residents to a heightened risk of coronavirus contagion, a "bodily injury," and thus led to *extra* deaths?

If the public could understand extra deaths in the facilities, past or present, as an eldercide, that understanding would be an additional impetus to transform the system, and a welcome development of agewise consciousness. The lethality of compound ageism could be a revelation as great as that of lethal police racism, in the same period. The residents' painful history is of the highest political importance, and it should be of concern to everyone who has a keen sense of social justice or a fear of growing old poor.

CHAPTER 4

A CHASM OPENS

Vital Youth vs. Moribund Age

The issue wasn't only that older *residents* were dying or that "the Old" living in the community were also dying in startling numbers. "The Old die" had become the globe's most incontestable fact. The issue of concern was what those deaths meant, or if they signified anything. This book has started to explain the rise and spread of a damning belief—that suddenly, as the president of the British Society of Gerontologists, Thomas Scharf, put it in June 2020, "old people's lives appear[ed] not to matter." Of course, they did matter to old people themselves and to their loved ones. After 2021, they mattered to governors who decided to vaccinate the surviving residents and older adults first, even if their motive for doing so was to empty their hospitals or undo the political damage of having too many nursing-facility deaths on their watch. What truly devalued older lives was a blatant contrast: Youth was almost idolized.

Nothing significant happens to one age group without affecting other age groups. Certainly not when the worst epidemic in one hundred years strikes and—unlike the flu of 1918–1919, which killed all ages indiscriminately—especially strikes older adults. Year One of the COVID Era brought sudden, historic, and irrational alterations in the way ordinary people thought about a host of intimate beliefs—specifically, those concerning "the Old" and "Youth." Such collectives are imaginary, but the chasm opened between them had real effects. In different ways, it harmed everyone.

"THE OLD" BECAME HYPERVISIBLE

Age had captured the spotlight to such a degree that it obscured other distinctions. Race and class took a back seat. Even though death tolls were disproportionately mounting in communities of color, it took much longer for the media and state officials to *notice*. COVID had been devastating a much bigger second group that lived outside care facilities: midlife and older people, white and of color, many of them immigrants, including those working as aides in the same facilities, as well as indigenous people, the undocumented, the unhoused, workers in meat-processing plants, and prisoners.

Many members of that second group of outsiders overlapped with people in nursing facilities, not least in terms of lesser access to resources such as savings. Members of both high-risk groups (whether the residents or community-dwelling white, Black, indigenous, or other people of color) had in common that they been worn down bodily by psychosocial factors—*social* determinants of health. As noted earlier—a scandal among rich nations—almost half of all Americans were living with serious chronic conditions, and 53 percent were below sixty years of age. Almost 20 percent suffered from such conditions (diabetes, hypertension, asthma) young, in their twenties.

Even when deaths became highlighted, as of Black and Latinx community dwellers, people rarely noticed how relatively young the dying were. By May 2020, the CDC's data, indicated that more than one-third of Hispanic [*sic*] decedents (34.9 percent), nearly one-third (29.5 percent) of nonwhite decedents, and 13.2 percent of white non-Hispanic decedents were *under* sixty-five. African Americans were dying from COVID at roughly the same rate as white people—but the former were dying a decade younger. Tribal Americans, whose health services have long been underfunded, were even worse off. Racism and classism lessen life chances, starting in utero. Come the epidemic, suddenly "life chances" meant better or worse odds of literal survival. Prejudice is more dangerous to *everyone* whom society has left vulnerable.

Despite overlaps among these two vulnerable groups, I noticed that news stories oddly tended to segregate them. There would be articles about "the Old" in the facilities, and separate articles about people of color. This pattern suggests a conceptual wall between community dwellers and care-home residents, as if they were categorically distinct, as if people of color didn't *also* live in nursing facilities. As if people dwelling at home were all young, healthy, and able to go out working. As if nursing-home aides did not go back and forth between the two locations.

Community dwellers were correctly reported as being at high risk from comorbidities but not as if *biology* were their foremost enemy. No. Unlike residents, their death toll was explained mainly by socioeconomic circumstances. True, but incomplete. Often they were constrained to live in cramped multigenerational households, especially in high-rent cities. Some community dwellers of so-called retirement age were forced by need of a paycheck to work outside their own homes. Many families found it difficult to take precautions or isolate those who were sick.

Overriding distinctions of age, race, and class, transcending the surges and lulls, another number, growing only in one fierce and fatal direction, mesmerized the population. By the first autumn, there had been two hundred thousand US deaths, and by the new year, almost four hundred thousand. Thinking about death could be forced on anyone, daily. A writer in the *Boston Globe* condensed common impressions from that period:

It's hard to remember a year when death was so in your face from morning to night—from pages of obituaries in the morning paper to the nightly news with its images of mobile morgues parked outside overwhelmed hospitals and cemetery workers burying bodies as fast as possible with few mourners present.

Who were they, in the mobile morgues and cemeteries? As early as July 2020, a new statistic circulated, that 80 percent of the US dead were over the age of sixty-five. The headline "1 of Every 100 Older Americans Has Perished" appeared on the front page of the *New York Times* in 2021. The early blare of announcements that residents composed 40 percent of the dead, and in some states over half, was overshadowed. Obviously not all who died had lived in nursing facilities. Residents had made up only 0.42 percent of the population. Everyone over sixty-five constituted *16* percent. Receiving less attention, the residents' dire conditions may have caused less concern or regret. The most succinct definition of "the expendables" I have found is "people whose disappearance wouldn't draw attention." With the onset of a more encompassing dread, that small hapless group was exiled, farther still, from the social embrace.

"GOD'S WAITING ROOM" GETS MORE CROWDED

The definition of "the Old" had expanded; all older adults in their millions were fused as an imperiled or dying mass. As early as April 2020, a distinguished critical gerontologist at the University of Manchester, Chris Phillipson, wrote me about a disturbing trend in the UK that I was also seeing in the US: "'Frailty' and 'vulnerability.' Much used pre-Covid-19[, the labels are] now applied routinely to anyone over 65/70; profoundly disempowering without question." Across the nation, a miasma of doom was spreading around the entire group of older adults, often as young as fifty.

Long in advance of the pandemic, our economy and society had cast troubling doubts on the value of growing older. The life-course narrative was characterized by warring descriptions, often set up between "positive aging" and "the truth" of inevitable age-related decline. "Aging," or more exactly, aging past youth, becomes hypervisible on "our surface edges" (Ralph Waldo Emerson's keen metaphor of embodiment), on hair and skin. Past some uncertain age, being viewed as "aging"—meaning growing beyond midlife, or toward old age—could already become a trigger for ageism, as I observed in a

2017 book. The war of interpretations, however, although apparently tilting steadily toward inequality and life-course decline, had had no settled outcome.

With COVID the emphasis on elders' risk and death marked an escalation toward settling that outcome in the worst way. The "eight out of ten" statistic bandied about suddenly made susceptibility to the deadly disease a frightening, incontrovertible fact about the entire midlife group, people in the so-called Third Age, many of whom had considered themselves in their prime: busy, humming, healthy, and active. *Everyone* above a certain age became one of those-who-tend-to-die. . . . *can't be helped.*

Statistically, as I noted, early data had revealed that frailty and co-morbidities determined death *more* than age alone did. Over and over, however, graphs widened the gap between "the Young" and everybody else, merely by showing number of deaths rising by age. If the danger was said to start at age *fifty*, the anonymizing category, "old and high risk," expanded even more. In August 2020, the scientific journal *Nature* divided the population into two groups: those under and those over fifty. "For every 1,000 people infected with the coronavirus who are under the age of 50, almost none will die," reporter Smriti Mallapaty asserted. "For people in their fifties and early sixties, about five will die—more men than women." A full third of Americans were over fifty. The unhealthy half of Americans, often uninsured, were particularly vulnerable.

Such facts should have been understood as part of a huge risk shift away from simple age toward socioeconomic causes. The Centers for Disease Control, providing the government data, nevertheless remained focused on age as the mightiest risk factor. "Risk increases with age" was still the CDC warning. Getting "very sick" meant "hospitalization, intensive care, or a ventilator to help them breathe, or they might even die," the website said. Risk "increases for people in their 50s."

"God's waiting room," as Governor Ron DeSantis called his state, Florida, was actually a derisive metaphor rather than a spiritual location. In a state known for its many retirees, the image referred to the entire older population.

(Apocalyptic data left out the most important condition of survivability. Thinking affectionately of my aunt, my mother's sister, living at home vaxxed and boosted, who turned 102 in February 2023, I venture to say that before vaccinations the greatest risk factor was inability to protect oneself.) In any case, it would have taken far more than reasoning or wonky research to make headway against the COVID Era data whirlwinds.

In the US, God's waiting room was getting mighty crowded. The effect was to confirm the frailty of older adults. Negative feelings for care-home residents, ranging from distress to squeamish avoidance to indifference, had always been based on accepting their deaths as natural. Now such feelings could be transferred to cover any community dweller seen as no longer young. To such sentiments were sometimes added calls for sacrificing "the Old." The blatant rhetoric of the COVID Era was a pernicious result of scarce resources and bitter arguments about lockdowns and the economy, or individual rights versus the collective good.

How did such a broad, destructive, age-based construction of doom spread, overthrowing our "prime of life" discourses, undermining pride in longevity, and even overriding the scatter of our polarized, multi-platformed socio-technological networks? In ancient Rome, condemned criminals were called the *morituri*, "those who were about to die" in plain sight in the public arena. The mortality data alone could not have led us to this bitter polarization. It was the new cultural canyon between the two main age groups that helped construct all older adults as *morituri*.

VITAL PARTY PEOPLE AND THOSE WHO EMULATED THEM

The crevasse took only a few weeks to open. After the WHO announced a global pandemic on March 10, the Centers for Disease Control and Prevention advised people to avoid gathering in groups of ten or more. Some institutions took quick action. They canceled sporting and theatrical events. Starting as early as mid-March (in normal times, spring break), colleges and universities released students from their perilous congregate settings. Some went home. Others left for the beach. Trump, lying, had told younger adults that their marvelous immune systems made them safer. Believing their president, some risked living normally when there was no new normal in sight.

College-age students, seen as the potential of the future, often serve as an imagined proxy for youth in general. They are a special, elite, precious group, often indulged. That same month, the governors of warm states, reviving tourism, invited students to come out to play. Miami Beach canceled spring break by prudently declaring a state of emergency. Students, presumably funded by inattentive parents, headed to other vacation spots, like Daytona Beach in Florida. In the midst of early panic and precautions, many in the media covered that subgroup of students who chose to take vacations rather than those who went home to shelter with their families, wash their hands with antiseptic cleanser, and protect others. My undergraduate Brandeis researcher, Vishni Samaraweera, told me, "I remember all the [party] stories and thinking how terrible and selfish all the students going on these spring breaks were. I was being sent home from school and having to pack everything up."

The news filled up with multiplied images of near-naked bodies. In our visual culture, it was hardly possible at that time *not* to see images of young people, mostly white, clustered on beaches, bodies exposed. They were shown grinning (mask-less) at bars, boys shirtless, girls in bikinis, holding beers; head-to-head, shouting in each other's ears. In a related development, many people stocked up on liquor; binge drinking went up; references on social media to "blackout drinking" rose.

Photos of kids on beaches at spring break had been an annual sight. But in 2020 the deathly danger gave formerly unimaginable meaningfulness to the students' attitudes, their defiance, their revelry. Politicians were pilloried for partying (UK prime minister Boris Johnson was drummed out of office). Reporters, however, must have liked the apparent normalcy of spring break, a fragment of the Old Normal. They enjoyed quoting male bravado, its insistent nonchalance. Twenty-one-year-old Jawontae Rodgers in Florida told a local news outlet he didn't think the virus was a "big deal." He knew he could die, but "you only live once. YOLO." Brady Sluder of Ohio told Reuters, "We're just out here having a good time. Whatever happens, happens."

One message was universally available, whatever your judgment about student behavior. Youth seemed *young*—healthy, immune, liberated, sportive—"free." The giddy visuals and the intense controversy concentrated the image. Youthsex was implicitly on display. Speaking to eugenics and the will to hope, such physicality signified exemption from death. A Canadian age critic, Sarah Falcus, says nubile bodies assure us there will be a future, "for the community, nation and planet. As their shadow side, (non-reproductive) older people symbolize the past, representing what has gone, not what is to come."

Youth was conceived in what sociologists call an "ideal" form, losing all the diverse and complex attributes younger people possessed (or lacked) in the real social world. Some were dying but they were not *shown* dying. What they represented mattered: not only the pleasures of life (as the photos showed) but Life itself—*survivability*. Dominance in that single thing was without doubt a precious unconscious advantage amid the carnage.

YOUTHINESS 2020

Certainly, long before the pandemic, a high valuation of those who are currently young had been an intrinsic part of American reality. Just as obstinate, for some, was a nostalgic high evaluation of their own time of having been young. After a certain age, many chose to "pass" for younger. In private life, this choice may be foolish or sad, or even rational—as when made, for example, to get a job as age discrimination worsened after 1980—but the harm to others was contained.

Not so with Donald Trump as president. His behavior and speech during the COVID crisis shows that the flip side of his calamitous ageism was his youth-cult complex. Trump's fantasy of youthfulness was dangerous because it was shared by many. The prolongation of what he thought of as successful, youthful, male behavior was simply more visible in his case. As he grew older, afraid of germs, blood, and needles, his desire to escape the signs of aging drove significant behaviors: owning the Miss America pageant from 1996 to 2015; re-marrying younger women several times; fathering a child at age sixty; and speaking with boisterous boastful bluster of his sexual assaults on *Access Hollywood.*

Ovid's Narcissus myth is about a young man who drowns when he falls in love with an image of himself in the mirroring water of a lake, kissing a face he doesn't recognize as his own. But in real life, Narcis-sus doesn't die young. Psychoanalytic theory infused with age theory follows him as he grows older and still wants to kiss his own face. He flees his intimate sense of growing bodily weakness, his distaste at what his culture forces him to see in the mirror.

Some men assume conventional stances of youthfulness in order to look fearless. Trump had refused to mask; his employees were unable to use a mask in his presence. In October he got COVID. Throwing off his mask with disdain was only one of his theatrical shams when he emerged from Walter Reed Hospital after spending days in the ICU and getting multiple treatments unavailable to the public. He tweeted boastfully, using relative youth as his standard: "I feel better than I did 20 years ago!" It was the performance of a man who believed COVID would not kill youth-identified macho men like him.

Anti-government groups and individuals welcomed the March–April partying. Like Trump, they called COVID fear "a hoax." Their conscious reasons for risky practices included disinformation, ma-chismo, or fear of government. They claimed ideological correctness and economic savvy. They politicized as "authoritarian" official orders to mask and maintain six feet of distance from others' bodies. Toxic individualism was trying to shift the balance from "social solidarity" to "liberty" (defined as doing as one pleases, risking even one's life). Many, I conclude, identified with youth's recklessness and alleged physiological immunity.

The COVID Era concocted a strange new fantasy, that feeling and acting *like* the young (by refusing to wear masks or get vaccinated) would spare your life. This fantasy appeared to be widely shared—especially by Republicans, rural men, police, and older men. (It is not irrelevant that the greatest number of ads on Fox News, a right-wing site that promoted Trump's opinions, offer to treat erectile dysfunction.) But in Year Two of the pandemic, 2021, the year of vaccinations when the Delta variant arrived, avoidance of vaccinations caused a surge of sickness and death and overwhelmed the hospitals again.

Self-destructive behaviors on so wide a scale beg for explanations. The history of the emotions, a scholarly field that looks below rationales like winning elections or keeping businesses open, suggests looking at how people both evade negative feelings and seek pleasant or exciting ones. In a prose poem written pre-COVID, Joyce Carol Oates captured the giddy identification with toxic masculinity.

> Because the recklessness of adolescence is such elation, the heart is
> filled to bursting
> Because recklessness is the happy quotient of desperation, and
> contiguous with shame, and
> yet it is neither of these, and greater than the sum of these. . . .
> Because there is a savage delight in loss, and in the finality of loss.

The ambivalent ferocity of these lines—"the happy quotient of desperation"—helps explains why many (I don't entirely exempt myself) were captivated by the holiday imagery on the beaches.

Martha Nussbaum, a highly regarded professor of philosophy, has described the nexus of fear, bravado, and solipsism. "Fear is a 'dimming preoccupation': an intense focus on the self that casts others into darkness." Young people in crowds, and the many more who identified with them, seemed to lack "fear *for* the other," the foundation of an ethics of responsibility. The two scholars who quote Nussbaum, in a discussion of Emmanuel Levinas, call this caution about others "being fearful of all the violence and murder my existing can bring about."

The fantasy that Trump and others held was latent in America's obsession with "the Young." Risky behaviors on the part of teens and younger adults (with sex, alcohol, drugs, and smoking, for example) had already been correlated with ageism. By distancing oneself from adulthood, caution, and self-care, danger-seeking *proves* that one is young. That intriguing conclusion (published in *Death Studies* a decade before the COVID spring break) was consistent with terror management theory's view of ageism as a buffer against death anxiety. In 2020, there was a lot more need of buffers.

Robert Jay Lifton coined the term "symbolic immortality" to explain the yearning to escape universal death after the fearful nuclear proofs of Hiroshima and Nagasaki. With COVID a global horror, endlessly (as it appeared) killing "the Old," identifying with the imagined youthful survivors may have provided some sense of secular immortality—even for people utterly free of Trump's exaggerated youth complex.

I am piecing together in alternative ways COVID Era events and their unexpected affects. Some people avoided dread by taking precautions to make themselves as safe as possible. But in a crisis where millions were closeted by fear, it's not hard to see the irrational but powerful appeal of Youthiness 2020. Envying those who appeared to escape fearfulness, wishing to emulate them, appears to have been common. In a time of panic and death, magical thinking floats around. Superstition seemed to gain power. Younger people gained no *other* supremacy in this period, but survivability had become a supreme value, and it was attached to Youth as tightly as skin to flesh.

ALTERNATIVE HISTORIES

A century before, around World War I, the value of younger adults had also exploded. Even before the losses of 1914–1918, the eugenics movement had explicitly idealized the (white) young for their procreative potential. During the long war, millions of beloved, achingly young men died horribly, of mustard gas and trench warfare. Prizing young people grew out of emotional pain. Older adults—generals, heads of government, jingoistic parents who had rallied so strongly—were damned for the war, the military conduct of the war, the bad peace. Blame could have been apportioned differently—as it was by historians who thought in terms of treaties, trade, imperial rivalries. Seeing the war through a generational lens was by no means inevitable.

A century later, in Year One of the COVID Era, 2020, also marked by intense grief, age relations were again characterized by a wild swing. But this time, in the Year of the Grim Reaper, the seesaw mechanism worked peculiarly. It was "the *Old*" who were dying in horrifying circumstances and terrifying numbers but "the Young" who (again) became overvalued.

The social imaginary of vital Young versus the moribund and undervalued Old did not have to crack apart in just the sharp way it did. One New York father forbade his son to come inside after Matt's Texas beach vacation. Matt's grandparents also lived in the house. His father, Peter, said, "There is no need to expose them to god knows what he had been exposed to!" Peter packed Matt's car for him and sent him back to school. Fear *of* one, and fear *for* beloved others, united in that household. And no doubt in millions of others.

People I knew "were assessing one another on the basis of the strictness of our quarantines," as Louise Erdrich put it in her COVID novel, *The Sentence*. Some, unlike Trump, were ashamed to have acquired COVID. Ama Saran, a colleague with a long, honored career in women's health advocacy, told me that one interviewee in her Geechee Gullah neighborhood asked the coroner not to put COVID on a relative's death certificate.

The fantasy that exaggerated the age gap proved lethal to some younger people. And they certainly could be vectors of disease. Cellphone data helped researchers prove that college students were spreading the disease to their families. Some were "super-spreaders." The notorious Biogen meeting in Boston led to an estimated three hundred thousand cases globally. "Youth" at play could have been considered reckless carriers, like the notorious vector Typhoid Mary was during the 1910s. (Immune herself, Mary Mallon, a young, single, Irish-born immigrant working woman—infected forty-seven people and spent twenty-six years in custody.) But opprobrium was unlikely to be directed toward the elite on vacation.

Spring break ended, but reveling in the public eye did not. Dr. Antony Fauci—still head of Infectious Diseases, the public health leader telling the truth as best he knew it—was the most trusted guide in the array of sycophants cowering or grimacing behind Trump at his news conferences. Fauci noticed the pathological behavior of the rebellious with a despairing laugh. In July 2020, with colleges now closed, Fauci explained why the US was faring so poorly in the daily case count of contagion. "The guidelines say, 'Don't go to bars. Wear a mask.' And you look at the pictures in the newspaper and on TV and you see large crowds of mostly young people, not wearing masks."

As the beaches filled with those vibrant, colorful, and prized young figures, actual older people were gone, literally. In the streets, if we were present at all, no smiles could be seen, because we were mostly masked below our widened eyes. (After returning from my hug-filled Milwaukee conference, I was still nervously sheltering in my chilly home in Massachusetts.) Older adults were certainly absent from Twitter; its ageist algorithms tend to crop out people in wheelchairs or people with white or gray hair. We could not be seen in lively groups because most who could, eschewed groups. We were not in motion. Not in color. Not outdoors. Not playful. Those most susceptible to the virus disappeared, except on gurneys. Could the public distinguish who lay on any given stretcher, a resident or any other pitiful older adult?

Anyone could overhear the language addressed to Youth. "The reassuring messages were definitely not intended for me or other old people," Sonia Kruks, a professor of politics, aged seventy-three, observed. "To the contrary, they were excluding us from 'the public.'"

If the age chasm was founded on actual mortality data, the end of the binary called "the Old" absorbed negatives from our actual invisibility and from the images and language labels that connoted futility. The opposite of vital Youth. Gerontologists and age critics like me, who had quickly started worrying about how ageism would manifest itself in conditions so rife with age difference, had at first no idea how hate-filled our society would become.

"ELDERLY" ALREADY?

People unexpectedly found themselves being considered "elderly" when they were still too young. "I turn 60 later this year so I noticed that acutely," said Chip Conley, founder of the Modern Elder Academy, told the *Washington Post* in June 2020. "It was all of a sudden: I'm in a high-risk group? I'm perceived as elderly?" He found the hop, skip, and jump from "high risk" to "elderly" ironic, almost funny. ("Elderly" is a label journalists should avoid, according to the *AP Stylebook* and the *Journalist's Resource*.) The interviewees quoted alongside Conley underestimated the demotion.

Taking ageism lightly was another bad habit of the former era of longevity and positive-aging propaganda. Like other systems of inequality, ageism as practiced can be painfully opaque to victims, if they do not know what forces whirl them around. Ageism exempts certain older adults from its devaluations (living ex-presidents, the ultra-rich, celebrities, etc.). Class, whiteness, and maleness had been protective up to a point. People declaring annual incomes above $60,000 and with more education had reported experiencing significantly less everyday ageism than their counterparts. "Ageism may be the first major type of discrimination some White adults experience," says Julie A. Ober, lead author of a major study on the subject. Women experience it earlier than men.

Now, ageism was obvious. An Austrian woman, only sixty-two, pithily described the change of social representation:

> The image of older people was turned around 180 degree[s], from those who like to consume, who like to go out for dinner and travel, and stay fit [. . .] and now, all of a sudden, they are completely fragile and at risk and are people who have to be cared for, and who are also somehow a burden to us, because we have to provide so much care, so much help for them and have to protect them so much.

This phenomenon could be called *simple ageism*, a pure form of bias based solely on age and not compounded by class, gender, race, or ethnicity. As Chip Conley noticed, the idea that "Sixty is the new forty" had evaporated. "Sixty is the new eighty" would have been more like it. People who had been living comfortably in the positive Third Age were suddenly removed wholesale from that desirable state of existence, transported overnight to the Fourth Age, abjectly near to death. Those who noticed felt the brutal transfer as a personal slight, when the deeper truth was that it made *all of us* seem expendable. Who could be exempt?

Startling, inaccurate confusions were being constructed or confirmed: not only that older adults (whatever age *that* means) die, but that we are indistinguishable from those in nursing homes, by also being frail, forlorn, merely "waiting to die." (No one was pointing out how many residents of nursing homes who contracted COVID survived. That fact was too incongruous.) Joining middle-agers to "the Old," as the group of those endangered and dying, added mass to the downhill narrative of life-course decline, as if a lava flow were unstoppably spreading.

THE BOOMER STIGMA

It was not good for the health or valuation of older adults that so many of those dying could be considered "Boomers," because long before 2020, people so labeled had become discredited. The cohort name had been conferred on the babies born between 1946 and 1964. They suffered a strangely narrated life course. Critics, including me, have dissected it. Starting as an "adorable baby bulge," they lost cachet as the oldest among them turned forty and fifty. On the Internet, the sardonic retort, "*Okay*, Boomer" had spread in the fall of 2019. The exasperated tone implied "Have it your own way, then, because you always have." Age cohorts are of course utterly heterogeneous. Generationalism had conferred conflicting stigmas on this cohort: being both wrongly powerful and rich, or over-the-hill.

Boomer-bashing, begun in the 1990s, let younger people sneer in Oedipal exasperation at their parents' unspecified faults or crimes—but it also enabled social opprobrium and nasty economic consequences. "Deadwood" discourse undermined the value of midlife workers, normalized job discrimination, and weakened unions that supported seniority and wage increases, and thus respect for growing older. AARP surveys showed how widespread age discrimination was. Youth bias led many, including the unskilled and people with only high school degrees, to involuntarily and prematurely drop out of the workforce even when they needed the income, stature in the family, and respectability. Middle ageism—as I call it, to refer to both the fictive characterization and its real effects—lowered worker expectations and wages. It rationalized employers' preferences for younger and cheaper workers. Excluding midlife and older adults was a main utility for capitalism. It was not a bug but a feature.

It should be clearly noted that before COVID, the "cult of youth" conferred few benefits on the temporarily young—first the so-called Gen Xers and then the so-called Millennials—aside from the prestige of cornering the market on sex and beauty, fresh ideas, tech savvy, and entertainments flagrantly aimed at their gendered demographic. All this prestige is not nothing, but it did not raise the first wages these young groups received on entering the workforce or lessen inequality. Any period of success and self-esteem was threatened by fear of turning thirty or forty, especially for women, suffering from the long tail of what Susan Sontag long ago called "the double standard of aging."

Middle ageism dismayed the excluded—through, for example, men's sexual or marital preferences for younger women, the growth of the dysfunction and uglification industries (selling rejuvenation by making growing older seem a shameful decline), and politically motivated intergenerational warfare. Opioid addiction can be linked to dour midlife job prospects in states where companies had gone overseas. Disability claims rose. Economic inequality was disabling. A growing half of the population, mostly marked by poverty, color, gender, and age, lost the chance to save, which makes a comfortable old age possible. That loss made winding up in a nursing facility more likely. Much human damage was accomplished by the cult of youth joined to Boomer-bashing.

Before COVID, however, middle ageism had weaknesses. The unattractiveness or economic disposability of older adults had been staunchly denied by popular writers and HR directors as an ignorant stereotype. Favoring, praising, hiring, and imitating youth was shown up as useful to the commerce in aging and to capitalist attempts to control the labor market. Such umbilical ties to ageism were so obvious that critics could debunk the ideology of life-course decline. The new distortions of Youth and Age, however, far from being obvious, have not been adequately noticed, described, or critiqued. They may prove much harder to undo.

Few but gerontologists sounded the alarm. Nobody was out on the street protesting that the astounding death rate in the nursing facilities was preventable, or carrying posters asserting that "Old Lives Matter," or shouting, "We won't be sacrificed for the economy, capitalism, youth, or other Americans' convenience." Instead, the not-so-very old were transformed as if overnight, with light hand-wringing but almost without resistance, into the *morituri* of 2020.

SHAKEN AND VULNERABLE

Within their own families, of course, many adult offspring had no truck with this ugly new social imaginary. Some moved in with their parents. Many closed the distances made by the quarantines. They called their parents. *Are you masking? Are you washing the packages from the supermarket? Can I order hand sanitizer for you? Test kits?* The anxious belief that age mattered more than other risk factors led to these worried (and sometimes harassing) questions posed to healthy community-dwelling parents able to quarantine. We sat out in the cold together. Some wore shields as well as masks. Acting lovingly, many maintained the family embrace and friendships.

But beyond such tightly knit units, unrecognized passions can have a detrimental effect on the *social* embrace. Feeling alienated from older adults one didn't know and never saw was likely. If no longer being young was a doom, blaming the system for the deaths of the no longer young became less thinkable.

SOMETHING WORSE THAN DYING?

Verbal barrages against older people were unleashed instantly. Hostile speech spurted out on Twitter and from officials possessed of blatant social bullhorns. On March 23, 2020, the Republican lieutenant governor in Texas, Dan Patrick, appeared on Fox News. Lurching forward with canny callousness, he said that "lots of grandparents" should be willing to "take a chance on your survival" for the sake of resurrecting the economy for grandchildren. At that point the economy had been partially closed, here and there, for about a week. Carlson followed up: "There's something that could be worse than dying?" Pause. "Yeah," Patrick responded. Either Patrick presumed that listeners his age (he was born in 1950) would be docile or he was signaling over our heads to younger people who agreed that we were expendable.

Some did agree. As early as March 2020, trolls on the Internet were jeering because they thought it was only Boomers, their name for the Old, who were dying. (The Boomers then ranged in age from fifty-six to seventy-four.) "Okay, Boomer" was replaced by the murderous hashtag #Boomerremover, trending on social media. Studying tweets from late March, Brad A. Meisner, an interdisciplinary gerontologist, found "clear themes of population cleansing." Not "cleansing" by ethnicity but by age. The blatant ageism gave a fresh twist to the term, "the enormous condescension of posterity."

Thousands signed the Great Barrington Declaration, sponsored by the American Institute for Economic Research, a libertarian think tank, and published in October 2020. The declaration's eugenicist goal, "herd immunity," proposes, as in animal husbandry, the culling of the least fit—presented innocuously as a scheme to isolate older adults. Others, the young and allegedly invulnerable, ought to be allowed to go about freely.

Other experts countered that trying to achieve herd immunity would be too dangerous. With almost half of Americans suffering from preexisting conditions, there was no way to segregate them all. Many signed the John Snow Memorandum, which countered the Great Barrington Declaration, as did the Infectious Diseases Society of America's twelve thousand scientists, physicians, and public health experts. The head of Medicine at Queens University in Ontario, Dr. Stephen L. Archer, summarized their arguments: "Their rhetoric invalidates public health policy and feeds the 19 per cent of North Americans who don't trust public health officials."

The cult of Vital Youth and the avoidance of "the Old" became further politicized over the 2021 vaccine. Bravado and ideology put the most defiant anti-vaxxers out in public. In 2021, when vaccine distribution had been going on for a few months, evidence indicated that that unvaccinated people, especially white male anti-vaxxers, were dying in greater numbers. Risking COVID, some lockdown skeptics toted guns, invaded state capitols. Protesters complained that their livelihoods were in danger, their fun curtailed, their children going uneducated, merely to protect "the Old." Protest signs evoked ideas of herd immunity with language like: "My virus, my choice"; "My right to die"; "Sign up to die for the economy"; "Natural immunity over manmade poison"; and even "Sacrifice the weak." Neither side "won," or could win. Government dysfunction won; chaos continued. States and cities went in and out of lockdowns.

The ageist, ableist hate speech was overheard by the vulnerable — adults locked into their nursing facilities, community-dwelling midlife and older people, people with disabilities. Dr. Lisa Iezzoni, a professor of medicine at Harvard, has multiple sclerosis; she has used a wheelchair for several decades. Iezzoni said:

> I remember so vividly the rest of us being told, "Don't worry. If you're young and healthy, you should do fine." And so, implicit in that kind of language that the rest of society was being told, was the message, "if you're older, if you're disabled, if you live in a nursing home, you're not going to do fine, but we're not going to talk about that."

Death was given gray hair, one particular — wrinkled — face, and a disabled body, like the silhouette seen on road signs in many countries to signal disabled or "elderly" people: a figure bent over with a cane. *"You're not going to do fine."* And an accompanying message flamed out, too: "We don't care."

Older readers wrote to AARP, resenting the attacks, intuiting the politics: "Trump believes the older generation should willingly die for the sake of the economy. It would solve a lot of problems. No need to worry about healthcare for the seniors and the load on Social Security will go away," said one. Another asserted: "All we get from this administration is 'Screw the geezers, the almighty dollar is more important.'" To find oneself overlooked proved easy when one's death was seen as inevitable, or, indeed, as desirable. Dr. Iezzoni—and others— perceived the underlying message of futility.

FUTILITY

The new national unconscious reached far beyond Internet trolls, the tens of thousands of signers of the Great Barrington Declaration, and the right wing. Already in 2020, trained observers could notice a momentous rearrangement of a nation's culture of feeling, and could begin to sort the consequences. The contrast between vital Young and moribund Old was distorted and tendentious, but it was hard to fight rationally. Other US binaries were explicitly sharpened, polarized by current events: Republicans versus Democrats, whites versus Blacks, men versus. women. Cases where Young versus Old rose to explicitness in public (as in Dan Patrick's pandering to the Republican base on Fox, or in rhetoric on a poster in an armed protest) were rare. Yet the abyss was ever-present. At deeper levels—for those youngsters flaunting a simple Get Out of Jail Free card, or people dealing with death anxiety or craving symbolic immortality; or, on the other side of the gulf, for those feeling helplessly endangered, or unloved and expendable, or overwhelmed by perceiving age hatred and feeling resentful— it was possibly inescapable.

Finally, the exaggerated belief in the biological susceptibility of the oldest third of the nation's people, along with the sense that old lives mattered less to so many other Americans, created hopelessness that rescue is possible. My shorthand for this whole phenomenon is "futility." In 2020, Age Platform Europe, a coalition of nonprofit organizations, had concluded, "Casting all older people as highly vulnerable and frail created an attitude that the deaths of such people could not be prevented and that the rest of us have no obligation to try to prevent their deaths."

As the "knowledge" of futility spread, it became life-threatening to people over a certain age, from within another hierarchy that dominated our precarious lives: medical personnel. The guardians of our health, dedicated to providing care for all, given inhuman responsibilities in a frightening time, were also exposed to the new chasm distinguishing Old from Young. While laypeople were free to withdraw emotionally from the potentially moribund, medical personnel suddenly confronted the exceptional urgencies of adults who were often obviously older than they. Many responded with discipline and self-abnegation. But the profession revealed that its Achilles' heel was age.

CHAPTER 5

CONSEQUENCES

TRIAGE BY AGE

In the COVID Era, the lessened value of older lives had dramatically graver consequences than it had in the Before Times. To begin with, criminal behavior—"elder abuse"—increased. Abuse at home, truly "domestic terrorism," soared in 2020 by as much as 84 percent, according to the *American Journal of Geriatric Psychiatry*. Aides and nurses stole prescription pain drugs from residents. Fraudulent behavior also rose, along with need, greed, selfish anger, and opportunism on the part of caregivers and "trusted others." Elder abuse ranks low in the field of family violence, which tends to concentrate on children.

Early in that hellish spring of 2020, however, the Federal Trade Commission and the American Bar Association, alarmed about the increases in crime, issued respective warnings. The IRS had to remind nursing facilities that Economic Impact Payments sent to residents— rare cash to add to the pitiful amount left them by Medicaid—belonged to them and could not be impounded.

The evils described in the rest of this chapter, however, arose not from outlaws but from a group of admired professionals whose ethics require they do no harm: the medical hierarchy on which, suddenly, our lives depended.

For residents of nursing homes, these protectors were the medical directors that facilities are required to hire. Ideally, experienced physicians or surgeons with five years of experience in management are meant to guarantee "the vital tasks of coordinating the medical care given in the facility." During the lockdowns, humane priorities should have put the weakest first—those who couldn't walk to the toilet or were not able to feed themselves because of low vision, depression, or severe cognitive impairment. Perhaps we don't really know what "dignity" means, although we use the word often. We had better think about what it *requires*.

In some facilities these medical guardians increased the dose of drugs they gave residents. If some residents are too comatose to express their needs, fewer aides can be hired. The growing use of "chemical restraints" such as Haldol was concealed by mislabeling victims as having schizophrenia. The World Health Organization and local media and family members described people who were dehydrated, malnourished, in fevers, their tongues dry, their skin open from pressure sores. In encounters from afar, family members observed painful declines in relatives they had seen as stable. Some who needed help with eating were left alone. Mary-Therese Connelly, a lawyer who led the drafting of the Elder Justice Act of 2010, believes that some residents starved. How could physicians, hired to monitor care, avoid observing humiliating stench or life-threatening neglect? If aides failed to hand out medications at properly scheduled intervals to control pain or symptoms, how did those medical directors miss seeing patients who were groaning in pain? The fact is: Directors were not always present. Eleven members of Congress had already realized by May 2020 that slack oversight had let some corporations hire only a single physician serving ten or more of their facilities. Some facilities had directors "in name only."

As the massive increase in abuse was occurring, abusers were less likely to be detected. The residents, now more completely incommunicado, were even less able than usual to fight back. With lockdown, concerned outsiders could not learn what was happening to their loved ones. Inspections, we know, were rare and limited. Residents had fewer face-to-face encounters with physical therapists, social workers, or community providers to whom to complain. The ombudsman could take complaints but was barred by lockdowns from visiting to investigate them. Reports to Adult Protective Services actually decreased.

TRIAGE: EXCLUDING "THE OLD" EXPLICITLY

Many of us learned a startling new keyword, formerly little-known: *triage*. Pre-COVID, older adults had already been regarded, by some with power to publish, as those who had a "duty to die." That injunction had been considered "only words." But in 2020 the focus on scarce ICU beds and Do Not Resuscitate orders gave the duty to die two fields of *action*—nursing facilities and hospitals.

If saving residents' lives had been their object, some state and national policies were disastrously wrong-headed. Elaine Ryan, the plain-speaking vice president of Government Affairs at AARP, suggested that the government focus on the needs of *hospitals* was itself odd and counterproductive: "Early on, there was a lack of prioritization for nursing homes. Hospitals were seen as the epicenter of the crisis—but the epicenter in deaths was nursing homes." The author of a Brandeis University thesis, describing the choices made by governors, agreed:

> As in many other states, the Baker Administration [in Massachusetts] prioritized hospitals in early response measures by helping them to secure resources, even though they were in a better position to bid for PPE than nursing home facilities, and by including hospital leadership in planning meetings during which the voice of nursing home leadership was not invited.

A journal for medical directors, summarizing the lacks, concluded, "Our cultural fear and societal revulsion around aging have simply rendered invisible the patient and resident population and the workforce of [Post-Acute and Long-Term Care]."

Doctors found ways to exclude older adults in general from the lifesaving measures considered most valuable at the time. This exclusion became explicit in April of 2020, in, of all places where medical science and public health concern should reign, hospitals. Scarcity of ventilator equipment in some hospital intensive care units, especially in New York City and Boston, the first epicenters, became the next media theme. That calamity turned into a rationale for age discrimination. In Bergamo, doctors had always taken "age and condition" into account; at the peak of the Italian crisis, Dr. Lorenzo d'Antiga feared having to "select" further because of lack of ventilators. Then US conditions, deteriorating, mirrored the Bergamo crisis. *Scarcity* is always an ominous term, an excuse for redistributing privilege. Scarcity means choices only for those with power to make them. Medical personnel made them, adversely, for "the Old," by favoring the young.

The Oath of Geneva was designed by the World Medical Association in 1948 after the depravity of experiments carried out by Nazi physicians was exposed. Not all US medical students swear oaths, but many now swear to avoid bias, by taking the Oath of Geneva. One clause stands out here: "I WILL NOT PERMIT considerations of age, disease or disability, creed, ethnic origin, gender, nationality, political affiliation, race, sexual orientation, social standing or any other factor to intervene between my duty and my patient." Age comes first in the list. Yet the Old became the biggest part of "the Viral Underclass."

Many doctors and nurses deserve our awed thanks. Like Dr. Okrent, the poet, they risked their lives before much was known about transmission, before any prophylaxis was available, and while PPE was scarce, fearing for their own lives and for their families. That said, evidence suggests that the death toll for older adults was almost certainly worsened by iatrogenic ageism: alienation from older and less able bodies and geriatric ignorance.

NO ONE OVER SIXTY-FIVE? FIFTY? FORTY?

The first evidence for prejudice appeared, in writing, in the explicit 2020 rules of ICU exclusion. In the crisis, various US medical centers, state health commissions, and bioethicists rushed to create triage guidelines or unearth existing ones. Triage means that some patients receive lesser or no access to treatment. Setting proper criteria for treatment is crucial for saving time and avoiding injustice, guilt, and tragedy. In the history of triage since the battlefields of the Napoleonic era, treatment priority—based on equity, a civic value of the French Enlightenment—was dictated by degree of need rather than, as earlier, by military rank or aristocratic title.

Guidelines appeared in April. The process of deselecting some patients was defended as setting "crisis standards of care." This language sounded high-minded though enigmatic, but it meant that standards were allowed to go lower. Since the US lacks a national health service that must adhere to one universal ethical standard (such as exists in France or the UK), triage guidelines are the only semi-official codes the US had (and still has). I decided to read the main triage guidelines. Like CMS's letter to the states, the incriminating documents were public. They horrified me. They still do.

Triage gives scores to the sickest, and ideally tries to save those whose scores suggest they have an equal likelihood of survival. The process is supposedly blind to age, race, level of ability, and gender. Once shortages of ventilators were anticipated, access turned out to be a proxy measure for "who counts" in American society. Unlike the cagy CMS letter, the University of Pittsburgh guidelines, a model for many states, did not mince words: The tiebreaker for access should be *age*. They use the term *life-cycle considerations*, but the guidelines give priority to younger patients within age groups: twelve to forty, forty-one to sixty, sixty-one to seventy-five, over seventy-five. ("Gut-wrenching," the *Boston Globe* commented.) If there were enough very sick younger adults, the likeliest outcome would be that no one over sixty, or over forty, would get access to a ventilator.

Guideline writers were legally forbidden to deploy other biases, but the age exclusion made that attempt incoherent. The Massachusetts guideline said that "disabilities" would not lead to exclusion, but then it put people over sixty-five, many of course with impairments, in the two lowest priority groups. A list of "factors that have no bearing," which starts with "race, disability" and includes "perceived social worth, perceived quality of life," omitted age.

"Age" had become another suspect criterion to those of us in the disability, poverty, anti-ageism, and civil rights movements. Dr. Michelle Holmes, a Harvard epidemiologist, pointed out that "schemes using point scales to penalize older Americans and prioritizing those in better prior physical condition automatically would put marginalized groups . . . at a huge disadvantage." We had in mind the nearly 50 percent of Americans, many of them people of color or working-class, who acquire chronic illnesses and disabilities at younger ages.

The NGO Justice in Aging astutely observed that some guides used "other factors that take age into account" without appearing to do so. Scorekeepers were asked to *estimate* an individual's remaining number of years of life. In a society that has lacked Medicare for All for people *younger* than sixty-five for the entire sixty years of Medicare's existence, burdened by racism, market-driven capitalism, and small-government ideology, injustice is built into any crisis standard of care that prioritizes highest long-term survival. The Johns Hopkins criteria for treatment in the COVID pandemic required no more than one year of potential life. This guideline respects strong people in later life. (I had in mind my dear aunt, then ninety-nine, who was quarantining. At seventy-nine, I felt that my life was worth no more than that of my aunt, nor less than that of a nineteen-year-old.)

Triage by age was not new. What is striking is that in the spring of 2020, when "the elderly" were suddenly, obviously, at highest risk, the groups producing the guidelines, who often included ethicists, did not *rethink* the ageist criteria. It seems no accident that the hospital guidelines prioritized younger people as the neediest or worthiest patients at the same time that the discourse of Youth ascendancy was prizing their vitality. The discourse of futility could become prophetic.

Dr. Lachlan Forrow, a senior fellow at the Harvard Medical School Center for Bioethics, told me that his team revised the Massachusetts guidelines not once but three times; they kept the age categories (first priority, ages birth to seventeen; second, eighteen to forty-nine; third, fifty to sixty-five; fourth, sixty-five to eighty; fifth, eighty and up). Forrow wrote me that he is currently sixty-six, but that if he were in his eighties, he would accept his low ranking:

If the other patient were someone in their early 20s, or perhaps even younger, and everything else about us was similar (for simplicity's sake, let's just stick to odds of surviving the hospitalization) I think it would be bizarre to offer me equal access to the single-available potentially life-saving intervention, and I would not consider a policy that directed that to be at all troublingly "ageist."

Favoring younger people could be argued aggressively, unapologetically. Early in the pandemic, on March 23, 2020, an article in the prestigious *New England Journal of Medicine* argued in favor of giving "priority to those who are worst off in the sense of being *at risk of dying young and not having a full life.*" Sick younger adults would receive a chance at "a full life" by taking it away from equally sick older adults; further, "we believe that removing patient from a ventilator or an ICU bed is also justifiable." The first *NEJM* author was Ezekiel Emanuel, a doctor and "bioethicist," already notorious for having announced in the *Atlantic Monthly* some years before that, once past age seventy-five, he would not think it worthwhile trying to live longer. He was then in his early sixties. Some people believe they will never reach seventy-five or ever change their mind.

Youth ascendancy came into media conversation instantly. A man described as a bioethicist in a March 3 *Washington Post* article objected to a "blanket stop to resuscitations for infected patients" because it was "too 'draconian' and may end up sacrificing a young person who is otherwise in good health." The word "sacrifice" always bears scrutiny. It was usually applied to older people.

"The life-cycle principle" sounds less lofty if it really means that no one over forty who might survive gets a chance. The argument in the Pittsburgh guideline is that it is *correct* to consider "extending the life of an elderly, disabled, or terminally ill individual *as of lower value* than extending the life of an individual who is younger, nondisabled, or not terminally ill." This estimate is called Quality-Adjusted Life Years (QALY). The National Council on Disability has documented "sufficient evidence of the discriminatory design and impact of the QALY."

Using QALY is as vicious as deciding Black people are less worthy than white people. CMS had banned QALY in Medicaid.

Fears of rationing led the Office for Civil Rights to issue a statement to prevent lifesaving medical care from being denied on the basis of disability *or* age. Other concerned practitioners offered a fair alternative. By May, Dr. Michelle Holmes, a friend and a diversity consultant, advocated a lottery for those patients whose scores were tied. Hundreds of physicians signed her petition. Tens of thousands, of course, never saw it.

Art Caplan, founding director of the Division of Medical Ethics at NYU's Grossman School of Medicine, seventy years old, is a trusted commentator. On April 1, 2020, when tensions were high in the city hospitals, Caplan told a reporter:

> The first thing you have to commit to is that you won't discriminate. . . . I wouldn't start with an age cutoff because we've seen healthy seventy year olds and very, very sick, compromised twenty year olds. But it would be fair to say if you can't sort them out by biology and physiology, then you go to age because age is somewhat of a predictor of who's going to do well.

Treating age as "somewhat of a predictor" rather than instituting a lottery is a license to exclude.

No doubt doctors intended the guidelines to help other doctors facing chaos: the racking noise, the patients in hallways, the lack of equipment, the inadequacy of Trump's administration of provisions, the tension of those who had never experienced rationing. With decisions made "efficient," a person who had faced some hideous choices that day could go home at night and sleep a bit. But if they ever saw the lineaments of their own parents in the patients turned away from the ICU, their stomachs must have turned.

Doctors feel "despair" at the futility of caring for older adults? It is *we*, simply by growing older, who may "despair" that authorities who relegate us to the bottom of the scale of human value consider doing so legitimate.

AN UGLY PAST?

Why should arguments against hospital triage by age still matter to-day? Isn't the emergency over? Presumably, ICUs are again trying to save people who are old or impaired and whose bodies are ravaged by poverty. Isn't this an ugly past we can forget about? On the contrary.

This nation swings in and out of emergencies. Other epidemics, other outbreaks of ageism, almost certainly await us. The frightening cultural change in the COVID Era is that the concept of age-graded triage, with racism, classism, ableism, and dementism baked into it, was hammered into the minds of every hospital doctor, financial manager, ICU pulmonologist, medical director and medical resident; many private physicians; and every EMT or nurse forced to decide, as happened in Los Angeles early in 2021 with the post-Christmas surge, whom to leave out as apparently having "virtually no chance of survival."

All these persons in command positions learned triage-by-age in the most exceptional circumstance, the kind that imprints bias as "knowledge" in the mind. They may not want to talk about it. They may excuse their colleagues. But no one who solidified their age prejudice at that conjuncture is likely to forget its rules as long as they live. Youth ascendancy, toxic and life-threatening to older adults but justified, may become unspoken, implicit, even without crisis conditions. Excluding older people is unjust and tragic. But day in and day out, many a solitary person with medical power is on their own and prejudices may rule unseen.

Signed Do Not Resuscitate (DNR) orders were the next medical practice to plunge the ethically challenged toward simple ageist bias.

MY MOTHER'S WISHES

One can live a long time before knowing anything, good or bad, about Do Not Resuscitate orders. I was in my late sixties, years before COVID. My mother, in good health and of sound mind, in her early nineties, made clear that she did not want to go to a hospital for any reason. A legally binding form helps ensure that such wishes are respected. My mother asked her doctor to sign the Comfort Care / DNR order.

The amiable, athletic Dr. Galgano always squatted in front of her for conversation, to get eye to eye. He gave her a big grin, bigger to her than to me. My charming mother smiled back, glad to see him. She was wearing a new black-and-white tweed jacket she had ordered from a catalogue. It was a well visit. My mother had no chronic conditions. She could stand up from his office chair without using the armrests. The good doctor knew she had had some loss of memory and executive ability; he admired her vivacity.

Dr. Galgano did not do the hard-sell *frailty discourse* for getting people to sign a DNR. Frailty discourse foregrounds an imagined decline narrative about the risks of cardiopulmonary resuscitation: broken ribs, hospitalization, intubation, surgery. The following is an excerpt from such an interview in a Toronto clinic, before COVID. One clinician gestured with his index finger down his throat, asking "So, for instance would you want to go to the ICU? Would you want a tube down your throat?" and thumped his chest, asking "Would you want electric shocks to bring you back to life"? Frailty discourse reminds people of the risks of survival. "What's the harm in trying to resuscitate when you're too frail?" a clinician asked, and answered: "Well, the harm is who is going to come back. So, the [Margaret Gullette] that we know is not necessarily the [Margaret Gullette] who comes back." The *more life* discourse instead reminds people of how well they are and how much medicine and surgery can still do for them.

Dr. Galgano did neither. He told us about his hospice team, providing comfort care or palliative care. That distant prospect was reassuring. My mother's order hung inside a cupboard. She never needed it. The quiet, gentle members of the team eventually did attend my dear mother in her last months. From reception, housekeeping, and administration, members of the staff who had enjoyed her jokes and fair treatment came in during her last four days of coma to sit beside her bed and privately say goodbye. With morphine alleviating her pain, her life ended in her own bed, with me at her side.

LAST ORDERS

End-of-life care is meant to offer people autonomy through options. Patient autonomy has become a primary value since 1914, when Justice Benjamin Cardozo wrote the opinion in *Schloendorff v. Society of New York Hospital* that "every person of adult years and sound mind has the right to determine what shall be done with his own body." Many people, not just in old age, ask for a DNR. They may do so before surgery, in case it fails. It is now possible to ask for a DNH (Do Not Hospitalize) or a DNI (Do Not Intubate).

Others want every chance to survive. They may have seen *ER* with George Clooney, the philandering Doc Doug, where the emergency room staff regularly slams defibrillator paddles on chests, springing patients back to breath. (It is coherent to choose both Full Code—everything—for yourself and vote for assisted dying for others.) A POLST—a Physician's Order for Life-Sustaining Treatment—is always voluntary and is meant to follow shared-decision-making conversations with a professional. The form varies. Some states make it possible to reject or to proactively choose from a range of measures: symptom-treatment only, intubation, ventilation, noninvasive ventilation, or AND (Allow Natural Death).

My mother's order mandated only that cardiopulmonary resuscitation (CPR) not be attempted "if my heart and/or breathing stops." There's a caution. DNR orders are not meant to be "a medical professional's assessment of a patient's chance of survival" in *other* circumstances. Signing does not justify ignoring other treatable issues like pneumonia, stroke, or COVID symptoms. A person with failing kidneys may sign a DNR while undergoing dialysis. A doctor can order oxygen, blood, antibiotics. DNR does not mean "Do Not Treat."

FROM UNDERTREATMENT TO NO TREATMENT

Unfortunately, some physicians don't know what "DNR" means. Some assume that people with DNR orders want to abstain from all other treatments as well. A survey of 155 medicine and surgery residents discovered what they would *not* do for you if you had a DNR. Some believed that diagnostic tests need not be ordered. Thirty-two percent would not give antibiotics; "many physicians . . . inappropriately extrapolate [from] DNR orders to limit other treatments." One former public official who had read similar studies in *Archives of Internal Medicine* and *Critical Care Medicine* said, caustically, that these practitioners "misconstrue DNR as Dying, Not Recovering." Many doctors are also ignorant of important differences between DNR and DNI (Do Not Intubate), a 2014 Harvard study showed. A patient can sign a DNI and benefit from noninvasive ventilation, like oxygen therapy. Hospitalists did not typically make clear the difference.

In New Hampshire in 2020, by the time Gene Randlett finally got a positive COVID test, he was in an ICU. Randlett at age eighty-eight had a DNR order. He wasn't put on a ventilator, his son Mark said. That felt wrong. He believes his father would have rescinded the DNR if Mark could have talked with him, but no one could visit. "I really strongly feel my dad could have been saved," Mark Randlett said. "Maybe I'm just saying that because I love and miss him."

The true and aggravated worry in the COVID Era had become undertreatment. *Undertreatment* had always been a euphemism. The blunt way to put it was *medical neglect and exclusion, inadequate treatment,* or *no treatment at all.* Two geriatricians and a family-practice doctor surveyed the 155 medical residents who would undertreat people with DNRs. They suggested other motives for such undertreatment. This situation is one of moral hazard. Medicine trains doctors to believe they know better than any patient what those patients *should want.* Professional arrogance may combine with ignorance and internalized age bias.

Eighty-eight percent of physicians say they would choose a DNR for themselves. Hospitalized, seriously ill patients often don't get the end-of-life care they ask for. But their doctors are more likely to honor their wishes if the patients have *rejected* CPR and are "older and ha[ve] a worse functional status and prognosis." In *Intimations of Mortality*, Barbara Reich, a lawyer, suggests that physicians are projecting their own low valuation of the appropriateness of resuscitation for such patients. By those who offer only the "frailty discourse," patients are characterized as "good" if they resist the offer of possible life-prolonging interventions and accept the end-of-life order.

Historically, fee-for-service incentives and pride in lifesaving might have overcome the frailty discourse and ageist, ableist attitudes. The prior charge against doctors had in fact been that they tried to save even the moribund: their fervid overtreatment caused pointless suffering and unnecessary expense. The norm had been sending a code team into action, using all means to save anyone. If a patient came in without a code like a DNR, withholding treatment, if discovered, was cause for license suspension. (This risk may have been a strong deterrent in some states. However, in Texas, "not coding" was a Class C misdemeanor, the least serious of charges, along with disorderly conduct and theft of under $50.) In any case, with COVID overwhelming hospitals and doctors and nurses across the country, the incentives turned against older adults.

AGEISM, A PREEXISTING CONDITION

Medical ageism too had preexisting features. Ignorance was one. Ignorance of geriatric medicine and of disability rulings had permeated the medical profession. The supply of students studying geriatrics and geriatric psychiatry had gone down—alarmingly, by almost a quarter—between 2001 and 2018, even as longevity grew and geriatricians would be in higher demand. Dr. Louise Aronson made a passionate case in *Elderhood* that all future doctors learn that specialty. Among specialists, she added, the happiest were geriatricians.

But Aronson knew why most medical students avoided older bodies. Salaries in geriatrics were 20 percent lower than for other medical specialties, according to Payscale. Many doctors-to-be considered older patients too scary. Multi-morbidity challenged their ignorance. Failure to teach geriatrics—a form of ageist disregard—characterized most medical schools. But even after taking geriatrics courses, Aronson pointed out, medical students admitted they felt "despair at the futility of care." *Despair.*

Ageism had always potentially interfered with clinical judgment. Older people almost always have doctors who are younger than they. The narrator of Ben Lerner's *10:04: A Novel*, believes that his doctors, precisely by being younger, "could no longer stand in benevolent paternal relation to my body because [they] would now see in my pathologized corpus their own future decline." Older adults had long complained that doctors used "Elderspeak" (baby talk uttered in a loud voice) or ignored them, instead addressing their adult offspring. Ageism already had fatal consequences if your doctor ignored your serious but treatable condition as inevitable "aging." But as in nursing facilities, the consequences occurred singly and thus invisibly—until COVID brought older adults into contact with doctors not one by one but in battalions.

The latent sense of futility about treating "the Old" was intensified— *justified*—in 2020 by the age chasm (the increased preciousness of young lives and the media blare that older adults composed 80 percent of those dying), by the well-publicized ICU guidelines, and by panic about their comrades in the hospitals being overwhelmed by dying old people.

ADVANCE-CARE PLANNING

Misuse of the DNR order is far more significant in practice than ICU triage, because the order affects many times more people. Triage directly affects only those sick enough to be admitted to tertiary care at a time of potentially inadequate resources. Excluding anyone was considered a desperate resort. The DNR, by contrast, is a normalized tool, familiar to all. Failure to honor a preference for end-of-life care has been considered a serious medical error. However, the DNR order is "misunderstood" frequently enough to be dangerous to any one of us who comes in contact with medical personnel—even nurses and EMTs—anywhere, for any reason, at any stage of any illness, inside a nursing home or in a hospital, now and hereafter.

In the spring of 2020, the pressure to lower the numbers of people needing CPR became intense. Once it was known that the virus was airborne, awareness grew that doing CPR exposed everyone around.

I was told that some doctors felt compelled to start CPR without suiting up. One fear expressed by doctors was that hospitals with few intensive-care beds would be "instantly overwhelmed when coronavirus got into the local nursing home, *leaving no capacity for community cases, imperiling local healthcare workers.*" Since workers would be equally imperiled by multiple community cases, only compound ageism explained preferring to be overwhelmed by *them.*

There were sound, resident-centered reasons to treat those with COVID "in place" if they didn't need supports available only in ICUs. Hospitals were dangerous places for residents in normal times (from infections, falls, confusion, pressure ulcers); now sick people had to endure long waiting periods in ERs and hallways, often without attendance.

Medical directors in nursing facilities could best avoid hospitalizing residents by protecting them from COVID: getting PPE, paying staff for sick leave, offering higher wages, etc. There was a shortcut for them to achieve the same end: by getting potential patients to sign the unmistakable Do Not Hospitalize or a DNR. Doctors had often avoided "the Conversation" about end-of-life care, as Atul Gawande, the author of *Being Mortal*, complained. Suddenly advance-care planning was top of mind. An advance-care planning "Swat Team," working at Hebrew Senior Life in Boston between April 13, 2020, and May 26, 2020, to get residents' proxies to sign, considered the pandemic an "opportunity"—but it turned out to have limits: "There was substantial opportunity to increase the proportion of LTC [long-term care] residents with DNH orders during the COVID-19 pandemic."

Some owners of facilities no doubt immediately understood the financial advantages of having DNH/DNR orders on hand. Although outsiders may have believed that few *morituri* survived, medical directors and administrators could have observed that a great many did. But people who had formerly required slight help with Activities of Daily Life were turning into bed-bound patients. We now recognize many survivors as victims of long COVID. Staffing needs, expensive even at a miserable $13.02 an hour for aides, as the Labor Department found—would obviously rise. In the spring of 2020, Congress provided $4.9 billion without strings just to nursing facilities, as part of the $46 billion disbursed in the CARES Act. To owners, lesser function-ing and long COVID meant higher costs, cutting into assured profits.

Advance-care planning is not proof of "coercion." Any time before that fatal spring, ACP would have looked like doctors offering an-other chance at autonomy. As they should; people change their minds as the real comes closer. But in 2020 the nation had been invaded by an unknown virus; the overcrowded hospitals seemed terrifying. People were especially unprepared to undergo "The Conversation." Having a doctor initiate it suddenly, proactively, before a person had any symptoms—which is what was happening—could make it feel desperate rather than pro forma. DNAR—a new acronym, Do Not ATTEMPT Resuscitation—made CPR sound hopeless.

An end-of-life conversation could of course be fair by including both *frailty* discourse and *more-life* discourse. How would we know whether both discourses were used? In the spring of 2020, many doc-tors discussed advance choices with residents. In one instance, be-tween April 1 and May 30, 2020, twenty practitioners asked 963 Texas nursing-facility residents or their surrogates about advance wishes. Those doctors overcame their discomfort and the problem of not get-ting paid. Until then, 361 residents had wanted *everything* done. They "were full code status." But after the conversation, Do Not Hospitalize orders increased from less than a quarter of the group to almost half.

The situation in 2020 foreclosed options for those like Gene Randlett—people with prior or casual "just-in-case" DNH/DNR or-ders. The worst case meant a risky DNR could be imposed on patients who had never opted for it. A third of five thousand patients admit-ted to California hospitals after *successful* out-of-hospital resuscitation nevertheless had a DNR order imposed on them their first day. That third received less treatment and suffered worse outcomes.

OPERATIONALIZING ABANDONMENT II

In some hospitals, the unacknowledged prejudice against saving people who presented with DNRs quickly became overt. In triage, the quickest and easiest step, before the individual assessment of survival, was to apply automatic "exclusion criteria." Two Hastings Center ethicists discovered in April 2020 that "some existing and proposed guidelines ... put DNR status in the list of criteria for excluding patients ..." Such an exclusion signified that DNR was, indeed—as previously noted—taken to mean "Dying, Not Recovering." Would patients arriving with a DNR in other emergency rooms be asked again whether they wanted CPR or everything-but-CPR? *Bodies* change too. "A patient who would not have survived a cardiac arrest last week might do so today; a patient who could have initially survived a [full] code, now, after a week in hospital, with renal failure and hypoxia, is not likely to do so."

At the very moment that hospital decision-makers were setting triage rules, Dr. Joseph J. Fins, the head of the bioethics team at NY Presbyterian Hospital, said that doctors across his hospital "were imploring us to sanction [in the sense of approving] unilateral do-not-resuscitate (DNR) orders, something that is not permitted under New York State law." Other hospitals immediately considered conferring the DNR, on the judgment of the attending physician. Unilateral and blanket orders were unethical, often illegal. Fins said no.

The keyword aside from "DNR" is "during a public health emergency." One crucial fact about emergencies is that they *allow for involuntary* DNR protocols. In April 2020, the National Medical Association and the Rainbow Push Coalition co-produced a joint statement entitled "A Public Health Manifesto," reporting this alarming provision. Their warning was timely. On January 27, 2020, Trump's Health and Human Services secretary, Alex Azar, had declared a public health emergency for the entire US. Many saw the positive side: finally, government action! We didn't suspect that an "emergency" implicitly legalized a clinician or staff member (without prior consent of patient, family, or health advocate) to *withhold* basic life support, advanced cardiac life support, or extraordinary measures from people with DNRs who arrived with acute, life-threatening, or deteriorating conditions, or who then had DNRs imposed on them.

From a patient's point of view, of course, avoiding "the risk to [medical] workers" meant saving *someone else's life*. Some agreed. Residents at the VA Boston Healthcare System in West Roxbury, Massachusetts, being treated for COVID but not in intensive care, said they would forgo aggressive treatments if others might benefit.

Given unequal power dynamics, coercion in the hospital situation was even more desperately likely than with private patients. A surrogate who didn't know their loved one's end-of-life choices might be asked to decide. Dr. Richard Wunderink, an intensive-care medical director in an Illinois hospital, said that an interval of stability in admissions "allowed medical staff to talk with [some] families about the risk to workers and how having to put on protective gear delays a response and decreases the chance of saving someone's [someone else's] life." Dr. Wunderink told the *Washington Post* "that many family members are making the difficult choice to sign do-not-resuscitate orders."

DNRS: TOO DRACONIAN FOR "THE OLD"

Dr. Joseph Fins at NY Presbyterian had felt "a queasiness" about permitting unilateral DNR orders. But it was racism or xenophobia, not ageism, he worried about. One study he read had alerted him. At Massachusetts General Hospital, some surrogates had persisted in requesting resuscitation. Those who "persisted" in challenging the medical power structure for their loved one were disproportionately people of color, those for whom English was a second language, or the foreign born. They lacked trust. The question these findings raised for Fins was whether families might have reason to worry if their sick person was poorer, of less mental acuity, or of color.

Age, like race, is instantly visible in the ER. The supreme value put on "youth" as a proxy for health also implicitly favored patients less likely to look frail or wrinkled or small, or as if they had few years of life ahead. The worry about the "culling" of certain elders was no attenuated whisper. The National Medical Association, which represents forty-five thousand African American physicians, was perspicacious enough to imagine the grief and injustice that other biases, as well as racism, might lead to. The NMA acted quickly. They wanted it "to be required that state and local health departments collect and report all involuntary DNR orders, including data according to race, ethnicity, gender, and age." States do record all signed statements of DNR, DNH, or Medical Orders for Life-Sustaining Treatment (MOLST). But did any state create a register of involuntary DNRs?

NO SECOND CHANCE TO LIVE

So far, evidence points to some hospitals' *intent* to give physicians carte blanche to decide how to treat people who arrived in life-and-death situations without a DNR, by acting *as if they already had one, and that it meant asking to have all treatment withheld*. On April 17, 2020, first responders *outside* hospitals and clinics received a blanket do-not-resuscitate order, an instruction to desist from trying to revive patients who had no pulse. Multiple states adopted it.

Some paramedics were disturbed. Before the crisis, EMTs would instantly start chest compressions for a person in crisis without a visible DNR. That was what they were trained to do, according to the American College of Emergency Physicians, "when the patient's wishes are not known." The rule was to try to resuscitate a patient for up to twenty minutes. "They're not giving people a second chance to live anymore," said Oren Barzilay, the president of Local 2507, Uniformed EMTs, Paramedics, and Fire Inspectors Union, in New York City. The then-governor of New York, Andrew Cuomo—the early Cuomo of "my mother is not expendable"—rescinded the order five days later, on April 22, 2020. In 2021, Oren Barzilay told me,

> In New York we never complied. We were working in a war zone. But still we could be making an effort. We took an oath to preserve life, the Oath of Geneva. All medical professionals take that oath.

Barzilay went on, "There were some people on the field who felt that the order [not to try to save] was needed. But most disagreed. It was too soon. We still had options." I asked him about those who agreed. "They may agree with the order, but it may haunt them down the line. 'I could have saved that parent, that person of forty or fifty' ... And their child was there, watching us saying 'There's nothing we can do!'" He burst out, "Don't put it on the people on the bottom with the most traumatizing experience. Put it on the doctors in the hospitals, when we bring in the patients needing resuscitation. You can't let the people behind the desks make these decisions."

It *had been* the people behind the desks putting it on the EMTs. The list of endorsers announced by New York's health department's spokeswoman was long and eminent. "This guidance, proposed by physician leaders of the EMS Regional Medical Control Systems and the [New York] State Advisory Council—in accordance with American Heart Association guidance and based on standards recommended by the American College of Emergency Physicians—was issued at the recommendation of the Bureau of Emergency Medical Services."

A NEW NORMAL WE MAY REGRET

The eventual medical history of the COVID Era pandemic may well focus on the heroism in the hospitals, the rapid creation of the vaccine, and treatment breakthroughs like Paxlovid. A grateful and terrified nation lauded physicians and nurses and EMTs for their bravery, their inhuman work hours, their quick learning, and their own death toll. Recently I thanked a young doctor who told me, but only after I asked about his COVID experience, that he had worked in a hospital at a time when they needed 150 ventilators instead of the forty on hand. I said, sincerely but feebly, something about how hard it must have been. He said without hesitation, "You have no idea."

In the UK, where a National Health Service decides universal policies, during COVID some care homes were given blanket DNACPR (Do Not Attempt Cardiopulmonary Resuscitation) notices. Then the NHS delivered such a notice, "emblazoned with multiple bright, red-bordered boxes which you are requested to place in a visible spot in your home," to Lucy Jeal, an independent, mobile ninety-three-year-old. The contempt made her feel like "throwing herself off a bridge"; only thoughts of her children and grandchildren stopped her. In the UK, in the first wave, only a very small percentage of people over eighty— 2.5 percent—received top care: "the official version is that the old did less well in intensive care," but according to the book *Failures of State: The Inside Story of Britain's Battle with Coronavirus*, the survival rate for people over eighty who were admitted to ICUs was relatively high, at 40 percent. "Some form of triage was taking place."

A doctor who helped write the Massachusetts triage guidelines told me in writing that they were never operationalized in hospitals. How can he know? A comparable overview of US data is lacking. We need a large enough sample to indicate whether there was ageist or ableist ICU exclusion here. And we need some way to discover whether residents of homes were less likely to be sent to hospitals when intensive care was precisely what they needed.

The uproar in the UK over the NHS's bright, red-bordered boxes brought the issue of age discrimination even to the tabloids. In the US, Dr. Fins's anxiety about *racial* bias and xenophobia was published only in an academic ethics journal. Abandonment to death through DNRs now has become thinkable. COVID Era data on the oldest age group with comorbidities has been used to show something that has been sufficiently proved: they did disproportionally die. No one doubts that. The real question is how many more might have lived. Marie-Therese Connelly received a MacArthur Fellowship for her activism against abuse. Her soft features take on an earnest frown of concentration when she discusses abuse and neglect. "When older people die, others don't ask questions," Connelly grieves.

Can we ask some questions? Did some of "the Old" die from under-treatment, foisted on those who might have preferred to be treated? These would be *suspicious* extra deaths. Did an ailing resident chance upon EMTs who left him because he *looked* old and frail (as happened in California at one point when hospitals were full)? After transition to a facility, when an older woman was released with some inevitable brain fog, did her comfort and dignity depend on finding an aide there who did not assume her confusion was late-stage Alzheimer's? Or was she brought back to an understaffed facility owned by a private firm using it as a cash cow? Hidden aspects that we can only imagine (and should try to, because investigation depends on it) are likely to have caused or accompanied the Eldercide.

As normality returns, people are reminded of what lies on their conscience. One college youth who partied nonchalantly over spring break on the beaches of Florida ("If I get corona, I get corona") later dramatized a public apology on Instagram and CNN, announcing that he had in his life "elderly people who I adore more than anything in the world." After the scandal and searing investigation of the seventy-seven deaths at the Soldiers' Home in Holyoke, Massachusetts, an occupational therapist confessed deep remorse at "walking them to their death." Her facility, like so many, exposed employees to moral injury— to acting against their deeply held values. She felt as guilty as a soldier who follows a bad order, like some in the Vietnam War or Iraq.

Haunted medical personnel may confess or report what they detected. In nursing facilities, did those in charge fail to call 911 if a very sick resident had a DNR in her record? Is that why one woman I quoted earlier had to call 911 herself?

(I haven't signed any end-of-life order. I have trusted my primary care doctors to have my best interest at heart. Not deciding what to sign had been due mainly to my failure as a personal futurologist. I couldn't anticipate what I would wish for after some crisis of lungs or heart—how much impairment I might manage. Having stumbled on more evidence of simple ageism in my research, I now also consider the risk of falling under the care of a mind that, despite swearing an oath to do me no harm, would get a glimpse of my whitening hair, my date of birth and—if I had one, my DNR order—and opt not to treat me or even offer me tests.)

With or without an emergency, the sight of a DNR paper linked to certain bodies awakens a set of prejudices in some unknown percentage of physicians. In 2021, I asked a doctor who had served as a hospitalist in Queens, at the time that that borough had been an epicenter of disease, about whether he now believed there was a "risk of misuse" of the DNR. He paused long enough that I thought he might not answer.

I pondered his silence. Doctors may not like to snitch; too many stories to tell; too many complexities. He wasn't sworn to *tell*. But he had taken another oath. He responded shortly, "You're not wrong."

THE OPPOSITE OF "YOUNG": OBLITERATED

The pandemic exposed long-term failures of custodial care that had been partially recognized but not corrected. Dementism deserves its own hideous pages in the annals of explanation. In the COVID Era the belief may have solidified that the lives of those with cognitive impairments or with other mental-health issues matter less than the lives of others, *even to them*. Nurses know better: they tend to recognize the spectrum of abilities and respect those on it. All clients should be allowed to change their minds. A well-known training text from 2018 pushes back against doctors who would foist DNRs one-and-done on anyone. "It is ethically inappropriate to assign blanket 'incapacity to decide' to patients based on isolated incidents of irrationality."

Some blame the residents themselves for getting COVID. An occupational therapist told *Politico*, "You could put a mask on someone out in the hall 100 times, and it will be taken off 100 times." Analyzing the factors contributing to the "unusually high dementia death toll," the *Politico* analysis linked "missed Covid-19 diagnoses" to "lapses in nursing home care." Had people in later stages of cognitive impairment lived in better homes, they might not have needed masks. "Memory homes," where everyone needs respect and close attention and staff are highly trained, were like cautious family pods. Sixty-one percent saw *no* COVID-19-related deaths in the ten months of 2020. They protected their own.

Dementism can cause hospital medical personnel to ignore what even articulate and well-educated patients are trying to convey, if they are older or people of color or speak with an accent. The attendants sometimes assume such patients are confused and incorrect. It's likely that dementism sometimes operated like a blanket, permanent, misunderstood DNR order: AND, Allow Natural Death.

TELLING HISTORY

Mistrust of biased doctors and scientists has a sad, bitter, well-attested history in the United States. Clinical exclusions by age, class, gender, race, ability, or cognitive status menace trust in the profession. We can't afford to lengthen that sorry history. Americans have to be given good reason to trust again.

Many questions concern all older adults, if past is prologue. Was lethal exclusion-by-age, or by proxies for age, enacted widely in ICUs? Was hastily conferring DNR orders on people who had not asked for them an issue of early-2020 behavior, or does it go on even now? It may be time to ask of Congress a commission separate from CMS or HHS—perhaps NASEM, the highly respected National Academy of Science, Engineering, and Medicine, which provided a blueprint in 2022 for nursing-facility transformation—to investigate COVID Era US medical culture in relation to ageism.

The point of compiling facts and describing suspicions about triage and the DNR is not to indict governors, ethics teams, medical organizations, state health-department heads, hospitalists, physicians, or medical directors. We do need a fair-minded hearing for grim, unexpected, and unwanted information, to pave the way for transformations of minds and practices. Dr. Fins, the hospital leader who had worried about bias, came to a wary, anxious conclusion about the future of medicine: "The extreme conditions of a pandemic could easily become the template for a new normal that we might come to regret."

CHAPTER 6

ON FUTILITY AND "MIRACLES"

AT THE NINETIETH BIRTHDAY PARTY

In the fall of 2022, at an outdoor party, there was the typical amount of joking about old age, although my friend "the birthday boy" was an estate lawyer in active practice. Poised over the cake, he grinned handsomely and said, "Ninety, and still counting."

Someone jokingly yelled out the words on a wide banner stretched behind the head table. "*Holy shit! You're old!*"

"Ageism," I said, and rolled my eyes.

Standing near me was a woman with a pale narrow face and graying blonde hair smoothed behind her ears. She shook her head, sadly. "I work in a nursing home. When people talk about COVID deaths, they say to me . . . to *me*, 'They would have died anyway.'" She said this in amazement and pain. "It's cruel. I love my old people."

In a split second our exchange had leaped from everyday ageism, which may look like joking but is never entirely harmless, to the terminal discourse of futility. Nancy worked as a massage therapist at a good place, a nonprofit. She liked the administrator. She countered the cruelty by loving the despised residents she cared for, a bit proprietary about them but unashamed and unsentimental. Many who do this work feel chosen.

Competence and kindness were more deeply appreciated there, during COVID, when conditions had turned so desperate, than in any other work at any other time. In *Help*, a 2021 film set in a Liverpool facility in the harrowing spring of the first COVID year, Jodie Comer plays a teenage failure, Sarah, who finds herself adept at caring for the residents and then devoted to them. Suddenly some are wheezing. The plot depicts her anguish as she discovers that National Health Service ambulances are ignoring the residents at risk of dying. The script writer, Jack Thorne, said *Help* was his "love song to the care industry": He wrote *Help* "in extreme anger about the state of care—not just in the U.K. but around the world—and the lack of priority it was given around the world."

Nancy was surprised—"enlivened" was her word—to meet someone who cared enough to write about the catastrophe. I was excited to talk to someone with her wealth of experience.

"Are any of your people alive who were there through the first wave in 2020?" That was my first question.

"Oh yes, of course."

Of course.

"They would have died anyway." The obtuse callousness that Nancy met with reached beyond residents to older adults in general. Tara Swanigan, a grieving daughter, encountered it when she talked about her own father's recent COVID death at only seventy-five. He had been strong and healthy. "Well, your dad was super old," one man told her on social media. Perhaps he meant to be clumsily consoling. But Swanigan was incensed. "For seniors and the immunocompromised, it's almost like we're saying, 'You don't matter. We'd rather just not be inconvenienced.'"

Before COVID there had been walls protecting decent people from passing along ignorant hatred like the implications that care would be "futile" for "the Old." Those walls had been battered in the Before Time; now they seemed shattered, as the painful demise of older adults was rammed home by mortality statistics and age-focused graphs, flammable language, and photos of bodies in distress. People much younger than seventy-five had been turned into the "super old." In 2022 the Centers for Disease Control was *still* emphasizing age. They chose to announce that people fifty to sixty-four were twenty-five times as likely to die of COVID as eighteen- to twenty-nine-year-olds, the reference group of Youth. And those my own age? 140 times as likely. Doomed by nature. In the anxious general population, the futility of caring for us medically could pass for a truth.

WHEN I SAY "THIS"

As early as March 20, when the pandemic had barely started, Dr. John Okrent wrote:

> I can't wait for a time when I say "this"
> and you don't know what I mean.

To many people, older adults symbolized "this." By being the ones sickening and, in some minds, by being the cause of economic closures, older adults prevented "this" from ending. Human bodies had not changed in those few months of 2020. How the embodiment of older people was viewed—*that* changed.

2020 was a frightening and isolating time. No vaccine in sight. People had quickly tired of COVID restrictions—the lockdowns, the boredom, the six feet of separation, living in a separate room from the family, if you could, while you had COVID. They wanted the danger to be over. They *expected* it to be over. Facing their own endless problems, with friends or colleagues drifting away, they fought anxiety and depression, cut back emotionally. They donated much less to philanthropies. They bought guns. When the popular hospital-based TV show *Grey's Anatomy* opened its seventeenth season in 2020, 5.7 million viewers saw almost all the stressed-out doctors suffer breakdowns. Many people must have identified, feeling exhausted, at the end of their rope.

Cities and towns looked forlorn. No movies, no bowling alleys, no gyms, no restaurants. No schools. Little businesses shuttered for good were like missing teeth in a smile. Many "for rent" signs defaced the emptied windows. Almost no street life animated the sidewalks, even in Manhattan. Those who could work from home did so, avoiding contact. The symptoms were terrifying. In the ERs, a man would come in talking, even walking. *He's okay, no need for a bed.* Twenty minutes later he would have "crashed"—his oxygen levels had dropped staggeringly low on the pulse oximeter.

Then governors told all older people, *Best to stay away, keep apart.* Moribund Age had already been separated—as far as metaphors and mortality data could do it—from vital Youth. Now *physical* distancing separated us bodily as well. Age segregation had long been lamented as a source of ageism. Before, however, the only people *structurally* separated from the rest of us were the residents of nursing facilities. After March 2020, older adults in general (like me, with gray or silver hair) who appeared rarely in public tended to be masked, hiding the expressions that humanize a stranger's face. I say "we" as a woman nearing eighty that year.

It was a superstitious time, filled with bad magical thinking. Later, experts studying mortality salience discovered that non-Old adults began an unseen "self-defensive process of psychological distancing" from anyone who appeared to pose a danger. To them, danger emanated from "the Old." "After being reminded of their own death [college students] who previously reported feeling relatively similar to elderly [*sic*] people showed pronounced distancing from, and derogation" of older adults. An ingenious inquiry by gerontologists found that the more completely individuals agreed in March with the statement that "*only* old people died," the more likely it was that they reported feeling *younger* at a follow-up survey in late April. *They* were still alive!

Feeling "younger" because older people are dying sounds ghoulish but for some makes inner sense. The people who were crashing were supposed to be old. The surreal contagiousness of the coronavirus was also marked "old." I had seen the National Guard arrive to disinfect the Life Care nursing facility in Seattle; men swarmed out in hazmat suits—coveralls, safety boots, goggles—an image of threat scarily familiar from a film about an Ebola epidemic in Africa called *Contagion*. Reporters, TV hosts, Twitterers—everyone raising the alarm that "eight out of ten who die are over sixty-five"—may have spread this extra motive to edge farther from anyone who had reached the dangerous ages.

The quarantine advisories, by yet more firmly attaching the disease to older people, put a warning flag on us. Our not appearing anywhere must have meant that we were frail, sick, hospitalized, or had died. The distance from all older adults increased beyond prior ageisms into some realm of estrangement our cohorts had never known. "Futility" could mean that there was no way to prevent the deaths of "the Old"; the rest need not worry except about themselves. A United Nations issue brief in April warned that "social stigma in the context of a health outbreak can result in people being labelled, stereotyped, discriminated against, treated differently, and/or experience loss of status because of a perceived link with a disease."

In the weird seesaw of 2020, the people likeliest to be perceived as Typhoid Marys were not risk-taking teens but us "vulnerable" old folks. Simply by wearing a mask to protect myself, I could signal to others that they needed protection *from* me—and from the millions of people who looked, more or less, just like me.

"LIKE A DOOR IN A HORROR MOVIE"

I had not the faintest idea of the personal relevance of these unexpected, and, at the time, unreported and simply unimaginable phenomena in fall 2020 when I finally returned with trepidation to a grocery store, shopping list in hand. I hadn't had COVID. Officials called such social spaces "petri dishes" for contagion. My N95 mask was strapped tight to my face.

As a doctor with a family, when John Okrent heard "the economy, the economy," he foresaw the dangers in terms of cases, suffering, death. He wrote:

The country is creeping
Back open. Like a door in a horror movie.

I walked through that door. Some markets had arranged a "senior hour" for people over fifty-five or sixty and the immuno-compromised, opened to us from 6:00 to 7:00 or 7:30 a.m. I arrived during the early daylight hours preferentially reserved for older adults. My dream would have been an empty supermarket, but the store I entered was, unfortunately, crowded; surprisingly, there were few "seniors" present. There were a number of low-income workers whose job was shopping for seniors. Everybody was younger than I. In my town, although there was no stigma about wearing a mask, some didn't bother. Hastily I turned back from any aisle containing the barefaced—the under-the-nose slacker, the guys wearing mask-as-chin-warmer.

In no time at all I felt hypervisible. Where I live, age segregation had become an invisible daily norm. No one expected to see us. I was found out, out of place. In the market, in that fall of COVID fatigue and apprehensiveness, people gave me the quick side-eye and stayed away. *Fragile, frail, infectious*—even lacking a cane or walker, all those *f* words were now attached to the likes of me. The glances told me I was a marked "old woman" instead of just another anonymous person striding quickly down the produce aisle to outrun contagion. My froth of white hair above my mask, my lined forehead, were a signal of something fearful: *immuno-compromised, liable to collapse: "Will I have to call 911 for her?"*

This was the new age gaze of the COVID Era. The pre-COVID variety had become tediously familiar. I'd seen the male age gaze rake my body quickly and move off, seeking a younger shape. I'd seen the age gaze at the drinks party glide toward a younger, louder laugher behind me. I'd reported the shame felt by people who experienced similar cruelties. In my seventies I already recognized how powerful epidermalization is toward me: Others took one look at my surface edges and automatically decided my status in relation to themselves.

To aid my thinking about how the gaze works in age relations, I had adjusted W. E. B. DuBois's theory from his doleful and riveting 1903 classic, *The Souls of Black Folk*. Black people often gained "second sight" into the racist white gaze. I had incorporated Laura Mulvey's theory, from her 1975 essay "Visual Pleasure and Narrative Cinema," about the power of *"the male gaze"* on women. DuBois and Mulvey were reporting, not projecting, an affect that had not been well articulated.

Age, like race, is only skin deep. On that micro layer, degrees of emotion have been erected. I didn't see kinship looks in the supermarket. *The age gaze* connotes distance. It can be unseeingly indifferent. In that crowded supermarket, understanding the vibe took me no time. It was a simple question of figuring out which age and gender clichés those strangers were likely bringing to bear in the terrified context of 2020. Once they noticed me, the younger shoppers were battling between feeling fear *for* the Other and fear *of* the Other. Had I coughed and fallen down, some would have called 911. Others would have turned away. People looking like me meant contamination, trouble, misery, sickness, ICUs, funerals. "The Old."

By now many have forgotten how fear inhabited them in 2020, or whether they became superstitious. (They want to forget.) The emergency officially ended, although people are still dying. Special hours for "the Old" ended. We turn up unmasked in shops, movies, bowling alleys, bars. Yet COVID Era ageism doesn't end. In 2022 a woman wrote to the *Boston Globe*, "Whether I am in a store or buying a car or in a social situation, I am made to feel self-conscious about my age. And superfluous!" Much later it occurred to me that the physical separations worked somewhat the way "Colored Only" and" White Only" signs did in the Jim Crow era: they nailed difference into all our psyches, for a long time after the spaces had been desegregated.

HAYWIRE

The pandemic, like a war or a revolution, shifted national moods. Anxiety to be done with fear skewed feelings, beliefs, and behavior. The whole twenty-first-century life-course narrative had gone haywire in some ways that were known and others that were unsuspected. Longevity had been an important mark of US optimism, the source of numerous pop screeds on how to live longer and healthier. But the run of rising longevity had dropped a full 1.5 years in 2020. The tally of US excess dead put us in second place: just after Russia, ranking at the top, and just before Bulgaria, ranking third. Adding to the register of shame, the fall was unequal racially. The National Center for

Health Statistics reported that white Americans' life expectancy had declined by 1.2 years; for Black Americans, 2.9 years. Even after the vaccine was distributed, life expectancy continued to drop. It dropped less for Black people (0.7 years) than white (a full year)—a tribute to the commitment with which Black community organizers worked to get people vaccinated. It dropped more for Native Americans—two years—than for any other group.

Age ought not to have been, ever, the single category to focus on. The claim that *old people died prematurely* should be altered to *the racially oppressed, the impoverished, and the environmentally neglected die prematurely*. The value of being young—framed as immunity from illness—having grown exponentially higher, however, it seemed as if later life was no longer worth a plug nickel. In the sad, brutal Year One of the COVID Era, that was central to the vague, resigned public sense of the concept of futility.

IN THE ICU: A GRIM TEMPLATE

Hospitals mattered—far more than nursing facilities, as we now know. In the entire country, hospitals had 68,558 adult beds and 42,562 airborne-infection isolation rooms (with negative pressure). That total was inadequate and inadequately shared. In intensive care units across the US, every medical determination of "futility" solved an urgent practical problem in the midst of wartime conditions. Hospital managers were desperate to get as many patients as possible out of their intensive care beds. That urgency—known as "through-put pressure"—made some hospitals cancel non-emergency surgery and even postpone necessary cancer and heart treatments. Even without a governor's evil mandate, they tried to discharge "bed blockers"—crude hospital slang—to nursing facilities, even though most facilities were unprepared or unwilling to accept the influx. But dangers to residents were easy to forget, because hospitals were where desperation concentrated.

How would the expected overflows of COVID patients be sorted? Medical discrimination against older adults became inevitable. The scores of those likeliest to benefit from interventions were based on tests and clinical judgment. Some patients, clearly dying, would get comfort care. The rest would get "the most aggressive possible care." It was at these insistent points of medical decision-making that two questions that should arise to consciousness did not. Now they must. *Whose care was considered probably futile?* That question translated as *Whose body would not heal itself, given help?*

To put it bluntly, ageism based on chronology was useful. For guidance in chaos, as we've seen, only one bias was formalized in public guidelines, undoing fairer norms of equal treatment. Only triage *by age*—despite its illegal penumbras of ableism and racism and dementism—was felt to be justifiable. The Do Not Resuscitate order helped to exclude some older or more impaired patients. The more patients presented with a DNR, the fewer who might require CPR or intubation. Whether doctors were ignorant of the legal limits of the DNR or willing to hand them out unwanted, the situation of scarcity allowed that group to feel proud of rescuing their cherished colleagues, rather than guilty about inadequately attending strangers.

The kindest cover story for those who undervalued old lives is that the pandemic stress-tested traditional ethical, interpersonal, religious, and democratic values and professional knowledge under the aegis of "crisis medicine." Haste leads to cognitive failures. Bias also thrives on haste. It can operate automatically, experts tell us, through sins of omission or fleeting justifications that just pass muster.

Most doctors start practice ignorant about multi-morbidity and also about the resilience of older or disabled adults, the ability of their bodies to heal. A despairing attitude about treating them was in fact inculcated implicitly by most medical schools. Some schools teach geriatrics well, offering mentoring and well-patient encounters; the subject is taught as part of primary care and residents may hear reprimands for insensitivity. ("This patient could be your family member.") But students shun geriatrics, as Dr. Louise Aronson showed in *Elderhood*; the mere sniff of the field they get before they flee is depressing. A geriatrician gave me two additional reasons for their despair. In hospital departments, his specialty can be housed next to palliative care—

unmistakably associating later life with death. The thimble of wisdom a geriatrician opts to impart, when asked to give only a single lecture or two, tends to be about end-of-life care. Many people with MD after their name emerge functionally blind to the needs of patients in all their holistic variety—people who may grow old long before they face dying, who may want "more life" rather than to have a MOLST order slipped in front of them.

Given that professional deformation, amid mathematically incontrovertible mortality data, older adults arriving in hospitals could readily be categorized as *morituri*. To prevent these compound-ageist calamities of the COVID Era from becoming permanent, our society needs to debunk the perilous idea that the deaths of older adults "couldn't be helped." Better thinking may emerge from a perspective yet to be considered—that of someone old enough to be a counterstory, emerging out of the tubes, cacophony, expertise, unconscious predispositions, and ethical conflicts of the ICU itself.

MIRACLES

It was best of times amid the worst of times in one of the epicenters of COVID, in New York City, on July 23, 2020. Lawrence (Larry) Kelly, a sixty-four-year-old retired New York assistant principal with a vocation for helping underachieving students, walked unsteadily but on his own legs out of a Manhattan hospital, alive, after 128 days, fifty-one of which he had spent on a ventilator in a drug-induced coma.

"Miracle Larry," he was called. Nobody can recover who needs intensive care and isn't admitted to the ICU. The first "miracle" I notice was that Kelly got admitted in the first place. He didn't have a DNR. He was sixty-four, not sixty-five: according to some triage guidelines, at sixty-five Kelly would have been relegated to a lower priority group. But in mid-March, Kelly was lucky. He was one of the first COVID patients at Mt. Sinai, by some considered the best hospital in the city. The operating principle there remained "first come, first served."

Kelly cried after being discharged. Through tears, he explained why, as best he could. "It's overwhelming. My wife . . . she saved my life. She wouldn't let them pull the plug. Thank you, Honey."

Kelly's wife had told him that after eleven days "they"—medical authorities—had called her: further treatment seemed futile. The ventilator would go to another patient in the queue. One ethicist who helped write Massachusetts's guidelines has "the impression" that clinicians continued to operate on the principle of "first come, first served." But in the very words of those Massachusetts guidelines, that principle may be termed "an unjust allocation of resources" if patients "demonstrate a failure to progress towards discharge." That determination permits them to take a ventilator away. Hospitals were supposed to create "Oversight and Review Committees" to hear appeals from "tertiary triage" about whether and when to switch a ventilator. Kelly had had seizures and a brain hemorrhage, and Mt. Sinai had suffered the brunt of a spring surge. "At this point, with Covid-19," a physician assistant noted, "it was a rare occurrence that a person was [kept] on a ventilator for so long."

They needed his wife's permission to take him off life support. Dawn Kelly said no. The last text her husband sent her had said, "I promise I'll never stop fighting." "I said he would want to live," Dawn Kelly told the doctors. She persisted in challenging medical power and clinical "knowledge"—that fateful alliance whose pervasive force Michel Foucault famously analyzed. But it did not prevail just then. The second miracle is that the medical team gave Larry a reprieve. They must have agreed that *every other possible non-ventilator approach to saving his life, which they would have undertaken aggressively,* would not work as well.

What can best fight the idea of futility? In Kelly's case, it seems to be just the words the team heard: "I'll never stop fighting" or "he'd want to live." Dawn Kelly's conditional tense implies, "If he only knew what you were planning, and could speak for himself. . . ." The review committee had to be convinced that this person, aged sixty-four, treacherously ill, about whose inner life they knew nothing, *wanted* to live. Something so fundamental . . . Yet I would wager that without needing any verbal proof from a silenced recumbent or their articulate loved one, the committee members all believed a priori that *younger* adults want to live. Perhaps they had always believed it. But in the COVID Era the new gulf between Youth and Age, QALY, the sense of futility about saving old bodies, greater public indifference to people in later life, the ageist guidelines—these forces were toweringly constructed on top of that assumption. It is curious, unexamined, exclusionary, discriminatory, and false, but it inspires the miraculous drive to save.

Kelly left amid a crowd cheering, holding congratulatory signs. His sobbing expressed conflicting emotions that survivors rarely have occasion to feel so deeply in their viscera. He surely felt the value of being alive, out in the sunshine, with his wife and daughter. Tears may spring out of joy. They rain out of relief. The involuntary heaving of his solar plexus taught him the tremulous alternative—the danger he might have succumbed to if not for his wife's insistence. He had lain limp and ignorant as a newborn baby of what was going on, in the hands of the medical hierarchy. Momentarily, after eleven days, they had felt, toward his one and only struggling body, something like efficient pitilessness. They had exercised their magic only after having threatened "to pull the plug." What welled up into tears was Kelly's natural, existential, self-pity at the thought of having almost been abandoned by those responsible for him when he *mutely* had so ferocious a desire to live.

Lawrence Kelly's sobs, as I hear them, might have welled up from people living in the nursing facilities—threatened by COVID—coming down with symptoms—enduring scary sickness—silenced by inattention. Their tears would have been addressed to a medical world that didn't believe they had five more years to live, or even one.

The world was wrong. "As we started to see the first patients waking up after successful COVID-19 ICU treatments, we also encountered many patients who remained comatose for days and weeks and then regained consciousness to become fully oriented," said Dr. Nicholas D. Schiff, a professor of neurology and neuroscience. In a study of 795 comatose patients, 72 percent woke to be discharged. "Our findings suggest that for patients with severe COVID, the decision to withdraw life support shouldn't be based solely on prolonged periods of unconsciousness, as these patients may eventually recover."

Pre-COVID, even the "oldest elderly" did well when treated in ICUs: as many as 74 percent survived. (For researchers, unlike the writers of the triage guidelines, survival is achieved at ninety days.) That quite-old people frequently survive will be no surprise to readers of this book, who have known from the beginning that over 80 percent of the nursing home residents who were infected with COVID in 2020 lived into 2021. In the context of "miracles," it is a good time to marvel anew that so many of these older and disabled people, often considered frail, *recovered*. That fact might help overthrow ignorance and negligent systems. The real question—social as well as scientific—should be, *What made their survivals possible?*

With amazing speed, COVID forced the creation of important knowledge that will serve us well: new vaccines, new prophylactics like Paxlovid, and healing techniques like proning, turning patients onto their stomach for some hours to increase oxygen flow to their lungs. Science changes, science teaches. ICU doctors gave Larry a long second chance. Now, asking new questions and finding fresh answers may amaze physicians who still hold the lethal stereotype of aged "futility." The medical profession would do well to take note: The assumption needed to inspire the miraculous drive to save must be, simply, pro-aging. *People may be old, sick, frail, or confused but still earnestly want to live.*

THE HEALING POWER

> All medicine wants
> Is pain to cure.
>
> JELALUDDIN RUMI, "Cry Out in Your Weakness"

"I do believe that it is possible to struggle against [lies], and that this is essentially a *moral* effort," was Orwell's way of encouraging us in the struggle.

In this postmortem, it was first necessary to compile facts about triage, the DNR, and geriatrics teaching; to share suspicions; and then to tell Larry's story, in order to overturn the sly, burly, underground concept of futility in the COVID Era. Given the ethic of benevolence and the promise of impartiality, a better template is possible. Writing in his bighearted, honest book *Better*, Dr. Atul Gawande says that success in medicine requires not superior intelligence but "character . . . more than anything a willingness to recognize failure, to not paper over the cracks, and to change."

Retraining can happen quickly. It did, in hospitals in the first surge, when many nurses and doctors had to be taught when to use ventilators or other apparatuses. My dear friend, the late Archie Golden, a kindly, smiling, beloved pediatrician, not dauntingly much taller than his patients, who had worked in Peru and on a Navajo reservation in public health, was a pioneer in the 1980s, developing programs simulating doctor-patient interactions. His model trained students not to stand condescendingly above their future patients. Archie believed that comprehensive primary care is "whole person care," often psychosocial, in "a long-term close relationship," thus "allowing co–decision making with the patient and family whenever possible."

Writing in 2022, Laura Kolbe, a poet and a New York City hospitalist, believes that the uncertainties of fighting COVID brought those ideals closer. "Doctors have become people, imperfect and embodied and struggling to keep it together," she says. Kolbe herself admits, though, that "my way was smoother and my life more untrammeled under the old, hierarchical, paternal models of medicine."

To undo the trammels for underserved older adults specifically, all the recent developments in medical education—competency-based education, interprofessional education, and technology-facilitated education—can be turned to anti-ageist use. Geriatrics would be taught as part of the core curriculum of basic primary care. Learning would include awareness of the flash triggers—like date of birth or the appearance of agedness—that unleash a range of prejudices, in the supermarket and the consulting room alike. That process of reeducation would require a vast change—in medical school curricula, in Grand Rounds where a lecturer holds forth, in learned journals, in medical departments, in clinical settings, in nurses' meetings, and in virtual spaces. When manuals and curricula change, when role-playing expands empathy, when "aging" becomes less horrifying—that kind of shift can overturn deficient and, at worst, lethal, habits. It would be worth the effort.

Dr. Abraham Verghese has called a doctor's encounter with a stranger a "sacred space." Jane Mansbridge, a past president of the American Political Science Association, pointed out to me that an older doctor may be better at taking advantage of that space:

> An older physician who has shared experiences with her own friends and peers may understand more fully what an older patient is trying to say and ask relevant questions that come from a deeper base than academic study. The subtle signals of common experience may also encourage the patient to speak more freely, with a greater expectation of being understood.

Mansbridge has pointed out that "representation by people with similar life experiences" most matters for certain marginalized groups when their issues "have not previously been processed through elections and campaigns" and particularly "when there has been a history of communicative distrust between their group and the groups that most frequently rule." An older practitioner might not only listen better but also consider warning older patients that a certain percentage of physicians do not understand the DNR and that some may use a patient's DNR as an excuse to deny treatment. That's an honest way to begin the Conversation.

One rule might yet emerge from the COVID Era. All providers—female or male, regardless of background, freshly minted or experienced—should see next to them a person, not a body judged to be deficient (by contrast to a prized body more like their own), not a set of morbid intersections, not an overwhelming "case." The goal is philosopher John Rawls's thought experiment in his classic book *A Theory of Justice*: Imagine yourself as one who dwells at the bottom of the status pyramid and thus becomes intrinsically *unable* to give more weight to one life over another. If this experiment is a dream of conscience, let it give us strength to face the hard realities.

A HARD SHOVE

Take goodwill in the medical profession for granted; add anti-ageist geriatrics to primary care and specialties; invite retired physicians to model role-playing in doctor-patient communication.

Do all that and still, undoing compound ageism will be made harder by the structural and financial circumstances in which medical personnel now practice. Whatever other harms the COVID Era wrought, it made real scarcity more common. The dwindling norm of "overtreatment" has had to make room for the practices and values of scarcity medicine. Perilous preexisting shortages continue—not of ventilators, for the moment, but of hospital beds and hospitals; of geriatricians, nurses, and aides; of better pay for aides and more humane training for everyone. On the grounds of cost reduction (although there are better ways to reduce costs), private for-profit insurance companies increasingly are taking over Medicare through more expensive, privatized "Advantage" programs. Critiques of the trend are sharp. Private insurance reduces the power of physicians vis-à-vis paymasters. It ultimately raises costs. It divides haves from have-nots. It has the power to curtail needed care.

The "power of touch," advanced by renowned doctors, is a major diagnostic tool. At the same time, cost-reduction means that the annual physical—the "touch exam"—is disappearing from Medicare and Medicare Advantage, at just the stage of the life course when the likelihood of being considered touchable is sadly waning. (At my no-touch wellness visit last year, the very young assistant PCP said casually, "You don't need an annual physical." I opened my eyes wider; I saw the Inuit on the ice floe, a mythical figure of "primitive" scarcity, leap into the modern world.) Decades ago, one canny observer foresaw the future: "A system [for patients] based on trust in the competence and fiduciary ethic of individual physicians is being replaced by a system based on alternatives to trust."

"Scarcity" designed for profit expands the categories of losers in the social contest. "Futility" discourse fits all too tidily into the era of scarcity, managed care, and undertreatment. We know the practical, achievable alternative: Medicare and long-term care for all. Millions are panting to encounter the one message that Abraham Verghese in his TED talk believes doctors must promise: "I will never. Never. Never. Abandon you." For many structural, historical, and cultural reasons, however, the guardians of health and life, despite increased goodwill, may discover not only compound but simple ageism added on to bad templates of medical care.

LIKE THE AIR AROUND US

The desire for a rapidly formed, new culture of feeling around later life is not readily shared by everyone. Unanimity would be unlikely even in a less polarized country. Pro-aging voices are sweet but hard to distinguish amid the panicky laments, authoritative bureaucratic pronouncements, and inflamed hate speech. Baleful feelings, beliefs, and behavior need not be universal to be widespread and efficient in the worst way.

The canvas I've been painting, still incomplete, is broad and dark. On a vast national scale, detachment from constantly dying elders afflicted a range of powerful agents early in the COVID Era. Like the air around us, poisoned by petroleum distillates, methane, sulfur, and carbon monoxide, this form of ageism amid the fierce economic chaos infected some of the populace, all the way up to the top layers of government with their ruthless political agendas (a president; the head of the one agency most responsible for nursing homes residents; many governors and legislators), many nursing-facility owners, some medical personnel, some journalists, and all the way down to the dregs of social media with their hysterical public projections onto "Boomers" and "the elderly" at most risk.

Ageism had already infected the way people spoke, thought, acted or failed to act, rationalized their behavior, invented impunity, and decided whom to rescue. In George Orwell's words, I have been "trying to isolate and identify tendencies which exist in all our minds and pervert our thinking, without necessarily occurring in a pure state or operating continuously." To locate the *sources* that "pervert our thinking" and grasp their power, I had to find the notable historical precursors that made the particular harms of the COVID Era possible. The next chapter goes back to the Before Time. The juvenile allure of pop-culture sites, the show-offs of mainstream punditry, literary and theatrical texts from know-it-all younger people, sly partisan attacks on the popular safety nets, a culture war over which "generation" was most responsible for global warming: The common viruses of ageist / ableist injustice were being produced around us and harbored inside the rest of us, too. COVID arrived as the clincher.

CHAPTER 7

THE BEFORE TIME

FIRST THEY INVENTED THE "DUTY TO DIE"

The *Before Time*. People say these words with a peculiar nostalgia, as if everything had been better then. *If only we could get back there*. Yet once we understand the historical backdrop, we see all too clearly the sour sources of the Eldercide and grasp the tenacity of "futility."

What was perhaps most insidious about the new COVID Era was that "the most obvious fact in the world," our smooth slide into sickness and death, strikingly *overturned* one of the fundamental aspects of the pre-COVID era. The worry in prominent quarters and running deep in the conventional imaginary had then been that "the aging" might be sickly, to be sure, but that far from being ready to die, older adults were likely to live *too long*.

Before 2020, Americans still inhabited the proud Age of Longevity. For some, longevity would be automatic. A stage I call "the long midlife" was touted as vibrant, economically valuable, "younger"—"better than you think." Some cities and states were becoming age- and dementia-friendly. Fewer people were developing Alzheimer's disease. Dr. Peter Whitehouse, coauthor of *The Myth of Alzheimer's*, briskly summarized for me the mid-twentieth-century policies that "in service of public health are believed by most experts to have enhanced the resilience" of older adults against cognitive losses:

namely, increasing education via the GI Bill and investment in state colleges and universities, expanded healthcare and improved treatment of risk factors that affect the brain (i.e., vascular disease, high cholesterol, hypertension), remarkably successful smoking cessation programs, deleading gasoline, etc.

"Bonus years" seemed inevitable. Life insurance companies warned those with savings that they might outlive them. TIAA, a managed fund, offered a semi-promise that it would see enrollees not "*to* retirement" but "*through* retirement." When life extension involved better health, gerontologists had a name for it: "the compression of morbidity." The long midlife could extend into one's eighties. Rich hopes of four-generation families, encore careers, longer working lives, and leisure seemed possible. Life expectancy hadn't actually "doubled" in the twentieth century, but that glorious fake fact became conventional wisdom. Everybody—politicians proud of Medicaid, Medicare, and the Affordable Care Act; activists; gerontologists; public health advocates; medical researchers; pharmaceutical companies—liked to explain their creative share in increasing life expectancy for a diverse population. It looked like each thrilling US milestone would be followed by another.

Yet despite such achievements, influential others had feared our tenacious life spans instead of boasting about them. Americans were saturated with troubling ways to feel about the same trends. Fresh evidence shows how prejudicial coverage was. Looking back over decades at more than one billion entries in American and British media in "one of the first known studies to use large-scale and multi-sourced databases to provide a comprehensive view of ageism in the US and UK," Reuben Ng found that negative "aging" descriptions were six times higher than positives. The negatives obsessed over the older body's frailty. "Burden" became a common keyword applied to us elders. "Taxpayer" burden flared up as an obnoxious worry about the public costs of keeping alive those destined to live into deep old age. Because of triumphs of medicine and public health and Social Security's miserly average $1,400 a month keeping the wolf from the door, many of us stubbornly persisted. When the media ignored the enormous unhealthy population under fifty, that oversight made it appear there were too many of *us*, "the Old."

That focus was concretized in the catchphrase "aging America." A powerful medical model of the life course represented old age neither as an interesting part of life nor as a stereotypical decline story begging to be deconstructed, but as a set of expensive diseases, "aging." In 1988, editor John Baron was already telling members of the American Editorial Cartoonists Association, "I think the aging of America is going to be the largest single news story you're going to be concerned about in your careers."

Even the largest story need not have been one-sided. Resistance was available: HR departments urging business to recognize accrued acumen and loyalty. Grandparents, caring usefully for younger family members. Writers on the left, arguing against neoliberal scarcities. Some, including me, were attacking ascribed cohort identities ("Xers," "Millennials") as the basis of foolish generational wars, a cover for ills that have nothing to do with age. As the next chapter shows, some scholars were struggling to make *ageism* a familiar keyword. Critical gerontologists, feminists, sociologists, ethicists, and humanists opposed the medical model and scorned "voodoo demography." However, 6:1 is quite an imbalance. Here I collate some of the multiple sources shaping the powerful hostility toward aging-into-old-age in the years before COVID struck.

Many journalists, producers, and editors may see in hindsight how they failed to provide adequate medical, political, or ethical contextualization. Since the mid-1990s, it had become clear to anyone with a kindly interest in older, disabled, and sicker people that the discourse of Republicans, Tea Partyers, and their satellites was "an exaggeration of the size of the resources required to meet [older people's] needs or of the sacrifice required [from] the sixteen-to-sixty-four age group via taxation." The right-wing solution was austerity—a smaller government budget for so-called entitlements, but not for, say, defense or space.

Other solutions for the exorbitant costs of US health care certainly existed. Provide Medicare for All for a healthier country. Argue that older adults put a high value on our remaining years. If you must focus on eldercare, rein in costs by controlling overbilling and fraud. (Paul Goldberg, a satirical novelist, has a character say that Medicare and Medicaid are like "abandoned property." The government has committed "tributary negligence" of taxpayers by making it so easy to steal from them.)

By mid-2021, six hundred thousand premature deaths from COVID of people over sixty-five had slashed the costs of longevity. This fact should have soothed fiscal anxiety if it had been a real worry rather than a pretext. Louise Penny, the best-selling Canadian novelist, wrote a satire of the eugenic position in *The Madness of Crowds* (2021). "If what had happened by mistake in the pandemic, the wholesale deaths of hundreds of thousands of elderly men and women, were to become policy, wouldn't that be a mercy? A kindness? Humane even? . . . society would be spared the expense. The burden." Bald-faced ageism should have been abashed into silence.

Far from it. In August of 2021, a writer for the *New Yorker* blithely mentioned as "fact" that "we really do spend too much money [*sic*] on health care in the last few years of life." "Last few years of life" was a dog whistle audible over those six hundred thousand death rattles. His editors must have taken for granted that a million *New Yorker* readers would *still* agree. These tastemakers may well have been under the sway of the growing social Darwinism of the COVID Era. When people agreed, in a US correlational study conducted in May 2020, that "*the physically strongest always survive, while the weakest are eliminated*," the authors assert that "lack of support for the policies that prioritize the redistribution of the budget . . . in favor of older adults" then becomes "more likely." My point in this chapter is that long before, many American minds had been prepared to recognize "the Old" as a "burden" that could be laid down. What dangerous stories could get told about older adults, who was speaking for whom, and what else got silenced in the public conversation?

MEDICAL CARE JUST PROLONGS THEIR DYING

Before 2020, the complaint was that we beneficiaries of longevity only *delayed our dying* by seeking health care, as if everyone who wanted a medical intervention had an illusion of immortality and was wrongly postponing that desirable goal, Death. Ingenious ageist solutions to the complaint could be found not only in churlish Reddit threads and trollish tweets, but also in articles in respectable publications.

In 2006, Dr. Ezekiel Emanuel and his coauthor Alan Wertheimer had decided out of the blue (there was no flu emergency) who should be denied the flu vaccine "when"—they assumed this would happen— there were not enough doses to go around. The two complained that government guidelines put sicker and older people—with lives likely to be lost to vaccine scarcity—near the head of the line. They felt the government should opt first for thirteen- to forty-year-olds, then seven- to twelve-year olds, then forty-one- to fifty-year-olds. "Not be- cause the lives of older people are less valuable," they assured gullible readers. (I took this rhetoric personally. It was my very own mother— whose heart and lungs were in fact strong but who might get flu—that their polemics threatened.) This was the same Ezekiel Emanuel who in 2020 used the "fair innings" argument to try to hoard ventilators for young people.

Other 2020 efforts to exclude older people from consideration (the Trump government's rhetoric about reaching "herd immunity"; calls for "sacrifice" like the statement of the Texas lieutenant gover- nor; the violent protests of anti-vaxxers; the "budget-busting" costs of retiree health care) also had a longer, sadder history. "Unsustain- able" had been the word that then president Obama used in the *New York Times* when his grandmother, Madelyn Dunham, got a hip re- placement from Medicare. "Unsustainable" is another dog whistle that means "The government can't go on doing this." The remarks were unbecoming of a president who was promoting health care for people *younger* than sixty-five. Hinting at cutting Medicare benefits dropped ashes onto bent old heads.

Emanuel, although receiving "furious criticism" in philosophical journals for his *Atlantic* article "Why I Hope to Die at 75," led a public pack of the like-minded in the mainstream. (President Biden nevertheless invited Emanuel onto his COVID advisory council, which also failed to include a geriatrician.) The *Atlantic Monthly* had previously published a story entitled "The Coming Death Shortage: Why the Longevity Boom Will Make Us Sorry to Be Alive," by Charles C. Mann, then age fifty. His version pitted "us" meaning, again, *younger* people who need careers and families, against *them*, "rich oldsters . . . expending their disposable income" on "longevity treatments" (like heart-bypass operations or pacemakers). Mann imagined state interventions in a punitive form: "Governments would freely allow the birth of people with 'bad' genes but would let nature take its course on them [translation: refuse them lifesaving remedies] as they aged."

Some writers tried to guilt-trip older adults, casting us as irresponsibly disregarding the costs laid on "our grandchildren." In another *New York Times* column from 2013 (this one titled "On Dying after Your Time"), a known bioethicist, Daniel Callahan, also slid in the word "unsustainable." And if older folks were healthy enough to work, "we" also took jobs away from the young. Two reasons why, he wrote, "our *duty* may be . . . to let death have its day." *Duty* is a formidable word, like *sacrifice*.

The "duty-to-die" discourse aimed to solve a problem its masters had created, of "aging America." It delivered an irrational message: *Don't get old; or, if old, find a way to die cheaply.* Past some chronological age thought to be *too* old, we ought to have vanished bodily as we had been banished visually from ads, most movies, and, in some domains, jobs. Wanting to attain the US promise of longevity was made to seem not a natural human response—or more exactly, a historical privilege of our era that should be extended especially to people who had suffered life-shortening biases earlier in life—but a wrong.

Duty-to-die speech—published or twittery, naive or impure, intentional or ignorant—was not always addressed directly *to* older adults. Alongside the *New York Times*'s "New Old Age" column, a sidebar referred to us explicitly for a time as "a burden" for "you." "You" was a direct address to midlife offspring. Even if adult children liked their parents, this poison pill of "burden" lodged in their minds, or perhaps confirmed, a disagreeable personal, emotional, or financial concern. In either case, "influencers" presented a life-denying ageist ableism as if it were an unanswerable philosophy rather than a point of view aligned with a partisan campaign paid for by millionaires. If a cherished program like Medicare, now half-privatized through Advantage plans, undisguisedly went private, it would shunt everyone onto commercial health insurance. "Aging America" would become a bigger Wall Street bonanza.

A PRIDE THAT BLINDS

As I briefly recapitulate this sordid record now, in the era of the Eldercide, when we can't avoid seeing the consequences, what is most striking is the casual self-righteousness of some published utterances. The theory that "morbid fulness of pride" causes blindness to injustice is James Baldwin's. Explaining the emotions that made white Americans so dangerous to Black Americans in the Jim Crow era, Baldwin had an intuition of how racists felt after they acted on ideas that he, as a former boy preacher, but not they, could see as "wickedness." Pride encourages the morbid illusion that there is no other side, no one who matters. This kind of pride justifies blindness. Baldwin's insight can be applied to other forms of discrimination, including any archive of ageism.

People don't speak confidently in public without proudly aligning with what they consider the "good" side. Writers and doctors arguing for "fair innings" for the younger people who needed ventilators were sidling closer to the gloriously vibrant "Young." Seema Verma may have had front of mind the owners who kept nursing homes operating, not the residents liable to fall ill unseen. Governor DeSantis on "God's antechamber" was speaking Republican demographics in the language of evangelicals. Other thinkers who keep ageist ableism in mind will recall the sinister craze for eugenics.

THE "DUTY TO DIE" AND NAZI MATH

The duty to die had been partially based on carefully selected data. It was therefore not useful to tell Americans how many so-called Boomers or members of the Greatest Generation actually die in normal years: about 5 percent of Medicare beneficiaries. Most incur low costs. The costliest to treat were midlife men between ages sixty-four and seventy-five, trying to survive heart disease and cancers. (Republicans could save money by pressuring midlife men to reject "overtreatment," as opposed to women over eighty-five, who often die natural deaths.) "Cost" should never have been treated as an end-of-life problem.

The typical cost argument relied on futuristic estimates of how many more very old people would be *alive* in [name a year, like 2050] and how many trillions of dollars maintaining our health would then cost. Laura Appleton, a professor of law, shows that the US's limited, unequal "approach to this pandemic is not an aberration, but instead a reflection of our long-held but little discussed eugenic beliefs, established in the late nineteenth century and still endemic today." American eugenics theories had influenced Nazi policies toward older adults and people with disabilities. Nazi textbooks in the 1930s had asked students to calculate how much money could be better spent if not spent on the cognitively or physically impaired.

In the Before Time, US sources who should have known better provided sinister math, graphs, time projections, and scary language about "the Old." As a cultural critic, I need to move back and forth from the mainstream to "experts," from extremists to progressives, to see opinion congealing. The Pew Research Center likened "population aging" to a "tsunami." The US Census Bureau, estimating the numbers of elders from 2010 to 2050, harped on "dependency ratios." Repetition made sure various publics were taught the biased language being normalized: taxpayer "burden," "deficit," "artificial life support," "heroic measures," "persistent vegetative state." This spin presents those ratios as demonstrating that there will not be enough working-age people to support Social Security (although beneficiaries receive checks only after having contributed lifelong). This paradigm comes close to the Nazi construction of "parasites." The US resistance to saying one is "retired" reflects the stigma of being considered "unproductive" in capitalist-decline ideology.

Overlapping, the dominant narratives of "aging America"—medical, pharmaceutical, fiscal, and even literary—portrayed people in later life as sick, asexual, ugly, unhappy, unproductive, abject, and, at worst, disposable. People are often surprised to learn that people over sixty-five don't all live in nursing homes, unkempt or unhinged and waiting to die.

THE DUTY TO DIE FLOWS INTO THE ARTS

[Cultural Studies has] a privileged capacity . . . to analyze certain things about the constitutive and political nature of representation itself, about its complexity, about the effects of language, about textuality as the site of life and death.

STUART HALL, "Cultural Studies and Its Theoretical Legacies"

In the Before Time, people over sixty-five, seventy-five, or, for that matter, ninety-five, did not stop soliciting flu shots, antibiotics, prosthetic hips, pacemakers, heart transplants, or cancer treatments. Given such sturdy will-to-live, a kind of public fantasy had to be and was being constructed. "Rationing" expensive care would have to be voluntary. Suggesting that sick older people should choose to forgo life-extending care may seem absurd, except that Emanuel had suggested it and others had implied it.

Oppression does not work only from above, from a head of state like Trump or medical authorities. "Cultural forms of oppression are no less insidious than 'official' socio-political ones," notes cultural theorist and Americanist Rüdiger Kunow. Kunow points out that "it is both empirically (with regard to the historical record) and theoretically plausible to argue that norms need discursive conduits to be publicly present." Through Twitter, the *New Yorker*, the *Times*, the *Atlantic*, and equivalent sites as we've seen, power knowledge "begins to circulate in the capillaries" of society, shaping feelings and becoming conventional wisdom.

Judith Butler says well what many of us recognize, that "in the domain of representation . . . humanization and dehumanization occur ceaselessly." These processes can happen ceaselessly because Stuart Hall's bold claim that texts can be sites of life and death refers to language of all kinds. Ordinary language: bureaucratese in a CMS letter; reportage that made care for older adults seem futile because "eight out of ten" died; speech that, in the Conversation, made life after CPR seem not worth living.

Ageist, ableist, classist, sexist, and dementist blindness seeps its way into the *arts* as well. Literary fiction, nonfiction, and visual modes gain power over well-educated publics because they come framed as novel, fresh, truthful—news that stays news. Artists *make up* people. That's what they do, for good and ill. They have license to promote fantasies, convey misleading stereotypes, confirm hostile attitudes. Then these attitudes circulate into public policy.

The commandments relevant to the COVID Era are clear:

Honour thy parents; that is, all
From whom advancement may befall.
Thou shalt not kill; but need'st not strive
Officiously to keep alive.

Suicide provides another loophole. Before 2020, some "creatives" developed new forms of the "duty to die." I discern two stages of literary attacks on older people. Both stages represent some of "them," or, more exactly, many of "us," as not *wanting* to live. Could withering dementism make older adults feel "sorry to be alive"?

EUGENIC AGEISM

The first stage, which I call "eugenic" ageism, targeted a first set of the "unfit": people with cognitive impairments. *Still Alice*, a popular 2007 novel by Lisa Genova, the eponymous film made from it seven years later (which earned $44.8 million at the box office), and a clutch of plays about people with "dementia" all made a duty to die seem incumbent on older people, but only if they had a serious cognitive impairment. These adults could be represented as imposing an intolerable responsibility on their families as they lost their "selfhood."

What saved a few of these characters from the silent aversion of readers or viewers was their willingness to take dying into their own hands. Alice, a professor, a victim of early-onset Alzheimer's, is played in the film by Julianne Moore (then forty-six). Alice is considered "still" herself because she tries to follow the instructions about how to kill herself that she had thoughtfully left for later use. Alice could not be given a scene where she *creates* the document of instructions, because showing her feeling cast off or worthless would throw shame on her family. She is shown later, despite so much memory loss, purposefully rummaging to find the thumb drive containing the instructions. The "burden" Alice represented was not old age per se but "dirty" incapacity usually linked to age, confirmed by her peeing herself while looking for a bathroom that her family has failed to label as such. At that time (2007, 2014), writers had to show incontinence or another deficit to get away with the strong hint that people living with such diagnoses should kill themselves while they still had executive abilities.

Such "symbolic atrocities," to use Theodor Adorno's phrase from *Minima Moralia*, rose into public notice as the terror of Alzheimer's disease grew. Fear had been building since the 1980s, like an anchor dragging down hopes of healthy longevity. Discourses emphasizing the disease's prevalence—used by the Alzheimer's Association to raise money for research—wrongly implied that it afflicts most old people. Memory loss gets medicalized when there is no cure in sight. Neuroscience described the brain as losing bits but overlooked that it retained other bits, self-concepts, sensibility, talents. "Dementia" was characterized by metaphors like "zombies" or the most alienating symptoms on the spectrum: hallucinations, rage, parents forgetting their children's names and becoming non-persons.

Dehumanization worked, as it will. "Rational suicide" as a response to cognitive loss was much discussed in the media. It became a topic in social circles. Suicide appeared in a most rational form in the 2021 film *Supernova*. A cultivated writer, Tusker (played by Stanley Tucci at age sixty), decides that what he most needs from his loving life partner, Sam, a musician (played by Colin Firth) is company in their rented cottage when he takes the pills. Tusker, a novelist, sees himself becoming, as the cliché has it, "another person" he doesn't want to be "remembered" as.

Sam is scared about helping Tusker but is willing to accompany him. Tusker—Tucci's face is wonderful here—lovingly, ruefully, refuses to "burden" him. The film shows no ignominious deteriorations, aside from a shot of Sam's hand leafing through Tusker's notebook—mutely showing that his handwriting becomes a scribble. Indeed, Tusker is witty in public and lucid and beloved in private. This portrayal keeps our assent to his choice empathic. The film encourages us to accept early, willed exits as an easeful solution without having to consider the philosophical debates or the obstacles, psychological and practical, to arriving at such an intention and executing it.

In the states that provide physician-assisted suicide, no Tusker could qualify. He is not six months from dying, and if he were, he might well be incapable of informed consent. Felicia Nimue Ackerman, a philosophy professor at Brown University, an active anti-ageist, describes dementism as "cruel and discriminatory cognitive snobbery." Older adults too can be neuro-snobs. We may continue to enjoy a sense of our verbal competitiveness and cognitive privilege unthinkingly, as some people take pride in their whiteness or youth.

Supernova won an LGBTQ Film of the Year award, as a love story. Surprisingly, it also won an AARP Best Movies for Grownups award. *Nihil obstat.* It has apparently become possible for prize-givers and moviegoers to think collectively of persons diagnosed with increasing cognitive impairment as future non-persons.

I understand some motives for arranging to die at one's chosen time. A dear public health mentor whom I loved, dying of end-stage breast cancer in Europe, overcame the formidable obstacles and died with her adult children by her side. When people say, "Kill me if I get *like that,*" one can't discount, as factors in their stance, Tusker's edgy pride or the pain of social ostracism that dementism causes. The future self, unable to maintain its precarious equality with others, may be condescended to, even ruthlessly exposed — as in the Holyoke Soldiers' Home — to a potentially fatal illness.

Imagining people living with "dementia" does not have to go in this terrorizing way. The wholesome ideas of "person-directed care" and the "duty to care" re-humanize people living with cognitive impairments. Just as the neurodiversity movement has made strides in improving behavior toward people on the autism spectrum, the dementia care community has been trying to show how to kindly accompany people along the spectrum of cognitive loss. These ideas are promulgated through best practices that anyone can learn with relief, as I did.

Pia Kontos is a lead researcher in a Canadian collective that produced a humane and credible vision of accompaniment, a brilliant play called *Cracked*; the film is available for a donation on YouTube. Anne Basting is a US playwright and the first MacArthur Fellow in age studies. Her multimedia *Penelope*, a version of the *Odyssey*, involves entire nursing homes — residents with various impairments, staff, and family members — who spent months involved in singing and chanting in Greek. A clip showing residents in wheelchairs, performing, is available on YouTube. The casting, writing, and staging of both plays fully utilize the capacities of the residents.

This kind of social embrace brings relief, even joy; it successfully delays symptoms. But such reassuring reframing, so welcome to family and friends, seems not to have abated the terror of Alzheimer's in any broad-scale way. "Burden" remains the acceptable word used to burden with stigma people who become cognitively challenged.

Supernova and *Still Alice* leave one's own futility a subterranean affect, a vague doomy thought: *Would I* myself *choose death prematurely? At what point?* Popular culture, although quite conflicted about assisted dying, registers a minor but notable willingness to honor suicide as an option when it is for *those other people* — about six million in the US who have been diagnosed with Alzheimer's and related illnesses. I call Alice and Tusker, the relatively youthful outliers, fictional *volunteers of expendability.*

Before COVID struck, the volunteers had expanded to encompass an entire, much larger age class, full of healthy and productive people: people like you and me, in their middle years. This new turn of the literary screw was marked by the text of Lucy Kirkwood's acclaimed play *The Children.* Considered by the *Guardian* to be one of the fifty best theater productions of the twenty-first century, it received many productions and blindly favorable receptions. In this play, the superfluous people are compos mentis, fully capable of fulfilling their former high-level engineering roles. Robin and Hazel are, however, over sixty-five. For this blameless fact, they are asked to sacrifice their lives prematurely to save people half their age. It takes an ingenious plot, involving a Fukushima-like nuclear catastrophe on the English coast, to get audiences ready for that sacrifice. Just before COVID hit, I sat through the production in Boston, becoming more amazed and dismayed.

Rose, an old friend come to visit, tells Hazel and Robin, who live safely outside the "exclusionary zone" of the meltdown, that she has come looking for engineers over "sixty-five"—retired. Her request is that the couple go with her to the damaged power station, in order to replace the engineers who are still there, because they are "so young . . . under 35 . . . have families . . . their whole lives ahead . . . it's not fair . . . because we built it, didn't we? . . . we're responsible." "Responsible" has become another ageist keyword, invoked to create guilt toward the more highly valued Young.

Hazel vehemently objects. "I am 67." She hopes to live to 103 and die quietly like her grandmother, "not bleeding from her gums, not hair falling out, nausea, bloody vomit, diarrhea, leukemia." Since "old" is a synonym for "not being equally human," she must say that she is *not old*. Hazel blames "this bloody country" for ageism and stalks around doing a comic turn about pro-aging values. "In the Mediterranean" she would have been respected. "My age would be a badge, a badge of honor." Hazel's brief rant constitutes the only rebuttal to Rose's assumption that they have a duty to die in order to save younger others—even if the cost is their own life. QALY.

When Robin agrees to go with Rose, he believes he has cancer already. He feels he is past his "sell-by date." Rose has had breast cancer. Ableism supports ageism in Kirkwood's decision to confer terminal diseases on two out of the three. Some sops—*these retirees will die anyway*—are due to members of the audience who, though willing to suspend disbelief, might be shocked at seeing lethal ageism normalized.

Rose has proudly rushed back from America after thirty-eight years just to round up twenty retirees: "To take over and let the young ones go, while they still have the chance, while there's still the possibility of, well, life."

> ROSE: I still have contacts at the Science Council so I flew back and I took it to them and they, I think fast-tracked is the word and, so what happened is I've been in talks with the Government, and the operating company and two weeks ago they approved the proposal.

"The Government" agreed with alacrity to entrust this cockamamie replacement scheme to Rose's out-of-date engineering skills. This is official fascism, invented as a hefty legitimation of Rose's ageism.

State power historically scapegoats groups, but only if they have already been successfully demonized (the US internment of Japanese Americans in World War II is one grave instance). Some targeting is socially impossible. Would any playwright show Rose asking child-free adults to relieve people their age raising children, for the sake of the future? Given ageism, however, a call to voluntary sacrifice can be justified. The cultural escalation—from suicide for early Alzheimer's to healthy volunteers of expendability—was dumbfounding.

HOW A WIDER PUBLIC GETS THE MESSAGE

A theater performance, inevitably seen by relatively few, arises from a wider cultural discourse; then that discourse is transmitted through ads, pre-show feature articles, and Internet comments. Plenty of re-viewers were exposed to Kirkwood's bizarre donnée—that midlife adults should be enthusiastically urged to sacrifice their lives to save younger adults—because *The Children* opened in London in 2016, in New York and Toronto in 2017, and in Berkeley and Boston in 2020. Whatever its performative virtues, the play shows enormous insensitivity to the feelings of older people and people with cancer in the audience. But reviewers failed to utter trigger warnings. One briefly mentioned a "shocking request" but in a manner that might serve as titillation. One championed the play as an "eco-thriller." An announcement in New York City said only, with massive under-statement, that Rose asks Robin and Hazel "to make a life-altering decision."

Some reviewers saw the ageism in the fatal proposal but justified it—with venomous reasoning. The *Montreal Gazette* critic found the much-derided Boomers an easy target. The play provides "a tough reckoning *of the debt owed by baby boomers to those eponymous suc-ceeding generations* . . . three once-vital party people slipping, with varying degrees of equanimity, into oblivion." (It was vital party per-sons who frolicked without masks on beaches.) In its own promo-tional materials, the Berkeley theater company openly sided with Rose's ageism, saying: "Lucy Kirkwood's unique play is a beautifully written puzzle about *personal responsibility, guilt, and what today's el-ders owe the young.*"

New York Times reviewer Jesse Green lambasted people like Hazel, who does yoga and eats healthily, for "selfishly" not wanting to die: And if, as Hazel smugly insists, you must "leave a place cleaner than you found it," what does that mean about the earth "*we bequeath to our children, blotched as it is with our awful mistakes and overrun with centenarian yoginis? . . . . Who's selfish now?*"

"Selfish" is an ageist keyword. In fact, the public health field consid-ers Hazel's energetic sexagenarian health habits a model. An audience member asked Kirkwood whether Hazel is "selfish" compared to Rose. Kirkwood denied it. Hazel was "sort of the heroine"; she found Hazel "moving." No reviewer I read got that message. No reviewer hinted to theatergoers that they would find themselves paying good money to see retirees sacrifice themselves because of their age.

Kirkwood's plot makes sense only if audiences agree that Hazel and Robin are guilty of having been young engineers at time when nuclear plants were considered clean energy, and if Boomer-bashing is acceptable to pious environmentalists. "The lurid spectacle of intergenerational warfare," prophesied by Charles Mann in 2005, no longer seemed so lurid by 2018. Mann had wistfully imagined a US Republican government as a potential ally of Youth, willing to reduce health entitlements for everyone over sixty-five; Kirkwood's fascist England in crisis would sacrifice only twenty people of that age. A modest proposal.

It isn't just "bad art" or Twitter idiots who disseminate serious hate speech into British, Canadian, and US minds. *The Children* wasn't awful theater. It was cleverly plotted; it's a neat three-hander; the roles were juicy. Lucy Kirkwood was twenty-seven when Fukushima (she has said) inspired her. Whatever her motives—planetary ruin must have been top of mind—she was content to have her play be intensely youth-identified. Her ideas thrillingly matched the moment: its pathos about children-as-the-future, its cult of Youth as a vanguard class, its furor of cohort blaming.

THEIR ECO HIGH HORSE

Getting on your eco high horse had become another way to bash stigmatized age groups. Greta Thunberg, a natural leader, was the most prominent of the young cavalry joining the climate-change movement. "Young people are being let down by older generations and those in power," Thunberg said at Davos. Thunberg sensibly recognizes that *power, not age*, creates the obstacles to change. The young who follow this flag see themselves as unique victims of a toxic legacy, righteously vengeful and passionately respectable. Pride, we have seen in other worrisome contexts, often blocks the doors of empathy.

The grain of truth is that anyone born later is likely to suffer more of the increasing harms of global warming than people born earlier.

My granddaughters are likely to be among the half of Americans born since 2000 who will live to be one hundred. (Unless much changes, some will need comfortable nursing homes.) One counter-truth is that some in the maligned "older generations" have a long head start at joining fossil-fuel divestment movements, voting against legislators who get money from climate-denying PACS, buying EVs and solar panels, raging as nation-states dither, and, some since the first Earth Day in 1970, joining marches. Joy Williams's 2021 novel, *Harrow*, features members of a retirement community as angry avengers of the ravaged earth. They are "in the worst of health but with kamikaze hearts."

It is cowardly as well as unjust to blame older age cohorts, because it's hard for members of those cohorts to find equal space in mass culture to object. Anne Karpf, writing in the *Guardian* in 2020, is one who did find space. "Pop princess" Billie Eilish had chosen a vitriolic vein: "Hopefully the adults and the old people start listening to us [about climate change]. Old people are gonna die, and don't really care if we die, but we don't wanna die yet." Karpf, the author of *How to Age*, wrote:

> What's happening here, I think, is that some young climate activists have adopted the intergenerational unfairness narrative—the one that also blames old people for zero-hour jobs, and pretty much everything else that's bad.

In any one-sided "intergenerational unfairness" narrative, those with true power often get off scot-free. In global warming alone we find Exxon Mobil, which executed the cover-up despite knowing the science and still bets big on fossil fuels; the enfeebled US Environmental Protection Agency; the nation-states in Paris.

An argument can be made that the "intergenerational unfairness narrative" seeped into the harsh ventilator guidelines of 2020 and medical ageism more generally. Despite common sense and sound rebuttals, shifting blame to older adults or dismissing their equal rights in the name of "generational justice" remains a fact of common culture.

It may escalate. Jesse Ballenger is an anti-ageist who has published widely on the social and cultural history of "dementia." Ballenger writes, "Unless we develop a much more robust social framework of justice and inclusion, all of the savage inequalities and conflicts that COVID has laid bare will rip through society even more violently in the catastrophes that are coming. I fear that ageism and generational conflict will be prominent among them."

AS THE CULTURAL CENTER RELOCATES

Sometimes, if rarely, it is possible to notice the acceptable cultural "center" being relocated even as it moves. I use Kirkwood's play as an example. Unlike any age critic, no one concerned noticed the ageism inherent in the "shocking request"—neither the playwright (except in Hazel's diatribe against being harried into dying prematurely), nor the Tony Award judges, nor the producers or reviewers, who are typically alert to other prejudices. Satirizing Hazel for seeking a human gain, longevity, which many had congratulated twentieth-century science for procuring, suggests how much scorn had been built up in mainstream speech before *The Children* could be conceived, find willing theater producers, and be praised. By 2023 the deaths of eight hundred thousand people over sixty-five from COVID might have made *The Children* seem in poor taste, or, in a woke world, rebarbative, but a new production went up in Santa Barbara, California.

Midlife and older audiences are those who mainly keep live theater viable. Productions of obviously ageist plays become less perplexing as cultural facts if we notice the financially ailing art form doing what it thinks will attract younger audiences.

Sensitivity often seems lacking when playwrights choose cognitive impairment as their topic. In *Blackberry Winter* by Steve Yockey, a daughter reveals that she has thought of taking her impaired mother into the woods and "braining" her with a rock. The play, produced, like *The Children*, in many cities as a Rolling World Premiere, was described by its Boston producers as "a charming and witty new work" about a woman "grappling with the frightening thought of her mother's

Alzheimer's diagnosis." Showing the *mother's* own fears would have given the work deeper ethical and artistic dimensions but might have made it less "charming."

Núria Casado-Gual, a playwright and theater critic from Spain, sums up our contemporary conjuncture as an implicit conflict about representation. She writes:

> The so-called 'crisis of aging,' through which the unprecedented global situation of the aging population is often presented as a catastrophe, together with the pervasiveness of the narrative of decline (see Gullette, 2004), which continues to inform current understandings of old age, coalesce in a series of contemporary plays that associate the phenomenon of growing older with personal and social decadence, images of dismemberment, anxieties about dementia, and even the apocalypse.

THIS IS WHAT "SENIORS' LIVES DON'T MATTER" LOOKS LIKE

During the Age of Longevity, in the Before Time, public discourses about ushering us off the stage of life had sounded nasty but vacant. I did sense a weakening of social cohesion, with millions of older adults being dropped down, down, down, out of the social embrace. The ill will made me sad. Dying is tough enough without publicly humiliating a group—in this case, older people—by urging them to die cheaply, prematurely, and against their wishes. It makes human and societal sense to give people unforced choices at the end of life, manage their pain, accompany them in that final journey with duty or devotion, and have no posthumous regrets.

But *wishing older adults dead* was a contested, lampoonable wish; I thought nothing could operationalize the fantasy unless, say, Medicare and Medicaid were eliminated. I was wrong. Despite having written a book subtitled *How Not to Shoot Old People*, I underestimated the lethal potential of the duty-to-die campaign. Its entertaining literary forms, incorrect and misleading demographics, neoliberal financial arguments, promulgation of bioethicists' irrational claims of rationality, appeals to families to feel generational envy and create discord— they had seemed to me noxious but safely contained, like a virus in bat saliva. Stored in culture as in a warm cave, however, compound ageist lethality remains handy and transmissible. In the fluctuations of events, beware of harsh futures for particular groups that dominant public voices are allowed to wish for.

Where age is concerned, then, nostalgia for the Before Time is painful and alarming. The ageist, ableist, and dementist texts seem more shocking than they appeared when encountered one by one. Non-US readers may be staggered by their coarseness and by the evasions and euphemisms quoted here. In the US, year after year, the intellectual authors created an informal continuing education for us in learning to discount older selves. Other agents in addition had rendered us a society in training—prepared in multiple, profound, dispersed, confused, and overlapping ways, to pay scant heed to what had gone wrong with the public health system that anyone who needed a nursing facility would have to endure.

HIDDEN

The first important question for millions of outsiders, *us*, now, because only an informed public can make reform likelier, is why we knew next to nothing about the dispersed and hidden devastation going on before the all-too-public COVID Eldercide of 2020. Neglect of the residents had been occurring in the Before Time on an immense scale, not only under the Trump administration. Reformers knew it, but damning evidence, appearing piece by piece, never got the media attention it deserved.

This lack of attention was curious, because in many facilities the atrocity-producing system threatened middle-class convalescents on Medicare. (In 2019, transients had composed about a third of admissions to skilled facilities.) Medicare is relatively generous in paying for their care. Yet their higher status and ability to leave if displeased did not guarantee them good post-acute care. "Adverse events" (the bland term for falls, infections, missed medications, missed symptoms) occurred to one out of five of these convalescents within the first thirty-five days of admission, according to a 2017 report by the Inspector General of HHS. The IG suspected "abuse and neglect." The media and politicians tend to care about the middle class. Was this privileged group of temporary invalids dehumanized by mere contiguity with impoverished LTC residents?

Wherever understaffing is permitted, every inmate can suffer. Most nursing homes had fewer caretaking staff than they had (fraudulently) reported for years. Before 2010, Medicare had been rating staffing levels based on the owners' unverified reports, making it easy to game the system. Why had CMS trusted those reports for so long? Why had fines been reduced so absurdly that the for-profit chains or equity owners could make business decisions to ignore the standards? Why did CMS rarely terminate a license, even of facilities that had injured patients or close failing facilities? Before the pandemic, Indiana's nursing home system ranked forty-eighth in the nation for total nursing staff hours when adjusted for patient acuity, despite receiving more nursing-home Medicaid funds than nearly any other state. The state director of AARP Indiana, Sarah Waddle, asked a question anyone might ponder: "When we know that there are bad actors within that system, why are we so quick to always protect them?"

CMS's program for catching dangerously underperforming facilities had found a ridiculously small percentage of offenders—far from all the worst—but instead of closing or fining them significantly, the agency opted to provide "retraining." In 2017, 52 percent of the 528 homes that had graduated from the minuscule program, by "showing what CMS called 'significant improvements in quality of care,' were subsequently cited for causing serious harm or placing residents in immediate jeopardy." These homes were the incorrigibles. Why was there next-to-no action from state departments of health to take over at least the worst of them?

In polls, huge majorities approve of Medicaid. But recent history shows, with dreadful examples, that not even an eldercide deters disastrous public policies. In 2020, recall, some state legislatures actually cut nursing-facility budgets, and three-quarters of legislatures rapidly provided *relief from liability* for owners of hospitals and nursing facilities. You couldn't make this up.

The coronavirus, once admitted into the facilities, turned "the duty to die" into actual facts on the ground. Those first weeks and months of fatalities were agonizing to reformers and would have been agonizing to the public if they had known then what anyone can know now. My findings staggered me from the beginning, and then they got worse. Summarized in this book, they reveal something frightening about the twisted ways in which common othering functions. Thus compound ageism—ableist, sexist, classist, racist, and dementist—could operate in domain after domain in Year One of the new Era. These isms were not *intentionally* organized; the separate players simply converged.

THE MANY ATMOSPHERES OF THE COVID ERA

To be sure, the era of the Eldercide provided much unprogrammed loving-kindness to me (I was in my late seventies in 2020) and to others. Grandchildren said they loved us on FaceTime. Adult children gathered outside our homes and nursing facilities to blow kisses. Although sheltering in place was lonely, boring, and depressing, and in my case good only for concentrating on a book, it mostly made me feel protected (except, apparently, in my nightmares). But the segregated protections that made me feel safer, as a person over sixty-five, also elevated youth supremacy.

The horror of COVID asphyxiation and awe at the hecatomb may have prevented some expressions of ugliness. But the ageism machinery revved up quickly. At first, only a satirist dared to say publicly, "This pandemic dropped 800,000 old people off the Medicare/Medicaid rolls." Then, in September 2023, the *New York Times* reported exactly that, a fact they must have thought readers would welcome: "A Huge Threat to the U.S. Budget Has Receded."

Nancy, the massage therapist in the nursing home, heard, to her dismay—she said it was "cruel"—that many Americans had come to regard the deaths of residents and older people resignedly, if they think of them at all.

That atmosphere lends a menacing side to current age relations. When residents of nursing homes and older adults were officially favored with the first vaccine, did it make them seem more worthy? In some spheres, it did. But prioritizing by age did not always indicate reverence for aging. In the public Hall of Shame constructed by some media, since states were ranked by the number of COVID-19 deaths per hundred thousand, some governors set the goal of lowering "their" death rate by hook or by crook. And because everyone over sixty-five was again preferred when the booster shots of 2021–2022 became available, our physiological vulnerability became part of the new normal.

Whatever the good intention, vaccine priority by age may actually have reinforced a veteran form of ageist ableism. A *Saturday Night Live* skit, "Boomers Got the Vax"—featuring baby-faced stars in old-people drag, one sporting a cane—mocked the named cohort for getting yet another unwarranted freebie. By October 2022, the skit had been viewed 6,956,784 times. Employer dropping of midlife workers accelerated during COVID closures. In an economy marked by delirious back-patting over supposedly full employment, only 30 percent of those over fifty who lost jobs were re-employed by the end of 2022. "Gerontocracy" became a pejorative that licensed belittling anyone in office represented as over-the-hill. A *New Yorker* cover in October 2023 aimed to ridicule the ambitions of four politicians (Trump, Biden, Nancy Pelosi, and Mitch McConnell) by drawing them striding into "the race" on walkers.

The achievements of longevity and the promises of pro-aging power to "change the narrative" had indeed been historically thrilling constructions. But all along they had been suffering steady erosion in the face of devaluing campaigns. Is there a way back to reconsidering old folks as avidly life-loving and worthy of care? Susan Flory is a UK podcaster and anti-ageist. Early in the COVID Era, discussing with me the eruptions of age hatred and violence, Flory summed up our conjuncture with quiet objectivity: "We are far from having flattened the curve of the virus of ageism."

PART 3

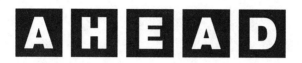

Toward a Fuller Social Embrace

CHAPTER 8

THE GUARDIANS OF LATER LIFE

How Anti-Ageism Tried to Wake America before COVID

AMERICAN SLUMBER

When Franz Kafka's character Gregor Samsa found himself turned into an insect—*treated* like an insect, avoided and abandoned alone in his filthy neglected bedroom—he found it incomprehensible. Kafka's astonishing novella *The Metamorphosis* has been interpreted in different ways by generations of rapt readers. For me, the tale of monstrous deformation begs to be read as an allegory of how debasing some forms of ageism suddenly, surprisingly, *feel* to the victim. "Inside" you are not old, ungainly, grotesque, forgettable! Perhaps not so hale or so keen, yes, okay, maybe, but since when despised? Being patronized, ignored, avoided, or laughed at—by adult offspring, a younger person at a get-together, a doctor, a clerk, a personnel director, a jogger—is painful. Pain goes with bewilderment. *Did that really happen? Why me? Will it happen again?*

WHAT DOES "AGEISM" EVEN MEAN?

Many older adults have no idea that ageism in its more hostile or deadly forms could injure them. Ageism, whether compound or simple, institutional or personal, overt or implicit, trivial or lethal, sneaks up on us after a lifetime free of it. People are not born "old" the way they are born with gender and skin color. We start as mere babies. Culturally speaking, people *become* old, but rather slowly. In the long midlife many feel it as their "Permanent Period," as the narrator of Richard Ford's novel *The Lay of the Land*, calls it. At fifty-five, Frank Bascomb considers himself "an actualized unchangeable non-becomer, as snugged into life as a planning board member." He's really not so snug. He fears the metamorphosis of aging, becoming "just an organism that for some reason can still make noise, but not much more than that."

It's possible to grow older without foreseeing so much descent. If women, people of color, or people with visible impairments become wised up to discrimination early in life, wincing personal exposures to ageism come later. Ageism may be the first bias some fortunate whites experience, Julie Ober Allen and her fellow researchers point out. People try to stick with their "Prime of Life" discourses. *I live* outside *a nursing home. I do yoga. I like sex. I have the right to rights.* As we age in appearance, we remain human, *of course we do.* Until the little dehumanizations begin to occur. And then what is to be done? Complaining seems humiliating, an admission of lost powers. Yelling "ageist"? Unlike the charge "racist," an accusation of ageism doesn't occasion fierce denials. Growing older with less money, social help, or legal backup, you may become humble and mute, feel yourself weakening, shrinking, shamed, a Gregor Samsa.

Now, after the sudden abandonment of the facility residents in the COVID Era, any definition of ageism necessarily includes the worst attacks. Before the Eldercide, the public at large was too innocent. This is one life-giving lesson that the twenty-first century had better learn: We weren't suspicious enough—nor alert enough to the brutal harms that compound ageism could inflict.

Many people could readily cite shorthand terms to tell you what *sexism* means: "#MeToo," "glass ceiling," "toxic masculinity." *Racism* also has a known backstory: "400 years of slavery," "Jim Crow," "redlining," "police violence." *Ageism* has few such ready connotations. Although some people have learned to resent sexism, racism, and homophobia even when they have not been targets themselves, they may entertain ageist prejudices unreflectively. "Implicit ageism" is the kind people deny they have. Yet 95 percent of the participants in a self-administered survey revealed they held negative views of older adults, a higher proportion than for implicit racism or sexism. Younger people sometimes even *say* they don't want to sit near unknown old folks, prefer not to talk to us, as if the stigmas staining nursing-home residents overflowed onto all older adults.

Bias means we can even be made to feel guilty about what othering does to us. A group led by Julie Ober Allen, studying internalized ageism, found that 80 percent of people aged fifty to eighty turned common stereotypes against themselves: *I'm ugly, sad, uninteresting . . . ashamed of being old*. Hating on old age may seem sadly normal, rather than being perceived as hate speech. Dumping on oneself is ill advised. Not just medical ageism but every kind raises the risk of bad physical and mental health outcomes and can even shorten lives.

Americans were aware of persistent job discrimination by age — deleting people from the workforce, especially people of color and white women — as AARP surveys showed. On my Google Alert, "ageism" started to appear more frequently, but without intensity. Hollywood's sexist ageism against photogenic stars was taken *very* seriously. The average person resented harsh birthday cards. But the average person was not likely to have shared intimate conversations with older victims, read exposés of ageist attitudes, or participated in activist resistance — those cultural assists that enlighten victims of other bigotry. People could not understand how grave, intersectional, and systemic a thousand age-related demotions are.

Given the 6:1 ratio of negatives to positives in a billion media entries, the public could hardly acquire much enlightenment. Other forces beside ignorance and fatalism (Arendt's "nobody worries about what cannot be changed") get in the way of unlearning age prejudice. Toni M. Calasanti, a sociologist and feminist gerontologist, holds the American ideology of self-reliance responsible: "Most people prefer to see aging as subject to personal control, with little concern, for example, for how Social Security privatization or other institutional policies could penalize most old people." Ashton Applewhite, the activist author of *This Chair Rocks*, thinks this narrow subjective position is common because "most Americans have yet to put their concerns about aging in a social or political context."

THE VACCINE FOR THE DISEASE OF AGEISM

In gerontology, cultural anthropology, and the multidisciplinary field of age studies, by contrast, everyone kept *age* at the center of their work. Age scholars (one name for the entire loose collective) considered intimate experiences of changes and continuities over the life course as social narratives. They shifted their readers' consciousness about what it means to be living in a body/mind whose life course takes place in a given culture and over historical time. They made *Aging* a burgeoning question, not a disaster foretold. Exposing these novelties to peers and students has been the collective's essential contribution to theory, model practices, emotional growth, and activism. Such enlightenment is a boon for which we are grateful.

In this milieu, ageism is considered another cultural disease. If someone has absorbed too high a dose of the social virus, anti-ageism is prescribed as the antidote. Yet our turn toward using the term came quite a while after previous cultural turns to confronting other *isms*: racism, ableism, sexism, homophobia, classism. When COVID began to kill, *ageism* had yet to become widely recognized as a keyword not only good to think with but necessary to act on. Those whom I consider the scholarly guardians of real-world age relations, including myself, were collectively unable to highlight ageism sufficiently for the public to have diminished its hostile social attitudes.

WHY SURVIVE?

Our weakness as influencers certainly did not come from believing that age-related prejudices (or hatred of old age and avoidance of older people) were harmless parts of US social, economic, psychic, and political life. Everyone knew better. Everyone knew Robert Butler, MD, who had famously coined the term *ageism* in 1969. At that time, a cruel crisis already existed around job discrimination in hiring, firing, and layoffs. Such discrimination was known to start as young as age forty; it was in effect already "middle ageism." The crisis was apparent to Congress when it passed the Age Discrimination in Employment Act in 1967, creating an agency, the Equal Opportunity Employment Commission, to levy fines against guilty employers.

Dr. Butler's standing was in medicine. He was the founding director of the National Institute on Aging, which landed under the National Institutes of Health. In 1990 he founded the International Longevity Center in New York City. In 1969 he had hoped that "age-ism might parallel or replace racism as the great issue of the next 20 to 30 years." Fifty years later, it hasn't done either. (He had presciently interpolated, "It might be wishful thinking to say, 'replace racism.'") In hindsight, "Aging and Disability" should have gotten a Cabinet seat—alongside Health, Housing, and Justice—as a space of rights. Butler might well have agreed. In 1975 he published a Pulitzer Prize–winning manifesto, *Why Survive? Being Old in America.* The acid question itself was an alert. Nicole Hollander, a satirical cartoon artist, inventor of the long-running strip, *Sylvia,* once quipped, "Getting old in America? Best to do it somewhere else."

Sadly, the US has not since then produced public intellectuals and activists with Butler's claim on public attention and his bitter urgency. Not for lack of individual efforts. Betty Friedan in *The Fountain of Age* (and, among others, Audre Lorde, Alex Comfort, Simone de Beauvoir, Barbara McDonald, and Margaret Atwood in her short story "Torching the Dusties") issued warnings. Ashton Applewhite gave a major TED talk on ageism and started Old School, a fast-growing online clearinghouse of resources. No movement existed, however, to spread across the land the foundational belief that age injustices were remediable, or the warning that they would hit residents of nursing facilities the hardest.

ROUGH TERRITORY FROM THE BEGINNING

Before ageism could be widely viewed as a social evil that could be dismantled like sexism and racism, "age" had to be understood as a category and set of experiences imposed by culture. The first necessity was to wrest age away from "the chronological and biological dimensions of aging—the arguably natural—to the arenas of artificial prejudice and social hierarchy, the incontrovertibly constructed," as historian Corinne T. Field succinctly puts it. A humble metaphor by Marguerite Yourcenar illustrates this truth: "Nothing is more stable than the curve of a heel, the location of a tendon or the form of a toe. There are eras where footwear deforms less." When might a society discover we are aged by culture? At times when the man-made shoe hurts *more*.

One obstacle to this profound discovery was that the study of "the Old"—gerontology—got its start in the eugenics era, when those perceived to be not-the-fittest were being selected and categorized. The field identified as its object a naturalized, dehistoricized body whose "aging" was defined as "*a collection of diseases*," ending in death. Elie Metchnikoff named the field in the early 1900s. Alois Alzheimer discovered the condition that bears his name in 1906. G. Stanley Hall's book *Senescence: The Last Half of Life* appeared in 1922. Science imperiously separated older people en masse from their other identities, from younger subjects (adolescents), and from their cultural contexts. As late as 1984–1985, Stephen Katz, a Canadian researcher who was to write a history (*Disciplining Old Age*), observed that "the critical forces revitalising other fields of knowledge had somehow bypassed gerontology." Those forces, often emerging from feminist and left theory, often coming from abroad, soon became influential.

US gerontology grew with the advent of government institutions, primarily for older adults, in the 1960s—Medicare, Medicaid, the Institute on Aging, the Administration on Aging, and eventually hundreds of Area Agencies on Aging. The field became professionalized when bachelor's, master's, and PhD degree programs were created, first at the University of Southern California, in 1975. By 2020, the Gerontological Society of America (GSA) alone had 5,500 members. Some members had been distinguishing themselves internally as critical, social, feminist, humanist, or literary/cultural in their approach— but they all sought to wrest age away from nature.

THE TENT GOT BIGGER

The tent got bigger. Theory-rich approaches in the study of gender and race inspired scholars with various professional degrees, of all ages, to make "age" a more provocative and alluring category. We realized that age had been understudied, under-theorized; its uses in common speech—and sometimes even in social science research—often went unexamined. The work that has followed, *thinking through age*, was not, despite what journalists like to say, an inevitable result of there being so many Boomers growing older. In 1993, I wishfully named the potential field "age studies." Age Studies earned a book series in the 1990s, published by the University of Virginia Press.

Dr. Butler invited me to his International Longevity Center in the 1990s. After my talk, he came toward me with his hand out to clasp mine, saying warmly, "We must think more about *culture*." The concept that people are "aged by culture" (the title of a book I published in 2004) spread. Those quick to understand the vast role of culture formed their own networks of age critics: the European Network in Aging Studies in Europe and the Middle East, and the North American Network in Aging Studies in North America. Exploring, as Stephen Katz's dragnet put it, "the alternative, performative, artistic, fictional, trans-sexual, poetic and futuristic conditions of aging," they drew on life-course studies, feminist theories of care, critical race theory, media studies, history, and philosophy.

The age mission felt thrilling and necessary. Our goal was not creating new departments, as women's or African American studies had done, but mainstreaming "age matters" into scholarship and teaching beyond the rare undergrad courses listed as covering the sociology or anthropology "of aging"—reaching students across all disciplines and sending them out able to confront the indifference, incomprehension, or hostility of the wider world.

The flourishing concept of intersectionality ought to have been adaptable to any of society's body-based prejudices—especially ageism, the one and only universal bane. But when it came to transferring new ideas of age across disciplinary boundaries, nomadic thinking went much more slowly than it did when people sought to denaturalize gender or race, and that work was slow enough. Erdman Palmore, the North American editor of the *Encyclopedia of Ageism*, suspected that the "lack of charisma" of the fields of gerontology and geriatrics slowed their uptake by liberal arts and science faculties. That claim seems an understatement. Even feminists and critical race and disability and queer theorists, allies whom we needed, mostly shied away. To them, remedying the dire problems of younger people was paramount. They could not see later life as something that mattered. Conservative minds remained arguably certain that "aging" was essentially about that squeaking organism. Perhaps it felt as if age scholars were mapping a distant galaxy, dark-sky regions that few on earth could perceive or care to know about—when *we* felt warmly certain that we were closing in on the experiences and imaginaries of older adults quite familiar and close by.

Some thinkers—in cultural studies, media critique, history, philosophy, business, law, architecture, psychology—welcomed age studies with a fresh cry of discovery. To those on the long march through the institutions, getting admitted into each of their flagship journals was a triumph. New journals also sprang up: the *Journal of Aging Studies* in 1987; *Medical Humanities* in 2000; *Age, Culture, Humanities* in 2014. The first book titled *Age Studies*, by British sociologist Susan Pickard, appeared in 2016. To train students and graduate students—and then to see some of them join us as colleagues—felt priceless.

If the Holberg Prize for development of a novel interdisciplinary field or the Berggruen Prize for advancing ideas that improve human self-understanding were ever given to a collective rather than to one lone individual, the international collective of hyphenated gerontologists and age critics would deserve the distinctions.

In hindsight, however, the worthy endeavor of integrating *age* in academe can be seen as a long distraction from addressing the well-hidden threats of ageism. (In 2008, I was still prodding people to ask, "What exactly has *age* got to do with it?") Mainstreaming age remains a slog through soggy fields. In her 2015 book *Age Becomes Us*, literary scholar Leni Marshall, having noticed that time and again new books on age or ageism were hailed in reviews as "groundbreaking," commented, "Forty years of scholarship and still we are just breaking ground—what rough territory this is!"

NO RIVALROUS JOCKEYING TO THINK IT NEW

Some of Butler's epigoni had in fact been moving the phenomena of *ageism* into the center of their work. "Scores of researchers have since followed Butler's lead in defining and measuring ageism," US historian W. Andrew Achenbaum averred in 2015. Despite this remarkable vanguard, the field was jarred by no creative disruption—not the kind of rivalrous jockeying to *think it new* that the inspiring British Jamaican cultural theorist Stuart Hall described so vividly, when the renowned Birmingham Centre for Contemporary Cultural Studies confronted its own sexism. In fact, the early genuflection of cultural studies to young people—treated as a vanguard class—was stunning.

Broad resistance to studying systemic ageism—rather than topics connected to the traditional keyword *aging*—was noticeable. The US author of *The Short Guide to Aging and Gerontology*, Kate de Medeiros, took on that reluctance. Writing in a flagship journal, the *Gerontologist*, de Medeiros argued in favor of our taking "a strong stand against ageism and ageist practices. *We should not view ageism as a separate topic of study within gerontology*, but rather as an essential element of all endeavor."

Clearly, a vanguard of anti-ageists was not enough. A century had passed since Metchnikoff, Alzheimer, and G. Stanley Hall. It took until 2015 before "Ageism Comes of Age," an overview in the GSA's *Journals of Gerontology*, agreed there was "enough research" to warrant a focused issue on the prejudice that most affected our subjects. In some quarters, any unified call may be resisted as "over-organization," as the twentieth-century sociologist Karl Mannheim declared, and thus "naturally undesirable." Treating ageism as an object of study, or as a cause, had not been made *naturally desirable*.

A GROUP OF EXPERTS EXPLAINS WHERE
WE SUCCEEDED AND WHY WE FAILED

There remained a lot to explain. As a cultural critic allied with the international field of age studies, I had read, admired, and quoted many of those vanguard thinkers about anti-ageism. In 2018 and 2019 I decided to interview some of the most eminent of these thinkers, from the US and abroad. They were keynoters, authors of major books. One or two were legendary. A few I knew personally. Everyone I asked was quick to reply. Self-criticism, which some thinkers eschew, came to them easily. Almost all the interviews quoted here were completed before the Eldercide. (I had in mind interviewing other experts, but the pandemic overturned my priorities. In March 2020 I started writing the articles that led to this book.)

The open-ended question I posed was to speculate on why anti-ageist work "had not packed a bigger wallop." My interviewees agreed that it hadn't. In an essay reviewing "Three Decades of Research on Ageism," Erdman Palmore had concluded that, "sad to say[,] . . . there is not yet any statistical evidence of reduction over time in prejudice and discrimination against elders." My informants might have agreed that ageism had in fact worsened. We were aware of the disappointing lack of impact of our joint endeavors. Speaking, I believe, for many, one said to me, "It's been a long struggle."

Stuart Hall wrote that, thanks to Foucault and Gramsci, "the sense of the concrete historical instance . . . has always been one of culturalism's principal strengths." I counted on my informants to be "culturalists"—in the broad interdisciplinary sense that includes symbolic and material factors and power relations and internalizations of stigma. Long reflection had led them to pithy summations of the weaknesses they considered most important. They took speculation on the concrete historical instance far beyond the question of belatedness. They pointed to "blinders" hanging on in the field, in the academy, in ourselves.

No one offered their POV as the single explanation, and I provide no single summation of their provocative critiques. The analyses organized here are multiple and complex. There will be later accounts; this one has the advantage of learned witnesses writing honestly about ageism before having endured the COVID Era. They offer an intellectual baseline.

SOME WRONG TURNS

Erdman Palmore was the first of my distinguished informants. His response was generously wide-ranging. He proposed that our blinders take many forms: "The same causes of ageism itself may also be causes of its belatedness." His list of causes included but did not privilege "death anxiety," as some psychoanalytically oriented thinkers have done. It included, on the individual level, ignorance and selective perception. He alone mentioned money power:

> Some gerontologists may find the study of ageism uncool because they . . . have a vested interest in continuing or exaggerating the "problems of aging." They may be getting research grants [or] speaking engagements, publishing articles, raising donations, etc. Just like the "anti-aging" medical and pharmacy industries profit from fanning fears of aging. Research and writing on ageism which counters these fears cuts into their profits.

Alzheimer's funding goes more toward solving the puzzle of causality than supporting the care of those who have it or improving their image.

To fight the stereotype of "the Old" as gaga and useless, some gerontologists had developed the concept of "positive" or "successful" aging. This reframing strategy represented everyone in the long midlife as healthy, active, socially engaged, knowledgeable, and financially secure consumers. A supportive fantasy held that they were capable of "changing aging"—certainly an excellent goal—just by expressing their desire to be treated better and hired.

The lavish focus on the privileged caused an internal split. Rüdiger Kunow, German Americanist and author of *Material Bodies: Biology and Culture in the United States*, pointed to the weakness in the strategy:

Some Age Studies work has in my view been muted, less effective as cultural critique because it has been sidelined by an ingenious redefinition of late life, [promoted] by the media and the business community. Splitting late life into two phases, the famed "Third Age" and the abject "Fourth Age" ([Paul] Baltes et al.), has offered material and symbolic rewards to people who appeared in the public as assertively not old.

Positive aging was critiqued as individualistic, gendered male, heteronormative, classist, and ableist. Anthropologist Sarah Lamb called it a global "contemporary obsession." Positivity could be toxic and naive, failing to attack the causes of lifelong inequalities in health and wealth. *Improvement* was wrong empirically. "The coming generation of elderly people will be considerably less privileged than their forebears, given the deterioration of the welfare system, the undervaluation of care work and the shuttering of nursing facilities," was the summation of two humanistic age critics, James Chappell and Sari Edelstein. Emphasizing the older adults who were not needy also put at risk beloved government programs.

Despite many counter-narratives, the traditional biomedical model of "aging" as an accumulation of diseases and deficits still darkened the image of older adults. "Aging and decline" and "aging and dying" were still tautly tied together. Many scholars doing fresh work retained phrases like "aging nations," which, even used critically, carried the neoliberal connotation of the burden of too many unproductive old people who cost too much to treat. (An essay I called "Against 'Aging'" was my attempt to explain the problems inherent in the continuing use of the term *aging*, a euphemism for old age, a decline term for growing older.)

Stephen Katz detailed the profession's avoidance of the real social conditions:

Gerontology conferences are about studying the ever finer molecular aspects of aging, care-industry products and therapies, and endless measurements around quality of life, daily activities, and, when

feeling a little more sociological, then family or generational relations. But there is little about how to . . . confront the prevalent suffering, disability, dependence, poverty, violence, and precarity that
come with it today. . . . [W]here critique becomes re-translated as
'negativity,' then ageism resurfaces.

Toni M. Calasanti, editor, with Kathleen Slevin, of the 2006 classic
Age Matters: Realigning Feminist Thinking, urged us to follow the example of Maggie Kuhn, a more radical thinker. Kuhn's Gray Panthers,
Calasanti wrote, "understood that we need to fight ageism by reclaiming old age as a valuable status, much as (some) women have argued
that women do not need to be like men to be valuable, or (some)
people of color would maintain that they needn't be 'more white.'"

THE TARGETS WE NEEDED TO HIT

The enormous and perplexing *spectrum* of ageisms was another obstacle to fully comprehending the bias. As early as 1990, British sociologist Alan Walker had argued that "age" was "*the unrecognised discrimination,*" in an anthology bearing that subtitle. Walker told me: "The
target is constantly shifting and taking on new forms, from politics to
the anti-ageing industry, and . . . it is highly gendered, that is, it is applied differently to men and women."

In the US, the mainstream media certainly shifted targets, and far
from reclaiming old age as a valuable status, the loudest voices were
undermining it. They harped on what was demeaning. Dreaded "dementia" remained shackled to "old-old age," despite our excellent rebuttals of alarmist data and our critiques of the way people with impairments were represented in film, fiction, TV, and theater. On Twitter,
Reddit, and other social media sites, youngsters posted ageist hate
speech in jokes and slurs. Partisan political agendas appeared in dis-
guise. Generational warfare got published in the popular press, ginned
up by decades of well-funded Republican propaganda to reduce social
programs and lower midlife salaries. When the nursing-facility lobby
influenced legislators to keep aides' wages low, or when nurses' unions

fought for reform, that news was scarcely reported, while neoliberal bias pounded out the notion that Medicare was not "sustainable." Few mainstream journalists concentrated on age issues. The media did not explain, could not perceive, how "just not caring" about residents of nursing facilities was operationalized in abusive and lethal ways, an analysis that takes up much of this book.

The public rarely heard *us*. Every kind of decline thinking claimed bigger audiences. We had rebuttals, but they appeared mainly in specialized journals and small-run presses. Few journalists interviewed us. Few of us spoke to or wrote for large or mixed-age audiences. There were never enough of us playing Whack-a-Mole in public, fighting for space against organized lobbies, ads for "anti-aging" rejuvenations, and neoliberalism's bias against later life. Alan Walker was brilliantly prescient in seeing the potential lethality of the tendencies; the ageist assumption, he noted, also "leads inexorably to arguments in favour of euthanasia or other ways of killing-off the burdensome old."

GRIT

Even before COVID, it took grit as well as new knowledge to face the injuries inflicted on older people. They are insulted, knocked down, immiserated, even killed, but in ways so subtle or apparently normalized that they rarely attract attention. Such sufferings have been less well publicized and discussed than the evils of misogyny and racism. "Ageism is often hard to prove, and may be more subtle than racism & sexism," Palmore wrote me.

Self-reflection on cognitive and emotional belatedness can be useful. I too was slow to recognize how dangerous ageism could be. My 2017 book *Ending Ageism, or How Not to Shoot Old People* recognized lethality in particular circumstances: suicides of unemployed midlife men; the risks to old bones of "walking while old"; instances of medical ageism; the danger of becoming terminally ill while married to an old man with a gun. It took years to decide that my strong and comprehensive keyword had to be *ageism*.

Deciding to use political vocabularies has been a problem for scholars, journalists, and citizens alike. Only in 2019 was the term *racism* decisively added to the *AP Stylebook*, the bible of journalists. Before, there were squirmy euphemisms: *racially-motivated* rather than *racist*. Many age scholars also used blurry euphemisms—like *age-related*— when *ageist* (*neuroageist, sexist ageist, middle ageist*) would have been more exact and persuasive.

In field after field—feminism, anti-racism, decolonial studies—it has taken theoretical effort to argue that analysis is not biased by being infused with feeling. (I lacked the "gladiatorial spirit" that Margaret Fuller, a dauntless nineteenth-century intellectual, rejoiced in at age fifteen. Temperamentally conflict-averse, I also had to fight my academic training to invent hashtags or call out "evils" rather than tamping down my feelings through blander language.) Explaining ageism can require locutions that at first sound odd: age injustice, "compound ageism," "replacement biases." We need to be nimble to link this-with-that across fields. Yet the approved genre of the monograph, the stylistic and content requirements of scholarly journals, and the demands of funding agencies have limited verbal innovation and creative interdisciplinarity. The siloes that have restrained us are baked into hierarchy and promotion.

NATIVES OF LATER LIFE

The experts I interviewed zeroed in on issues that went far beyond positive aging, the slippery multiplications of evidence, or linguistic and political timidity. Many went straight to our own biases. "One problem with gerontology, in my view," Stephen Katz wrote, "is that it assumes it is, by definition, anti-ageist, and that it has a homologous relationship with all older people as allies." Would we be more engaged if more age scholars were actual natives of later life, living with the painful effects of being inferiorized or knowing admired peers subjected to dehumanizations?

Age matters, as we saw with regard to physicians. Most age scholars tend to be non-old—far under sixty-five. In the academy, this lack of elders partly reflects subtle ageist pressures on tenured people to retire.

Harry (Rick) Moody described to me one result of relative youth. The editor of ten editions of *Aging: Concepts and Controversies*, Moody was formerly a vice president for Academic Affairs at AARP. One result of his professional "life review" was a realization about conferences:

> I've realized that professional and academic organizations in the field of aging, ostensibly concerned with the experience of aging, almost never have actual "elders" (I'm 74 now) speaking from personal experience about anything of relevance to the issues discussed. It's a bizarre situation. I've seen it over and over again in the 40 years I've been attending professional meetings. Can we imagine the NAACP having only white people as speakers? Or the National Organization of Women having only men on the program? . . . I've never seen it written or talked about. This is a systematic failure.

Thus, programs, surveys, ethnographies, theories, and public policy pronouncements tend to be about "others." (As I was writing a book in which I finally included myself in the "we" of old age, I began to notice scholars using "they" about the group to which they devote their professional activity.)

The "others," like the residents of nursing homes, are mostly older women. Perhaps in a research field that has been led by many non-old men, the "feminization" of longevity, poverty, and old age has been a problem. The low-wage service component in the agencies and nursing homes is also overwhelmingly female. Margaret Cruikshank, the author of *How to Grow Old*, commented, "Maybe if the field were woman-dominated [at the top], ageism would be a front and center issue." It might also help if more of us had a vested interest—owned up, as philosophers of disability Joel M. Reynolds and Anna Landre put it, to one of "the bodily variabilities we today categorize as 'disabilities.'" As late as 2018, Reynolds noted that "disability studies and gerontology would seem to have common interests and goals. However, there has been little discussion between these fields."

Privilege can be a blinder. In the US, academia is still overwhelmingly white. Men earn more than women as adjuncts or as ladder faculty. Among full professors, women's salaries are approximately 85 percent of men's. Many are insulated by tenure. If some age scholars, now healthy and fit, can look forward to an old age of engagement, respectability, and learning, they may find little reason to talk about decline, oppression, or violence.

Embracing intersectionality means opening up to the pain of others—a process that may incur a new pain that a scholar formerly preferred not to encounter. Although many researchers *survey* older adults, we do not always know the right ways to ferret out their emotions. Few are the interviewers willing to really listen to people who are slow of speech. On their side, the people who experience the coldness of polite impatience are used to blaming humiliations on their own defects. Undoing their inferiorization takes, to start with, participatory activist interviewing. Listening, as to an equal. Gerontological field practice and age scholarship (like social work, like good medical care, like visits from the ombudsman) is about making kindness available to others by way of inclusion.

To notice the failures of caring in our society, to name the malefactors, is to become indignant, puzzled, or outraged. In some people, however, newly stirred sensibilities lead to political engagement. The banked coals may derive from deep childhood awe at elders, and the tinder may catch from harsh firsthand experience, the revelations of empirical work, scholarship, empathy born of literary or cultural analysis, or the lightning flash of a new theory. About writers, Athol Fugard said: "The place from which you take your orders is probably the most secret place you have."

CHANGING SOCIETY?

Whether to bring activism into our work, and to what ends, have been daunting problems. Age scholars' remit certainly covered excluded people—Black, Asian Pacific, Native American, Latinx, and lower-income, and even people in nursing facilities and people with cognitive impairments. But studying subgroups and even serving them better "could happen without changing their marginal status," Peg Cruikshank noted in her frank, refreshing 2013 book, *Learning to Be Old*.

Martha Holstein, author of *Ethics, Aging, and Society: The Critical Turn*, said we needed an "alternative model" to change society. Martha died, to the deep regret of many of us, since my last email exchange with her. In that written conversation, she observed:

> Much of gerontology is about changing the individual. When the productive-aging folks started talking about an extended work life being not only desirable but normative, for example, they never asked the question of what changes would be required in the workplace or how to reduce [middle] ageism in the workplace, which individuals cannot do alone. . . . I think of the social model of disability as an alternative model: Don't ask *us* to change, but change society so we can function as well as possible within it.

Since ageism is a system built into institutions, laws, and norms, not only a result of personal hatred or ignorance, it is illuminating to connect the psychology and behavior of individuals, the micro level, with the economic and political, the macro level. Larry Polivka, winner of an award from the Association of Gerontology in Higher Education for contributions to education, saw much of our work "done without much regard for larger theoretical considerations, interdisciplinary connections, or political and public policy implications."

Some scholars shied away from exploring issues that their disciplines considered irrelevant or that required unknown research methods. Some felt anxiety about being attacked as partisan.

Progressives have leaped over that hurdle. But historically they have focused on the needs of labor, of people of working age. When "workers" moved on in the life course, into the category I have called "no-class-but-old," no longer allowed or able to produce, it was hard to see them still as victims of socioeconomic forces. Agewise progressives may wish that anti-ageism could become "The Next Big Social Movement," as *Tikkun* contemplated in 2017. Finding energy to resist ageism may be difficult for progressives, however, for a sterner political reason as well as traditional conceptual ones. In a society where each individual fends for themself, and with government dismantling the inadequate "safety nets," this sense of being alone intensifies. Progressives must fight their own skepticism about incorporating anti-ageism into precious existing movements, already stressed out by having to rebuff attacks from powerful, right-wing authoritarian forces.

INCHWISE

Looking back from the COVID Era, I see that some age scholars were inching closer to the most vulnerable people with each lens that focused on old women, veterans, people with physical and cognitive impairments, cumulative disadvantage, and class bias—or, more specifically, on the public health system, Medicaid pauperization, Small Houses, and staffing raises.

Others were engrossed by the mass of competing old-age topics. Community dwellers, millions in lieu of 1.4 million residents, had their own desperate issues: job loss and inability to save for old age, the privatization of Medicare, the expense of private long-term care insurance, Alzheimer's care at home, women as perpetual caregivers. This interview project took place before COVID, before 2020; perhaps it was to be expected that none of my experts mentioned nursing-facility residents. The index to my 2017 book—about not "killing" old people—had no entries for nursing facilities or the Centers for Medicare and Medicaid, even though I rebutted the "burden" and "euthanasia" and "dementia" rhetorics.

Yet I must have had a submerged sense of how deadly the discourses could become, because I reacted instantly and vehemently to the ventilator triage issue in March 2020. In the two weeks of my quarantine I wrote my first article critiquing the guidelines and joined Dr. Michelle Holmes's petition for a lottery. I gave up writing another book (a novel, *Confidences*, written in the form of emails between two old friends in long marriages, one of whom is coping with her partner's Alzheimer's-like diagnosis) and I never went back to it. I clung to the residents' stories even as they grew more heartrending and infuriating day by day.

An age critic could have visited a relative or friend in a nursing facility, as I had done—or have read a humanizing ethnographic account like Tracy Kidder's warmhearted, chatty, and admiring *Old Friends*, as I did—and not decide to investigate the residents' needs or try to alleviate the harms they endured.

Some critics did come closer. Some took giant steps. Anne Basting chose actors for her play *Penelope* from among nursing-home residents. "The person-comes-first" dementia networks and the explicators of "Fourth Ageism" (a keyword explained and promoted indefatigably by Chris Gilleard and Paul Higgs) tried to drag attention toward those whom society considered "abject." Leslie Pedtke, administrator of a facility, invented a program where young CNAs volunteered to live as residents (for example, blind, wheelchair-dependent, quarantined) for up to twelve days. The program was so successful in developing empathy that Pedtke required all her new employees to live with a resident for twenty-four hours. The ombudsman in the states visited the neglected in their tiny, crowded shared rooms and tried to resolve their complaints. Bill Thomas built the model Green Houses, loosely affiliated, independently owned, that did so well at making their lives enjoyable and then saved their inhabitants when COVID infiltrated elsewhere.

Long before 2020, of course, academic and medical reformers had loathed and decried the system that left many residents to filth, sickness, or early death. They were painstakingly documenting the common but often hidden wrongs we now know for sure: the buried violence of stingy state budgets and indifferent or overworked bureaucracies, understaffing and exploitative pay—providing information to undergird change. Improvements were not only hard to win but shaky. Reformers had, for instance, gotten government to eliminate the use of physical restraints—only to find that certain doctors were overprescribing antipsychotics, while some benighted places still tortured residents, especially people of color, with vests, straps, and tight sheets. Health policy experts, academic gerontologists, nonprofit administrators, and lawmakers championed improvements state by state and in Congress. Courage to critique the system did not fail.

But until the COVID dying mounted precipitously, even those who best knew the residents' risks could not make the dangers feel *urgent*. History—as detailed by Hannah Arendt and others—had confirmed that human rights could be abrogated by democratically elected regimes. Still, before the nation witnessed the carnage and suffering, the word "evil" might have seemed hyperbolic in regard to a US public health care system that despite its weaknesses prided itself on openness to (reluctant, gradual, inconsistent) improvement.

Could any of the reformers have anticipated a circumstance that would cause state power, under any conceivable US administration, to abandon the people in those licensed shelters? It took Simone Weil, in wartime, to note the latent menace of any institution with total power to decide the distribution of resources—that is, one's government. And she wrote in a style darker than some Americans can bear:

> How much more surprising in its effects is the other force, the force that does not kill; i.e., that does not kill just yet. It will surely kill, it will possibly kill, or perhaps it merely hangs, poised and ready, over the head of the creature it can kill, at any moment, which is to say, at every moment.

"HOW LITTLE WE'VE BEEN ABLE TO CHANGE ANYTHING"

Every happy man should have an unhappy man in his closet, with a hammer, to remind him with his constant tapping, that not everyone is happy.
ANTON CHEKHOV, *Selected Stories*

Had anti-ageism become a disciplinary necessity and a useful meme throughout the academy, it might still not have made a dent in a public-private health system for the poor that had become so entrenched. The victims' misery went deep, but the tapping of the victims' hammers didn't resound loudly. Anti-ageists don't do enough public advocacy, agreed. Cassandra shrieks in her classrooms. Teiresias is a whisperer in the central plaza of Babel. No matter how much more poignantly the age collective might have tried before March 2020 to bring the severest wrongs to public attention, we could no more have prevented the Eldercide than the most knowledgeable and active reformers in medicine, nursing, and public policy could. And then it came.

These are contexts, not exculpations. Stuart Hall, a wise and hardheaded guide, straightforwardly observed that when an emergency hits—he was talking about AIDS; many readers and researchers in a range of fields will now think of the catastrophe in the nursing homes—it is striking "how little [Cultural Studies] registers, how little we've been able to change anything or get anybody to do anything. If you don't feel that as one tension in the work that you are doing, then theory has let you off the hook."

By the end of 2020, many heads had swiveled sharply. I have quoted some. Scholars who focus particularly on ageism sharpened their analytic gaze and the items in their ethical toolbox to notice aspects of this historic moment that might otherwise have disappeared before they could become useful to the future.

CONSCIENCE RAISING

After the horrors of genocide and statelessness, Hannah Arendt sought attention for "the problem of conscience." Can conscience be redirected toward not only residents but older adults in general, after the long course of dehumanization that prefaced and aggravated the Eldercide?

Seamus Heaney somewhere writes, "Conscience, if we press on its etymology, can mean a capacity to know the same thing together." Years into the COVID Era, *knowing together* is harder. Something is even more salient than knowledge: Judith Butler says we have to take on faith "an internal desire" to subdue one's own sense of priority and superiority. If a desire for equality is not innate, how could it exist? I take it on faith that it is human to have that desire, but that it gets developed to different degrees. Yet the sources of simple and compound ageism and the afterimage of Youth ascendancy may linger like long COVID, or even strengthen like a new viral variant—so that one's egalitarian instinct must resist an engorged tendency to flee emotionally from old age and old people. The honest self-criticism, the persistent striving of the experts quoted here may help thoughtful people struggling right now against amorphous and partly internalized biases.

The lack of any diverse, intergenerational movement to expand ambitions and demand better outcomes has been, and remains, the biggest external obstacle to fighting ageism. In 2020, after the murder of George Floyd, the rise of a broad multiracial and multigenerational movement caused a personal, intellectual, and political revulsion against racism. Millions—Black, white, of color; fresh activists and older adults with experience from the civil rights or anti-war movements or the first Earth Day of 1970—hearteningly joined protests, safely masked and distancing themselves, for Black Lives Matter. There were recognitions that "Old Lives Matter" in that same dreadful year, but no similar mobilization.

Amid competing crises—economic insecurities; the structural violence of racism; the domestic terror of neo-Nazis; the escalating damage of global climate change—ending the Eldercide may not seem the most pressing concern. Indeed, it may delusively seem the one most easily ended by the magic wand of scientific management, governors' choices, and promised federal and state reforms.

SOLIDARITY

"Perhaps yet more strongly than other oppressed groups, the old need solidarity from others," political philosopher Sonia Kruks points out, because older adults are not "as likely to come together in common work or social spaces from where they could organize together politically." Israeli sociologist Liat Ayalon, lead editor of the volume *Contemporary Perspectives on Ageism*, wrote me,

I think ageism is slowly advancing to the front stage. But—the reason why [anti-ageism] is not really catching [on] is because young people need to fight the fight. When old people [alone] fight against ageism—the stigma is there and it always feels like young vs. old. When young people decide to carry the message against ageism—it will become a common problem of all of us and people will be interested in addressing it.

Many who teach students believe that their consciousness is ready to be raised and that the right pedagogy raises it. I agree; in Sarah Lamb's brilliantly designed course at Brandeis, I saw students rake through popular culture to dissect *Saturday Night Live* (Grandma's gonorrhea in a sketch called "Nursing Home," watched by 4,649,000 people); *SpongeBob SquarePants*; *Mean Girls*; the mock road sign "50-year-Old Xing." Everyone had produced a show-and-tell research exercise called "Finding Ageism." Such students may become conscientious guardians of age relations, bring outrage and intellectual renewal into mainstream writing, and develop into the cross-generational leaders a movement needs.

What does ageism mean in the new COVID Era? We need a societal shorthand, like those brought about by the anti-racism and anti-sexism movements. Can an answer now be unblinkingly attempted? *Dehumanizations. Job discrimination. Oblivion. Eldercide.*

Political leaders, historians, anthropologists, medical reformers, data analysts, and age critics will go on sorting through the wreckage. Acknowledging the agents with power and responsibility (the state's lethal failures of care, medical education, the political sources of aversion to old age and old people) would sharpen the will to rectify injustice. Even talking about social justice can increase the desire for social justice. A move toward *fearing ageism and distinguishing it from aging* marks progress, from overdetermined self-interest to changing our culture. The earlier this wisdom starts in an individual life and in the history of thought, the better. It falls to all of us to heed the residents, twist the truths of prejudice out of society's thickets of lies, be brave, *and care more.*

CHAPTER 9

IN SEARCH OF THE MISSING VOICES

"JUST TALK." PLEASE.

Asked what volunteers could best do to help residents of her nursing home, Dominga Marquez, seventy-eight, said, "Just talk. . . . We are lonely." Ms. Marquez, who was living in the New Jewish Home system in Manhattan, added, "I have a lot of friends that used to come every week to visit but, with the pandemic, nobody came."

Unlike Ishmael in Herman Melville's *Moby-Dick*—"And I only am escaped alone to tell thee"—plenty of residents survived to tell. A million or more. They were ordinary people caught in a doleful situation, shuttered within newly dread-filled facilities, not knowing who might die next, lacking ways to reach out to loved ones, missing the reassuring hum of voices in the corridors, the familiar soundscape. As we have heard, survivors had *stories*: going through hell, observing abuse, displaying remarkable qualities, recovering—even leading a normal life in an abnormal time. They needed to talk. When they were able to, their myriad of experiences was an inspiration.

One trouble with telling the residents' stories properly is that no exact historical parallel exists for their situation. There had not been a pandemic flu for a hundred years, since 1918–1919. It's hard to find a congregate living situation that is analogous. They were in facilities that were hosted by their own government. That should have meant more safety than it did. Their confinement was something like that in internment or refugee camps, where inmates are dependent on having food and medicine, or toilet paper, supplied—but it comes irregularly. The coronavirus rampaging outside the walls made them seem more like soldiers in bunkers, waiting to be struck down by incoming missiles. With communication choppy, their habitations also reminded me of remote space shuttles whose inhabitants carry on far away from us. (Would that the residents had been as well protected as astronauts from the atmosphere outside.)

But no ruling metaphor works. We haven't found the language for how different their experiences were from ours—we who were living outside. Writers have not thought enough about what the grave, exotic anomaly of the residents' conditions in that year demands. How should they be fairly written about? The nursing-facility fatalities of 2020 were the worst public health disaster in US history, beyond Hurricane Katrina in New Orleans. The Eldercide may yet be considered adequate cause for transforming the Centers for Medicare and Medicaid out of its current existence.

Certainly, "focusing only on cases and deaths, as is often the case with statistics related to the pandemic, does not capture the full impact of the pandemic on nursing home residents," according to the authors of a study of the health status of COVID survivors. The residents are the core of any history to be properly told and any future to be properly imagined.

Except that, surprisingly, few journalists were inquiring. The group of people who died in US nursing facilities in 2020—they may have numbered 112,300 or 128,000 or 152,000, depending on who was counting and who got counted, and on when others stopped counting— started to vanish from public consciousness. The media let the survivors' voices vanish almost entirely. This is an empirical fact.

IGNORING THE DEEP HUMAN STORY

"I think of journalism as a human story, first," Whitney Bryen told me. Bryen is an investigative journalist from the nonprofit news outfit *Oklahoma Watch*, which specializes in "high-impact journalism." She had succeeded in finding informants among the residents and publishing their interesting comments. Those articles led me to her.

Having questions that only residents could answer, hoping to find many illuminating viewpoints, I set up a Google Alert for stories using such keywords as "nursing homes," "interview," and "resident." Although hospital triage guidelines excluding people for age had shocked me, they had also provoked my curiosity about the feelings of people considered too old to keep alive. Questions obsessed me. I wanted to find reporters who had asked them directly, "The world is talking about your domicile as a death trap: How do you feel?"

The Alert brought in dozens of news articles daily, hundreds a month, and thousands through early 2021. I asked my intern, Vishni Samaraweera, to select only the articles that quoted residents—and to get every quotation verbatim. She was to stop early if she got inundated, as I assumed she would be. I sampled hundreds of articles as well.

But week after week brought both of us disappointment and head-scratching puzzlement. Gradually, and then suddenly, we recognized how very few firsthand quotations from residents there were. My indefatigable intern read 1,499 articles. She found only twenty stories that quoted residents at all. (No doubt we missed others; it was a sample taken at crucial time frames.) Only *twenty*: 1.3 percent of 1,499. A stunning disparity.

Honor is due. The writers capable of finding the 1.3 percent had actively sought residents despite all obstacles, treated them as equals and interesting informants, captured valuable stories. Some described how the interviewees looked, what they wore. Some major media did well but reporters in small papers or local TV stations also got what was wanted. They had connections, which saves time, or older relatives, which promotes caring. *They* would say they merely did their job. I name some. I relied on the interviews that my intern and I found. The residents' forceful stories educated me. I gained respect for their canny observations and heartfelt speech. These precious accounts should encourage others to dig deeper in the disdained milieu.

In the other 98.7 percent of articles that used those keywords, the people whom reporters quoted were *not* themselves residents: They were family members, administrators, nurses, doctors, aides, other professionals; officials in CDC or CMS—all talking *about* the residents. Authorities provided a sense of patterns. Medical personnel reported missing supplies, devoted care, or corruption. Once a relative has died, only family members, anguished and angry, were left to report their suspicions of wrongful deaths. So local investigations are a public service, saving health or lives and making prosecutions possible.

But however useful or urgent the copy, there could be no substitute for residents' testimony. "As we face the gloomy prospect of a pandemic winter," Dr. Eleanor Feldman Barbera, a psychologist, wrote in a 2020 blog entry, "I consulted some experts for suggestions on how to handle difficult periods in life—nursing home residents." People, with or without degrees, are indeed the only "experts" on their experiences. Many survivors were willing to talk virtually in 2020. They are waiting to be asked now. Although the entire communications industry was busy writing the first draft of crisis history, the media missed the essential story.

ONLY TWENTY RESIDENTS SPOKE

Ignoring the residents made no sense from a *news* point of view. In a tragedy, reporters usually flock to the victims. They thrust microphones under their noses. They pester them with queries. "What did you feel when the levee broke? When you saw the train derail?" They capture impressions, however painful, firsthand. Nor did ignoring the residents make sense for an oral history of COVID in the nursing homes. Whatever these resident experts said—brilliant or banal— would have to be the basis of such an account.

I had particular pressing questions in mind when I chose varying dates to home in on.

March–April 2020: "How did you feel when the murderousness of COVID was first discovered? What did you *do* when visits and excursions ended? Were you ever good with solitude?" The total shutdown coincided not only with college spring break but simultaneously with religious holidays—first Passover, then Easter and Ramadan. People in trouble may hold a particular ritual close and find a way to adapt it. "What did you do on the holiday?"

Summer 2020: "Did the Black Lives Matter protests engage you? Were you following the political campaigns?"

November 2020: "Did you vote for president? Did the facility make voting easy?"

Around Thanksgiving and Christmas, as the lockdown continued, when residents were about to lose the family festivities that marked the season: "Did your facility make virtual visits possible? Did you get enough to eat? Did you laugh or have any fun?"

And I wondered: "If you needed help with showering, did you get it regularly? Did your call button go unanswered for long times? Did you have a skin lesion not properly attended? Did a nurse or a medical director or a manager ever ask how you were doing? Did you or anyone you know write a letter of complaint? Did anyone answer?"

Only residents could give eyewitness evidence for the sake of accountability. Had anyone, for example, seen staff fail to put on clean gloves upon entry into residents' rooms—including rooms of residents infected with the coronavirus? Had they seen acquaintances deprived of necessary wound care or medications to control pain?

Survival was a man-bites-dog story of the kind journalists say they want. Once I figured out that hundreds of thousands of residents who contracted COVID had recovered, I had further questions that seemed obvious and fascinating. "Why do you think *you* survived? If you were very sick, did you want to be hospitalized? *Were* you hospitalized? Did you have a DNR or a DNH? Were you offered one? Who helped you recover?"

After vaccinations in 2021 would also have been a good time to ask, "How do you feel? Do you have long COVID? Had there been an arc to your year? Had fear or boredom or frustration been uppermost at different times? Did some relationships become more solid?"

When reporters did seek out a resident to talk to, they often quoted only one or two sentences. That fact, and not my editing, is why the quotations in this book are mostly so short. That brevity gives some quotations a lapidary quality—words ready to be incised in stone on a monument. *"I can't breathe."*

Unfortunately, few articles provided more than a sentence or two of a resident's speech. Short quotations could not indicate the way a person moves from idea to idea or expresses feelings. Such lacks made me grateful for a short cameo in a filmed TV interview or an impassioned excerpt from a 911 call. In order to suggest the human value of those who compose the group, I had to put skimpy stories together, reading between the lines to understand important context.

Family members will want to know what the media missed. As elsewhere in the narrative I am uncovering, much remains to be explained here. Looking back on the core story of the plague year, around which all others circle, what explains the general disregard of residents' first-person accounts? Why was it even *possible* for the media in general to fail so spectacularly?

A LAYERING OF EXCUSES AND OBSTACLES

Whitney Bryen of *Oklahoma Watch* described some logistical barriers she overcame. "There's no phone book in a nursing home. There's no way to know who lives there." She nevertheless persisted. "I found some families via social media. I went to Facebook, to posts with the name of a particular nursing home. I went to the Facebook page of the nursing home." One seasoned journalist asked a pastor if any of her parishioners were living in a nearby facility. Anyone could have done similar sleuthing. If a journalist found a daughter or son to interview, she didn't need to rely on a banal secondhand answer like, "Yes, my mother is unhappy not to see her grandchildren." Instead, it would have been possible to say, "Could I sit in on a call with your mom and ask her a few questions?"

There were problems on the supply side. If a reporter was on the phone, were inmates hesitant to share intimate or painful details? A journalist, excusing herself for not having interviewed any residents, suggested that residents feared retaliation from irritable administrators or frightened aides.

Family members shared this fear. "Adult children don't want to up-set the staff," Whitney Bryen told me. "They feel it could impact the care of their loved one. They are concerned that the staff might avoid that resident; spend less time with them." Before the lockdown, family members who visited and helped their loved ones incidentally served as undeclared surveillance. By freely walking around, even without being ombudsmen, they somewhat deterred bad practices. But with access ended, residents were totally reliant on overworked and anxious aides. It was impossible for families to check cleanliness or staffing levels. Infuriatingly, it was even hard for them to get facts about their loved ones' illness, treatment, or hospitalization.

As conditions worsened (whether by their fault or out of their control), some owners or administrators evaded oversight. Bryen, told me, "At one place, they hung up on me. They had hired a firm to handle communications." Health care workers, including registered nurses, may be willing to expose adverse conditions—and some bravely did, even when forbidden to talk to the press. In daily operations, however, administrators held the greatest powers: of life and death, and also of speech or silence, transparency or opacity.

One media old-timer I talked to, a former columnist, had guessed that even in 1,500 articles, few residents would be quoted. But when I mentioned the logistical excuses journalists gave for not reaching more residents, he made a rapid dismissive gesture, like a man brushing away gnats. Indeed, some TV videographers as well as reporters successfully entered the barred buildings during COVID. *Herzensbildung* begins by "wheeling a mile in another person's wheelchair." Those rare newshounds, masked, practicing social distancing, holding the mike down to a seated person, walked the mile that expands our understanding and leads to heart changes.

WHO IS NEWSWORTHY?

The real question—"Who is newsworthy?"—involves a demand-side problem for journalists and editors. Initially, many news outlets gave the young on the beaches and bars a media blitz that lifted the cult

of youth to formerly unimaginable heights. They gave ageist protesters against lockdowns more attention than their paltry numbers deserved. They failed to make heroes out of people who wore masks by
so frequently relaying the loud belligerence of hoaxers. They treated
residents and low-income community members as if they were separate groups.

If the goal had been to find touching first-person stories of at-risk
populations—as it often is—journalists found others who were hard to
reach, outside. Jails and prisons are forbiddingly self-protective even
in normal times. When prisoners were recognized as inadequately
protected and likely to die of COVID, some of them were nevertheless interviewed, although the obstacles to reaching them by phone
were even higher and more systemic than for nursing-home residents.
On the radio, one prisoner I heard memorably recounted his plausible terror. He put up a sign on his cell door—not that it would be
honored: "I am immune-compromised, stay away." One forty-eight-
year-old man was willing to be quoted by name, even though prisoners, like residents, might have wanted anonymity as protection from
retaliation. Prisoners were pitiable, especially those who had grown
old and ill in the decades since conviction and been refused medical
parole. If thousands were released, it was partly because media coverage suggested public indignation at their plight.

It hurts to draw out the comparison, but our matriarchs and patriarchs trying to survive COVID in old age, many with mobility issues,
also old and ill and locked in for the pandemic, were not so different from inmates. Few had a chance to win "compassionate release,"
because so many of them needed skilled care that no other place
could provide, or because they had no family with room or time or
resources—or health—to take them in and care for them properly. An
unknown number of residents remained in foul conditions, in institutions committed to silencing them.

Editors must not often have asked for investigative journalism that
included the survivors. It is worth noting that since 2004, the US has
lost more than 2,100 daily and weekly local newspapers. Downsizing,
a long-term trend, worsened after the 2008 long recession. In the dis-

integrating news fields of print and TV, many owners had eliminated older employees and "age beat" reporters who might have argued, as I do, that residents *were* the story. Caring more, knowing more, they might have been more adventurous.

Involved in "the age beat," about 1,000 journalists and academics receive *Generations Beat Online* (*GBO News*), a shrewdly annotated digest of current issues. *GBO*'s longtime curator, Paul Kleyman, calls the group "a slowly moving creek that gets refreshed on an ongoing basis." As of 2021, the Journalists in Aging Fellows, an annual funded collaboration of the Journalists Network on Generations and the Gerontological Society of America, had graduated 185 people dedicated to the age beat. Others on the beat may include graduates of the National Press Foundation programs on aging, Columbia's Age Boom Academy, and some of USC's Annenberg School of Journalism Health Journalism Fellows. The longest-known were columnists: the *New York Times*'s Paula Span, of "The New Old Age," and Kaiser Health News's Judith E. Graham, of "Navigating Aging." COVID brought Robert Weisman's reporting to the front pages of the *Boston Globe*.

Paul Kleyman filled me in on general coverage of age issues:

> The rise of the Internet has meant blogs and podcasts, often for specialized audiences, and more daily access for individuals to expert-sourced material on ethnic communities long underserved by mainstream outlets, and in journal studies. . . . The Association of Health Care Journalists regularly exposes its substantial membership to stories on the coverage of aging, written and edited by Liz Seegert.

(I've spoken at the annual conference of the Gerontological Society of America to a group of incoming Journalists in Aging Fellows. I have written for PBS's *Next Avenue* and for *Silver Century*, sources of news and freelance markets.)

Interest in older adults, however, as we have seen, doesn't necessarily translate into a focus on nursing-home residents. For journalists covering the age beat—"age" or "aging" or "old people," just as if they were studying a distant galaxy—specialization matters. There's a lot to know. Experts on Social Security may not understand the intricacies of Medicaid. Writers on the history of Medicaid may focus on low-income children but not know anyone in a nursing home. Or they may know only older adults living in communities. In 2020, the year when the nursing facilities became the tremendous, unavoidable story, of the seventeen new Journalists in Aging Fellows—all of whom had worth-while topics—only three were planning to tell nursing-home stories. In 2021, only one fellow—B. Denise Hawkins of the Trice Edney News Wire (a Black media news service)—was explicitly studying nursing homes. Hawkins's research concluded that places like the Maryland Baptist Aged Home, which I describe earlier as small and well-run, with no deaths in 2020, had a long history and also represent a new model of care.

Editors almost certainly sent out many journalists without special education on age matters. Most failed to search out the subdued voices.

CREDENTIALS

Bias may also help explain this state of affairs. If nursing-home residents had been considered credible witnesses, with evidence or feelings worth repeating, why would reporters have quoted others 98.7 percent of the time instead? This instance would not be the only time that the media's ability to get the big news first was compromised when reporters ignored the closest witnesses. The case of Flint, Michigan, was another. It was one of the worst environmental disasters in the US. In the story of corrosive, poisoned drinking water in Flint, long inaction on the part of officials resulted from want of attention to the complaints of activist residents who had been craving notice for their sick children and peculiar-smelling water starting in 2014. It was a seasoned Black reporter, Derrick Z. Jackson, who exposed that disregard of the urgent testimonies of low-income African Americans.

Jackson, who had been a *Boston Globe* columnist for decades, explained the wide detour around nursing-home residents as resulting partly from the same journalistic penchant for seeking witnesses with "credentials." Without cynicism, daily journalism could be understood as being essentially equivalent to the college term paper, developed with a sense of professional responsibility. In principle, this credential-seeking tendency is necessary in order to give an inevitably quick study some foundation. In practice, finding the right interviewees can become problematic. Jackson told me:

> Those [whom reporters] see as having sufficient right to opine tend to be white, male, professionals, people with degrees or titles. The people this tendency overlooks are often the Other. In your case, the residents. [Journalists] may have thought these people closest to the action would be unobservant—a priori "out of it."

Jackson brings out a fact about trust and information. Trusting a witness—in legal arenas, in the classroom, in news gathering, and even at parties with strangers—depends on their status in relation to you. My testimony may be thought less credible if I am perceived right off the bat as one of a category diminished by your stereotypes about age, gender, ethnicity, race, ability, or cognitive status. Miranda Fricker, an English philosopher who was president of the American Philosophical Association, calls this phenomenon "testimonial injustice."

I asked Judith E. Graham, Kaiser Health News columnist, for her understanding of the problem. She started by talking about access but then suggested stereotyping:

> It's very, very, very hard to find people to speak to in nursing homes. It takes a lot of time and effort—and luck. I'm fortunate enough to have a job that allows me to spend this kind of time. Many journalists don't. That said, it may well be that some reporters don't realize that everyone living in a nursing home isn't cognitively compromised.

Reporters who believed that resident eyewitnesses were impeded by strokes or Alzheimer's, unable to think clearly or speak lucidly, may have watched films like *Still Alice* or read articles that portray people as "zombies." They may have accepted as confirmed fact what had been a stereotype in the Before Time: that residents were soiled, "demented," moribund. If so, they were perpetrating the same testimonial injustice.

The 1.3 percent of residents who did get interviewed demonstrate that residents were credible to those who had ears to hear. (Some residents had exactly the credentials reporters sought. The man who reported that he couldn't take a shower because the stall was smeared with feces was a former hospital administrator, who spoke with authority, a sharp tongue. Another woman I quote had been a social worker for ex-inmates.) Transients in skilled nursing facilities who expect to leave, although turned into reluctant residents, may have felt less like lifers afraid of the guards. When I quote residents, I sometimes could not discern whether they were permanent or temporary. Even if reporters had assumed that transients were the only desirable interlocutors, they could have found such people to interview: About a third of inhabitants in 2019 fell into that category.

Some of those I quote had had strokes. Perhaps half of those in care homes have some level of cognitive impairment, but like the rest of us lucky enough to have grown old, they are "equipped with a repertoire of resources that are acquired" through earlier life, including sound observation and mechanisms for coping with trouble. Tom Kitwood, the guru of cultural approaches to cognitive impairments, calls this repertoire the "kitbag." Even as impairment deepens, much of the kit can remain. Gerontologists have stated repeatedly that people with a range of memory issues can and should be included in research.

It's true that, more than before, in 2020 some facilities took on "features of 'total' institutions," which, two gerontologists explain, tend to produce "patient-like role expectations" and undermine older people's sense of agency. Any of us might have become confused or traumatized if we too had been trapped, dreading what the next day might bring, our daily habits ruptured and our lives threatened. "Precisely because later life brings losses of unprecedented seriousness . . . it is a time of active challenge," wrote Paul Johnson, a British age critic; "older men and women have to be able to draw on their full resources, built up over a lifetime." Now, it is still wrong to think of residents only in group terms, as hapless victims rather than persons in travail, protagonists of their own lives. Some residents did better than I would have in the same circumstances, even though no one was offering *them* therapy.

TOO MUCH SUFFERING

We may be better able to realize the dreadful conditions by the fact that journalists suffered from vicarious vulnerability merely by spending some time learning what the residents endured for almost a year. Emily Hopkins was a data reporter for a team that produced a major series on the ways owners of Indiana's nursing facilities scammed Medicaid. The team interviewed family members who believed their relatives died of undertreatment. Hopkins told the *Journalist's Resource*:

> I got therapy at the end of year and it helped a lot. . . . And I don't think that any of us going through what we're going through right now should be scared or ashamed of doing that. . . . The pandemic, the isolation, and witnessing nursing home deaths took a heavy mental toll.

Did some part of the media failure come from an excess of sensitivity: reluctance to encounter survivors still threatened by death, just to ask invasive questions about private feelings? Or through feeling their own comparative safety on the other end of the phone as a source of guilt or shame? Reporters are usually trained to ignore their own invasiveness, as a necessary means to achieve an overriding Fourth Estate goal to inform the people. Such a motive would have been humane if reporters were considering informants as equally human in their susceptibility to suffering. *How would I bear it? Living in their shoes? Wheeling in their wheelchairs?*

Some situations were indeed so appalling as to be scarcely credible or bearable. Kianna Gardner, of Montana news service the *Daily Inter Lake*, reported on a female resident who had been interviewed on

April 7, 2020, by rescuers from the Montana Department of Health. The woman herself lucidly said, "I feel neglected, and scared. I could die in here and rigor mortis could set in before they find me." The report states that she was lying on a dark-blue air mattress with no bottom sheet and that "it was clear to see the skin flakes all over the mattress." She had not received a shower in thirty-five days. Soon after, the *Daily Inter Lake* reported that the state had stamped the facility at Whitefish Care with an "Immediate Jeopardy" rating, the worst possible. The IJ judgment came after a history of grave deficiencies discovered on inspections since its current owners took over in 2019.

A dead body "presents its case against the world with tremendous forensic power," Rebecca West wrote. I think of the limp body of the Syrian child at the water's edge, becoming a global emblem for the misery of millions. What about a living woman, trapped in a nursing facility, neglected and abused, who is discovered in time but then speaks slowly as she gathers her thoughts? She epitomizes all the "villains" of the social imaginary: ageism, neuroageism, sexism (given that the majority of nursing-home residents are women), ableism, and classism (given the high percentage of residents on Medicaid). In novels and films, horror is often associated with dirty old women, witches: their grotesque faces, their nails, their skin. This woman has a strong case "against the world" that is shared with everyone else relegated to understaffed buildings, but I fear she presents it less forcefully.

"That is another terrible thing about being a character in a tragedy," West writes elsewhere, with characteristic bluntness. "At the same time you become a character in a farce. . . . Three calamities are felt to be too many, and when four are reported, or five, the thing becomes ludicrous. . . . God has only to strike one again and again for one to become a clown."

AVERSION

There is one last hypothesis worth considering: the effect on journalists themselves of the media's obsessive focus on counting anonymous bodies and producing mortality data. While they were still being counted (however inaccurately), every numbing statistic ghosted the residents. Enumerators effectively blurred the mass by eliminating signs of belonging like gender or race. The residents became Othered at the time they still dominated the COVID news. Incomplete sociologically, counting also myopically pushed aside residents' parlous existential states. The restricted media focus may explain why no one thought to count, and then pursue the import of, having so many *survivors.*

Outsiders dying in the nation at large were also counted, but some were personalized. PBS's *News Hour,* for example, then delicately moderated by Judy Woodruff, began offering mini-biographies of those who died. They were not celebrities, but they had photos, names, a gender, races and ethnicities, ages, hobbies, work, and family members who characterized them lovingly. Music played behind the voice-overs, in a touching piece of journalistic remembrance.

Once it appeared that older adults in general could not be saved, I have suggested, preoccupied Americans turned away from the category—with pity or relief. Applying those psychological theories to the media context, alienation may derive from imagining "the horror, the horror" of the plague inside the facilities, as Jacqueline Rose implied. ("Counting is a system for classifying the horror and bundling it away.") Forced by their jobs to spend time in close mental contact with the leprosariums, why would journalists assigned to that beat, but not wise enough to know to seek therapy, not also be swept up in the general psychic retreat? If, to most of them, the residents' subjectivity did not exist, this perspective offers another hypothesis about why so many reporters interviewed family members, aides, and administrators *instead.*

As the pandemic continued, the results of compound ageism—forgetfulness, disregard, psychic withdrawal, the sense of futility about residents' lives—unobserved, became deeper-seated and more widespread. When the survivors got vaccinated, their dying ceased, as it were, to have a social existence. Without explanation, the *Boston Globe,* which had regularly distinguished the plethora of deaths of residents from outsiders' deaths, stopped providing disaggregated data.

Despite the continuing carnage, its perfunctory articles provided only all-state totals. Did that change mean the residents were finally being better protected? Or was the Department of Public Health protecting itself by burying that information, because the number of residents dying was still disproportionate? The only thing worse than being counted is no longer counting enough to be counted.

A LIFE OF RESPONSIBILITY

Will we ever know why the media mostly missed the crucial story of that lethal year, 2020? Only if journalists speak to the point. Anyone who wrote often about nursing homes, but who rarely or never quoted a resident, might well now ask themselves "Why?" This question could be the basis for an interview project: What do editors and journalists themselves believe caused the hole in the record? At times of historical crisis, as it has done with biased war reporting, not one writer or two or three but the profession as a whole needs to inspect its particular blinders. Flawed reporting begs not for finger-pointing, which can lead to denial, but for honest, patient self-reflection and the undoing of every implicit bias.

That "deliberate, even obsessive reflection" that we undergo in order to live "a life of responsibility" (in Atul Gawande's words) can be difficult, embarrassing, humbling. But in a collective, reflection and self-correction can become a matter of self-reinforcing practice. Those virtues are needed by journalists, policymakers, doctors and EMTs, and anyone in political life or with influence over the public.

If the media fail, we all lose. Throughout that clamorous first year, readers or TV viewers may not have noticed the absence of residents' voices. When first responders, doctors, pundits, and essential workers of color were the focus, they were of course interviewed. That goes without saying. The residents didn't know they were once again being degraded, as they were being socially silenced in their distant cells. No one could know how completely their testimony was being disregarded before my intern and I figured it out. Then that story of inaudibility and invisibility had to be put in its contexts: among other factors, testimonial bias; dementism; fear of close contact with the grimness; overlooking all the residents who survived.

Omitting residents' testimonies injured the health of the nation at the time. If more of their stories of actual horrors had been relayed to the public (by CMS surveyors and the media) with "forensic" power, in the first months of 2020 when the focus on the residents was briefly intense, remedies might have begun earlier. The Trump administration might have felt pressure to act protectively, without delay. More of the residents' unnumbered lives could have been saved, and almost certainly more lives of others among the more than 1,100,000 US dead.

ESSENTIAL STORIES

Representation confers self-esteem. It's why minorities and others want to see and read about people who "look like them." Lack of representation has dire consequences. Judith Butler, in *Precarious Life*, states plainly what is most at stake:

> Those who gain representation, especially self-representation, have a better chance of being humanized, and those who have no chance to represent themselves run a greater risk of being treated as less than human, regarded as less than human, or indeed, not regarded at all.

Repair of the violence of the Eldercide may be hampered if Americans do not listen to powerful personal stories and undo the worst failures of attention and empathy.

Bringing the residents back into society and history is still just possible. Some people do care. Age critics, sociologists, historians, lawyers, and psychologists, will want to gather more primary-source documents. A few investigators are extracting these missing stories, collecting "history from the bottom up," as oral historians say. In July and August 2020, the nonprofit Altarum Institute conducted interviews with 365 nursing home residents in thirty-six states. Altarum found those residents through its interviewers' friends and colleagues, aging associations, ombudsmen, and long-term care associations. They proudly call it the "first known poll of its kind to directly ask nursing home residents about their personal experiences during COVID-19." (The interviewees were anonymous; as a result, follow-up may not be possible.)

The New York Public Library started a program in 2020 to collect pandemic "audio diaries." Julie Golia, associate director of the Manuscripts, Archives, and Rare Books Division, wrote me in July 2021, "I couldn't agree more that these are essential and untold stories of this period that must be chronicled." After a full audit (about 350 hours of listening), however, Golia reported to me a year later that they had received no audio diaries from residents. She speculates that the library's crowd-sourcing design did not locate enough effective networks to get news of the project to the residents, and that residents may not have had the technology, or facility with the technology, or help with the technology, to have submitted their stories.

It's not too late to get more witnesses on tape. Future researchers should not have to go on ransacking thousands of articles and TV videos to find snippets of the missing voices and faces of the people whom the government first abandoned and the media then scanted.

We onlookers and outsiders want to know their narratives. Our desire rises from humane curiosity about people who have so much to tell. Without quick efforts, our lost relatives—and those strangers we need to understand—may remain a faceless, voiceless mass. But curiosity is not merely personal. Society could benefit. The residents would bring brighter lights from behind tightly closed doors. Their testimonies would give urgency to legal suits for corporate negligence or wrongful death. Most residents still suffer from understaffing. They and their families and the reformers are anxious for radical change. We need confessions; enforcement of protections; new geriatric curricula; a recognized connection to public health; Congressional action to restructure the system.

Our own future old age may depend on what we learn next. Everyone must be able to judge what went right inside grim walls and what went so badly wrong. The nation will not get the transformed system it needs unless we start by "knowing, understanding and listening to residents, and honoring their experiences and perspectives," two members of the nursing-home culture-change movement say. It's a fact: "There but for fortune go you or go I." Fresh testimonies in the press would also assure survivors and their families that they were worth rescuing. Amplifying the voices of survivors who rejoice in being alive would help undo the demoralizing belief that all older adults are doomed. The silencing bodes ill in the critical fight against futility.

Age justice demands fairer archives. Then it wants more. Homages. Commemoration of those the nation lost.

CHAPTER 10

THE COVID MONUMENT WE NEED

SWEEPING UP THE HEART, THE MORNING AFTER DEATH

Death needs rituals that recognize the value of a life. Rituals reknit the fabric of a community that has been shredded. They soothe our deeper dread that we may vanish from the earth without being missed. In a cross-country survey, 45 percent of nursing facility residents lamented that there was no acknowledgment of lost peers. No wake or sitting shiva, no bringing comfort food, liquor, a long hug. No memorial service (*that*, one could understand during the pandemic); but no vigil either, not even a photo in the person's last home.

The bereaved may suffer exceptionally strong grief reactions because of the lockdown isolation and then the lack of social solidarity. Dr. Toni Miles of the University of Georgia, who studies the health effects of grief, says we must do better: "Bereavement is this feeling of profound loss; it's having a giant hole in your soul." The painful losses of doctors, hospital workers and nursing facility aides had been sympathetically noticed. Not so the traumas of the residents who survived. Many may need counseling for PTSD after being quarantined in an endangered place, witnessing mysterious vanishings day after day; facing an empty bed, an empty chair; missing a familiar voice that inquired, "How'd ya sleep?"

Only in May 2020 did the media recognize a need to mourn collectively for the massive numbers of US COVID dead. A grim, until that-moment-unthinkable landmark of one hundred thousand deaths was approaching. "AN INCALCULABLE LOSS," read the *New York Times* headline above nearly a thousand names and one-sentence descriptions. As the numbers rose, the public record was about to fail. Obituary pages register only notables or those who pay for space. The public record could not register so many separate losses or handle communal horror.

Emily Dickinson told us how hard it is to mourn for strangers. She thought only "Immortal Friends" could provide that "vital kinsmanship":

> Bereavement in their death to feel
> Whom we have never seen—
> A Vital Kinsmanship import
> Our Soul and theirs—between—

By 2021, President-elect Joe Biden wanted to be such a kinsman. He sensed that the nation had been reeling. The vaccine worked, but continuing losses in lives and the economy had sapped faith in American can-do, in the belief that such things "could not happen *here*." On the eve of his inauguration, January 19, 2021, Biden chose to commemorate the COVID dead: at that time, four hundred thousand people.

As Dickinson wrote, remembering the dead is the "solemnest of industries, enacted upon Earth." Biden's evening ceremony, appearing on TV, was solemnest. A myriad of tall white lanterns lit up the darkness along the sides of the Lincoln Memorial reflecting pool. Deep bells rang out. Communities across the country lit buildings and rang bells to mark a "national moment of unity and remembrance." The austere national ceremony, the first act of the new presidency to come, symbolically repudiated a previous administration that had worsened the pandemic, divided the nation emotionally, homicidally made light of the danger of death, and callously ignored the mourning of millions.

"HARD TO REMEMBER"

Unfortunately, at that beautiful lighting ceremony, when the dead of the nursing facilities already amounted to at least 112,000 people, Biden did not specifically mention them. They were, disproportionately, staggeringly, *still*, over a fourth of the four hundred thousand dead. He forgot them again in the next ceremony, held in February 2021 when the toll from COVID had reached five hundred thousand— but now the residents had become his administration's special responsibility. A sentence—a single sentence—would have reverberated: "We particularly remember our parents and spouses and friends who have died in government-funded residences."

"To heal, we must remember. It's hard sometimes to remember," Biden said on January 19, 2021. Biden's forgetfulness on those crucial ceremonial occasions could have derived from his wanting to heal the political divisions inherited from Trump. When unity is the intended message, an already marginalized subgroup may vanish without being noticed. Our highest political authority failed to use his pulpit to influence the nation by lifting up the lost, devalued people as worthy of attention. He could have acknowledged the pain of mourners and of the residents who had survived. He could have kept in mind what an organizer said at a Gray Panthers NYC webinar that discussed the healing of mourners: "I guarantee you they are thinking about this every single day."

In unifying ceremonies, residents were ignored again and again. In September 2021, a public art installation by Suzanne Brennan Firstenberg in Washington, DC, featured seven hundred thousand flags that honored, again, *all* the people in the US who had died. One woman said, after dedicating a flag to her mother, "After months of mourning, I finally, finally feel the weight beginning to lift from my shoulders." In twenty acres of waving white flags under the title "In America: Remember," those who died in the facilities were indistinguishable. Where was the solace for those who grieve or rage especially for them?

The public was led to look away. News about the count, or about the abusive and potentially deadly conditions in the facilities, was no longer front and center. With so many other Americans dying—soon half a million—and the 2020 election and the January 6 attempted coup and the closed schools and the flailing economy and virtual life, many people (not only those involved in the machinery of ongoing abandonment, but also we others, lacking any such powers to rescue or abandon) succumbed to a different level of unconscious avoidance. Not perhaps the earlier instinctual psychic withdrawal from bodily misery and death, but sheer not-thinking about nursing facilities or residents.

How could they be lamented if the media did not make clear that they were still dying? Impersonal and political causes made it hard for officials, Democratic or Republican, to "remember" the residents' deaths, which would have required *bringing attention back to them* and accepting responsibility. People in charge don't like to remember what might open them to legal penalties, public shame, political fallout. Governments choose their time to express contrition, usually after a problem has been mastered. Here, it had barely been identified.

SHELVED

In public health, after the first vaccination crusade, the number of residents dying in 2021 was still almost as great as in 2020; the continuing emergency seemed not to add urgency to saving their lives. Vaccinations came to them early in 2021. The CDC Advisory Committee on Immunization Practices put frontline medical personnel first, surviving residents second. States decided their own priorities.

Most residents accepted the shots with alacrity. Prevention could have saved many more. The residents' continuing mortality, now obviously unnecessary, should have made prime objects for vaccination of everyone who entered the buildings: cooks, janitors, social workers, administrators, aides moving from job to job. In relatively small numbers, these people were also dying. Some aides were reluctant to get the jab, and bosses often encouraged them to turn up to work no matter how sick they were.

Prevention didn't happen, for lack of a mandate. Concerned advocates watched, incredulously, impotently, as months of delay to save the residents turned into years. Future historians can explain the slow-motion cowardice of the Biden administration, confronted with Trumpian shouts of "hoax" and rumors that the shot caused autism. It wasn't until September of 2021 that Biden required certain workers, in large firms, to get vaccinated or tested, and then, instead of the motive being presented as securing the residents' safety, the requirement was treated as a general labor-safety mandate, to be overseen by Occupational Health and Safety. (The Veterans Administration had issued a mandate to its health care employees in July 2021. The Supreme Court caused part of the delay in the issuance of Biden's mandate.) When Health and Human Services, not OSHA, became the enforcer, the Centers of Medicare and Medicaid under Biden produced a mandate only on November 5, 2021; it was not implemented until early 2022.

After vaccinations, the big nursing-facility story was the smiley-face of family reunions. This angle satisfied people's hunger for good news but encouraged everyone to overlook the real story: the ongoing danger to residents. Some facilities were taking new admissions, despite trouble finding staff and the reasonable objection (heard earlier from Chuck Sadlacek's daughter) to adding new patients as long as the danger was great. Although some people were able to move out of poorly staffed and risky locales, the majority had to remain, subject to the hazards.

The momentous disease has a long afterlife. The secondary curse of long COVID especially afflicted older people and those who had been hospitalized. Because hundreds of thousands of residents survived, many must suffer from serious symptoms: "brain fog," delirium, labored breathing, fatigue, headache, persistent cough, abdominal pain, diarrhea, chest pain, loss of smell, loss of appetite, unusual muscle pains. Their welfare ought to have remained a health issue and a matter of humanitarian concern. It did not. A social worker wrote to the *Boston Globe* in 2022:

> The group that I believe has been hit hardest by the coronavirus pandemic does not even get a mention in the front-page article "Tracking lingering effects of COVID-19," and one wonders whether this group is getting any care at all for long COVID illnesses. If 10 percent to 30 percent of the survivors have long COVID, who is caring for them?

Unanswered research questions abound about the post-acute sequelae of SARS-CoV-2 infection, or PASC, the acronym for long COVID. Residents are a locatable, trackable population, but they are as likely to be omitted from PASC research protocols as from getting therapy or, incredible as it may appear, antiviral medications.

"The massive underuse of [the antiviral medication] Paxlovid particularly in nursing homes almost certainly led to a lot of avoidable mortality," Dr. Michael Barnett of Harvard noted. Residents were "exactly . . . the intended demographic for these types of medications," said Brian McGarry, a professor of geriatrics and aging at the University of Rochester. My friends, and others in the community, were receiving Paxlovid instantly. But 40 percent of nursing homes reported not having any residents who received antivirals. In a *JAMA* study, McGarry and his associates struggled to explain the extra deaths and so widespread an omission of care. Access to good doctors was one cause. "A lot goes onto the shoulders of clinicians not staying on top of the guidelines . . . and [the facilities not having] clinicians who are up to date," McGarry suggested.

The majority of Americans apparently could not wait to forget the nursing facility catastrophe of 2020. (Some may recall isolated particulars: atrocities like the Holyoke Soldiers' Home in Massachusetts. Or the attempts of Governors Andrew Cuomo and Charlie Baker to lower the tally of the nursing-home dead so it would reflect less dishonor on their administrations.) The general impression: *The facilities are terrible, a fate worse than death. An appalling number, unfortunately, died there*. Our information about the survivors remains impoverished, and our feelings as detached as before. What good outcomes can any next phase bring until we find ways to undo society's seemingly ineradicable forgetfulness?

HOW CAN WE GRIEVE BEFORE WE HAVE BEEN TAUGHT TO CARE?

Forgetting takes one form when it concerns a new father who puts his baby in her car seat on top of the car while finding his keys, and then drives off without noticing until the car seat lands on the asphalt. (This really happened. One time I read about, the baby was unhurt.) The father lacks the *habit* of care, but he is aghast: His wife will "kill" him. Society treats babies' lives as precious; it is he, and only he, who "failed to care." Shaken, scared, remorseful, he vows never to repeat his mistake. Why he made it once is left for him and his wife to deal with; his memory lapse is that family's problem.

Forgetting the residents is *our* problem as a nation, because the Eldercide goes on. Such forgetting is not a uniquely US blindness, pace Hannah Arendt, because eldercides occur elsewhere. Our collective failure to care comes from a habit of carelessness about "the Old" in general (simple ageism), or about older adults who are infirm and indigent (compound ageism). Despite US laws and ethics, this cultural deformity is scarcely noticed when it results in day-to-day eldercide. Aversion—the most extreme form of alienation from victims, with dementism as its typical hellish basis—doesn't cover all cases. Philosophers and psychoanalysts help us *understand* forgetfulness of the Other. But, like any bias one does not share, compound ageism remains finally incomprehensible.

We struggle for language. How to explain ageist, ableist, classist, carelessness when it emerges officially, from responsible bodies? In 2020, the *Boston Globe* called residents "a comparative afterthought" for Governor Charlie Baker's administration in Massachusetts. "State leaders, who are ultimately responsible for protecting 42,000 elderly people unable to care for themselves, were so inattentive to the elders' plight that they thought it appropriate to claim nursing home beds as reserve space for the predicted flood of recovering hospital patients," one article in a series asserted. Governor Mitt Romney had let the Executive Office of Elder Affairs drop in the organizational chart, making it harder for him or for the public to hear the best spokesperson for those forty-two thousand residents, in a system weakly monitored by the Department of Public Health. No governor undid that demotion. No one can "say their names." My state must at a pinch be able to locate their names (cities and towns report all the dead) but has shown it prefers not to count them all.

And the public? Can we explain our forgetfulness by the hardships and turning-inward of the COVID Era? Partly, but this excuse doesn't explain enough. In the COVID Era, forgetfulness required, as we have seen, a host of unprecedented descents into ageism. We've encountered people who "felt" younger as mortality statistics rose in the spring of 2020, and young adults who dared riskier behaviors than Youth had ever been permitted in a public health crisis. Many groups dove deeper into obsession with being youthful. Silence and absence regarding an inferiorized group are productive as social phenomena: They dehumanize. Animalistic similes abounded, naturalizing residents' deaths as a regrettable Darwinian selection of the least fit, a sudden thinning of the herd. Discourses of futility reinforced the mountainous stereotypes. Numb resignation to "what cannot be helped" created a category of unmournable American bodies.

Grieving is human, but who is worthy of grief is something a society learns. Many categories of people can be constructed as unmournable. The processes that are sometimes moved forward only by remorse cannot begin if certain categories of human beings are considered of less worth—whether young men of color, people with physical and cognitive impairments, women, immigrants, older adults in general—or (overlapping in category with some of these groups) residents in care homes.

Unlike other protests against deadly systemic bias, the residents' conglomerate fate, brutally determined by their happening to be caught in a pandemic in nursing facilities overseen by the government, brought forth no mind-changing slogans or heart-stirring marches. At this distance of silent years, can almost two hundred thousand deaths be made to seem a vast communal loss, worthy of grief? "Sweeping up" the morning after is no simple process. It is the collective heart, not a dusty hearth or a chipped bowl, that calls out for restoration.

A SACRED GROVE FOR THOSE WHO
HAVE BEEN WRONGED

In *Oedipus at Colonus*, the suspense depends on whether the old man will be buried as a polluted and feared immigrant outsider or with honorable commemoration. Sophocles wrote the final play of his trilogy shortly before he died, at the age of ninety. "The end" for Oedipus refers not to the moment when his breath stops and his lifetime can retroactively be judged "happy" or miserable, as in his stricken outcry in *Oedipus the King*, "Call no man happy . . ." It is what happens *after* death that determines a final verdict.

Sophocles turns Oedipus from a miserable, self-blinded man, inadvertently guilty of parricide and incest, into a powerful protagonist with a just grievance. My interpretation of the play is strongly influenced by the brilliant acting of Frankie Faison as the old Oedipus in the Theater of War Zoom production of *Colonus*. With an astonishing ability to build credibly from intensity to greater intensity, Faison showed Oedipus successfully redescribing his ferocious lifelong suffering as *unjustified*. The wrong done him can be assuaged only by proper recognition of his posthumous standing.

A *good burial* rather than a good death had been on Sophocles's mind at least since he wrote the *Antigone*, a play that forcefully argued for the ethics (and human instinct, and religious necessity) of offering a posthumous ritual to a dead brother even after he has been proscribed as an enemy of the state. Now, in old age, writing a play about a hapless old man who had been afflicted with wretchedness all his life, Sophocles must have felt the desire for a righteous, state-sponsored, ritual pressing on him even more urgently. He made Oedipus mournable. He rewrote the king's life story to make an oracle agree that

Oedipus was worthy of being buried in a sacred grove. The resting place and the rites promised by the government will allow him to end his life as a benediction to the state that welcomes him.

In the COVID Era, the *Colonus* is more movingly relevant than the *Oedipus*. Like so much in the classic literature of grief, the concept of a good death and the propriety of commemoration have a new resonance now. We need to attune ourselves. Omitting the residents from grand public ceremonies, as Biden did twice, leaves us little imaginative choice but to think of the residents, most separated from their loved ones while they were dying, as pained and lonely, passive and bereft. As a result of the Eldercide, they may be judged to have had a miserable end. A "bad death." It would be purblind and cruel to leave this judgment as the last word on the group. Collecting the oral histories of the survivors may help make the group live. Remembering the dead residents appropriately is the next ritual the nation needs to offer.

"NEVER AGAIN"

I borrow "never again" as an oath for preventing another US Eldercide and making remembrance permanent. It was originally a vow made by survivors of the Buchenwald concentration camp after they were liberated by American troops in 1945. The vow has been used since—in particular, after other genocides—to ward off repetition of the intolerable.

It is possible to make those two words of defiance and determination refer, unmistakably, to those killed prematurely by the Eldercide. The goal must be, by honoring the missing elders collectively, to permanently record the government wrong and prevent the next catastrophe. As a matter of justice and solidarity, it is correct but inadequate for families to sue one by one to get blood money from their state—as Regina Costantino Discenza did. Discenza's parents had been living at Menlo Park Veterans Memorial Home in Edison, New Jersey, before they were exposed to COVID; after that, "it was a horror show," said Ms. Discenza. The state agreed to settle out of court and awarded each family of survivors on average $445,000. Similar lawsuits are pending.

In a capital dedicated to powerful remembrances of those whose bodies are buried elsewhere—from George Washington on—the residents deserve to have a permanent national cenotaph. History teaches how much it takes to eradicate a systemic social evil. The Eldercide has yet to receive communal consensus that its deaths were avoidable and their causes worthy of investigation. A special monument for the residents would signal not only remorse but the assumption of carefull responsibility for the poorest, sickest, and most disabled people in the nation's charge. If public will could be created, Congress would approve the concept and provide the land and funding and the president would sign.

In the next section, I take a closer look at the steps needed to turn a group that is today stigmatized or forgotten—the lost residents— into becoming central to our vision of a better future for all older Americans.

EMBRACING THE OUTCASTS

We can move past intolerable images in part by creating an architectural tribute—a permanent statement that the state has renewed its social embrace. Such structures attract visitors in perpetuity. We see such tributes in countries that have a genocide museum (Cambodia) or other concrete recognition of state criminality (Chile).

It's amazing that some memorials ever get built. The obstacles are high. To gain public-agenda status, an issue must be the subject of widespread attention and be perceived by a sizable public and influential officials as an appropriate national concern. The very idea of demonstrating government bias or negligent policy can raise up Eldercide deniers and protectors of the status quo. Recognizing the equal humanity of an abjected group may involve effortful stages of *unlearning*: shaking off the habit of indifference, accepting better information, and regretting past attitudes, in order to decide the loss in question *is* a grievance worth redressing. Or, more precisely, deciding *that the outcasts were always worthy*. A monument is a material symbol that a broad transvaluation has occurred. To the inevitable laggards and future generations, it continues to teach the new values and history that had been denied. Achieving such a monument is therefore intensely important—and predictably controversial.

To make the case for a monument to nursing-facility residents plausible, I trace the histories of two very different cenotaphs. One commemorates the Japanese American internees and soldiers of WWII. The other commemorates Black US citizens who were lynched during a savagely long period of American history in which the government looked away. These persuasive structures were successfully created even though they confirmed the guilt of the nation. At such remarkable sites, if not so readily elsewhere, the last can be first.

THE CRANES FLY, AGAINST ALL ODDS

With its soaring sculpted cranes and tablets of names, the graceful Japanese American monument in Washington, DC, recognizes a group of victims who feared they would be stereotyped as enemies forever. It explicitly recognizes a grave injustice inflicted on them in 1942. Soon after the Japanese military's attack on Pearl Harbor, Hawaii, President Franklin Delano Roosevelt ordered the internment of persons of Japanese ancestry on the West Coast. 120,000 people were hastily moved to concentration camps, losing homes, jobs, businesses, possessions, friends, family members, neighborhoods, and a sense of self-worth and progress for themselves and their children.

In her book *Letters to Memory*, Karen Tei Yamashita, a prizewinning writer, describes the misery of her outcast family and the "mean and hostile" treatment they received. The family saved the letters because "they knew what was happening to them was significant and wrong, that justice might not happen in their lifetimes." One woman, by then a hundred years old, told Yamashita, "Oh those were terrible times. You have no idea."

Most of the Japanese were kept incarcerated until after the war ended because the Supreme Court (in a six-to-three decision) ratified the federal government's prejudice in 1944. Like the infamous 1857 decision in *Dred Scott* about enslaved African Americans, *Korematsu v. US* denied rights to a racialized group. Those opinions are widely regarded as two of the most disgraceful Supreme Court decisions ever.

In 1982, Grant Ujifusa, a volunteer who became the Strategy Chair of the Japanese American Citizens League, joined the effort to get an apology and redress from the government. He was then forty years old, a Harvard graduate who was working full time in publishing. In a 2013 interview, Ujifusa declared:

> Broad public support was never going to develop. On talk radio, the callers would ask, "Would you believe that the politicians are going to give $20,000 to people who bombed Pearl Harbor?" We don't live in a direct democracy, so we took our case to the House, where we needed the votes of 218 people; the Senate, of 51 people; and the White House, of one person. . . . our success in Washington—[was] something the Kennedy School called "against all odds."

It took nearly forty years before the government formally acknowledged that "race prejudice, war hysteria, and a failure of political leadership" motivated this mass incarceration—not "military necessity." A Reagan-Bush Congress passed the Civil Liberties Act, which acknowledged the injustice, apologized, and did in fact provide $20,000 to each person surviving the camps as a reparation. The effort was worth the risk of failing. When I interviewed him in 2021, Grant Ujifusa surmised:

> Let's say we got it through Congress, but it got vetoed by Reagan. The exercise would [still] have produced a feeling among Japanese Americans that we gave it our best shot, and while doing it we educated the country about not repeating what happened.

After Ujifusa convinced him of its worth, Reagan signed the bill on August 10, 1988.

Strikingly, despite having received an apology and financial redress, no one abandoned the idea of a getting a monument. Certainly not Ujifusa. He is tall, white-haired. He wears round glasses. He told me, "The idea of a monument may even have preceded the idea of redress, I'm not sure."

Why did a monument matter so much?

Ujifusa explained this point in his grave, calm way:

> It would have been a monument to all those who went to the camp, to those who died there, the elderly, and those who died from lack of care. Their names are inscribed on it. There is a Japanese expression, *gaman*. "We endure." It is one of the principal virtues of Japanese American life to this day. Also, as we endure, we say, "We do this for the sake of the children," so they may have a better life. So then, out of gratitude, the children say, "We do better, and we thank you."

Gaman is a Zen Buddhist term that can be translated as "enduring the seemingly unbearable with patience and dignity."

He paused. "We are still with you."

Congress gave money to buy the land from the District of Columbia and provide Park Service maintenance in perpetuity. It was left to the foundation to raise funding for the monument's design and construction, $13 million. Although the Citizens League had envisioned the monument as honoring only the internees, who had suffered the "seemingly unbearable," that vision was not realized. In order to make a monument to victims of US prejudice politically acceptable, Congress submerged the mistreated group, by manifesting pride in another, more highly valued group. The DC "Japanese American Memorial to Patriotism during World War II" displays the names of all the members of the 442nd regiment of Japanese American volunteers who died fighting in Italy and France. They were the most decorated unit for its size in US military history. The passive prisoners and the military heroes were linked as "American citizens of Japanese ancestry and their parents," as President George H. W. Bush described them in

1992, "who patriotically supported this country despite their unjust treatment during World War II."

To receive the social embrace that originally failed them, it should not be necessary for a group of victims to include heroes or members of more acceptable groups. It makes civic sense to recognize the formerly maligned simply as human beings with equal rights. In the next cenotaph story, too, hard ideological work has also been necessary.

A HALL OF DARK STELAE

The Lynching Memorial in Montgomery, Alabama—officially titled the National Memorial for Peace and Justice—makes that civic point emphatically, by honoring the most dehumanized, abused, tortured, and murdered Black Americans. It was initiated, funded, and built not by the US government but by the Equal Justice Initiative, a nonprofit legal organization in Montgomery directed by a single-minded and indefatigable lawyer, orator, writer, and fundraiser named Bryan Stevenson. The Lynching Memorial is the nation's first monument to all the victims of racial terrorism.

Lynching, a vigilante action that eschewed trials, was presented by white perpetrators and supporters as a spontaneous response to a perceived "crime" so heinous as to be subject to death. These putative offenses were often trumped up, like fourteen-year-old Emmett Till's purported whistling at a white woman. A lynching often attracted large groups of whites, not excluding children, as witnesses to torture and execution. Postcards of the corpse or corpses that openly showed the faces of local whites were shared or sold like souvenirs. Local police and FBI did nothing to stop the extrajudicial murders. The perpetrators—often Ku Klux Klan members—were rarely tried and when tried were found not guilty. A history produced by the Equal Justice Initiative (EJI) notes, "Most communities [where lynchings occurred] do not actively or visibly recognize how their race relations were shaped by terror lynching." The EJI called the lack of effort "to acknowledge, discuss, or address lynching" an "astonishing absence." The Institute has tried to make the nation feel that absence as astonishing.

"The last shall be first" must be a spiritual injunction that Bryan Stevenson also follows. Stevenson has worked for decades to undo racism in the American legal system. His 2012 TED lecture, called "We Need to Talk about Injustice," has been watched over eight million times. His moving book *Just Mercy: A Story of Justice and Redemption*, about his original legal practice trying to save death-row inmates, became a milestone in the criminal-justice reform movement. The Equal Justice Initiative expanded into the larger mission of correcting the history of racism.

Counting victims matters differently depending on the crime. In 2020, the act of *counting* the dead nursing-facility residents displayed shock or sorrow but did not thereby signal the negligence, abuse, prejudice, or crime that *American Eldercide* aims to demonstrate. Almost the first step the EJI took was to collect correct data for their 2015 report *Lynching in America: Confronting the Legacy of Racial Terror*. Like the internment of Japanese Americans or the genocide of Native Americans, lynching had not been taught in history books. Accurately counting the four thousand "African American victims of racial terror lynching" and naming the locations where they died uncovered long-concealed facts, a preliminary to getting white communities to recognize the hideousness of their racist system. The powerful memorial opened in Montgomery in 2018.

The open-air pavilion of the National Memorial is a haunting hall of six-foot-tall Corten steel blocks hanging from the rafters, heavy dark stelae inscribed with the names of over four thousand victims. Eight hundred stelae name each US county where one or more lynchings occurred. As visitors walk down the sloping floor of the pavilion, symbolic coffins appear to move upward toward the sky. The stelae hang overhead like "the strange fruit" that Abel Meeropol described in a song that Billie Holiday made unforgettable.

The pavilion experience could feel oppressive and horrifying or bewildering. Or life-changing. In 2022, I interviewed Sia Sanneh, a senior lawyer at EJI, deeply involved in the projects, whose "life was changed" by taking a course at Yale on capital punishment. Sanneh told me:

> Over seven hundred thousand visitors have come, maybe more. That's incredible, because Montgomery is not central, it's not Atlanta. Afterward, they really understand the *scale* of the loss. . . . We observe the reactions. . . . It is moving to watch people making the pilgrimage. People leave with hope. As you leave, you pass a sculpture of the women who led the Montgomery bus boycott, one of the most successful social justice movements in history.

The initiators did wonder if the memorial would bring too much sorrow to Black people, especially descendants. "We tried to think about that," Sanneh said. "We waited 'til people could understand that the building would speak of solemnity, hope, power. . . . We did community outreach in Montgomery and put up some markers first. There was trust in our identity [as EJI]: that we had been providing [legal] services for such a long time. And we put effort into the opening. We invited John Lewis, C. T. Vivian [an ally of Martin Luther King, Jr.], *pillars*. All that helped people coming from a variety of mental spaces."

Any building to honor the nursing facility residents should "speak of solemnity, hope, power" rather than the horrors of the public health system in nursing facilities. And like the Lynching Memorial, the residents' memorial should not be a simple stand-alone monument but rather the material symbol of an ongoing process of truth-telling and transformation.

Bryan Stevenson and his growing staff at EJI are engaged in creating many nationwide rituals of commemoration. Eventually each atrocity will be marked by a plaque at the place of execution and by a bottle of soil from the place of death. "There was blood in that soil, there's DNA in that soil," Stevenson has said. Individuals volunteer to visit the site and, with a trowel, awe, and sometimes fear of retaliation, gather the soil. The secular hands-on process EJI invented confers on that anonymous dust an almost sacred character, the aura of a martyr's relic. A shop at the museum sells an artist's image of the stately, soberly lit soil-collection wall. An EJI group in Athens, Ohio, three hundred strong, put up a detailed marker on the site of an 1881 murder. The marker includes a remorseful deathbed cry from one of the killers who had been given legal impunity: "Take Christ off of me!"

I asked Sanneh whether they had asked Congress for funding. She said:

> The report of 2015 got so much publicity that descendants of people who had been lynched reached out to us with that idea. One of the most moving parts of the work was that there's a generation of people who lived through the violence. One woman was a hundred years old; her note to us was so affirming. . . . We did not, however, contemplate going that lengthy route. That might have compromised the story we wanted to tell.

Stevenson started the project himself—buying land, starting design—using his MacArthur Fellowship money and speaker's fees. (I heard him speak at Boston College, where he filled a hockey stadium and brought the audience to their feet and many, including me, to tears.)

Funding was unlikely to come from the cities or states where lynchings had occurred. A journalist from the *Guardian*, asking locals about the memorial, encountered outright hostility: "Some conservatives in Alabama rolled their eyes at the project, saying they were more concerned with saving Confederate monuments, now under threat from leftwing activists."

I had read about the many small donations the project received. Sanneh confirmed that: "Yes, over the last ten years, well more than 50 percent of the funding has come from small donors—gifts of $20 and $30 and $100. People send notes: 'My church group decided to do this.' It [the funding] was unusual." Later, EJI raised more than $20 million from foundations. Sanneh added, "I learned this from Bryan, that people believe in your idea after you have done it."

A DESTINATION AND A STARTING POINT

Transformational change can begin only with proper remembrance. The National Eldercide Memorial for Nursing-Facility Residents Who Died of COVID would commemorate the two hundred thousand, so far, who should have been protected and treated with every possible care.

What special work does a public building do that restitution in the courts or stories told in books and films, for instance, can't do? Bryan Stevenson believes that a memorial carries more conviction:

> Who is honored, what is remembered, and what is memorialized tell a story about a society that can't be reflected in other ways. Monuments and memorials speak to the truths about a community, about history in a way that everyone is forced to acknowledge. In that way, I think they occupy an important space for truth-telling that can't be replicated.

A distinguished edifice becomes a destination not only for the ingroup that identifies with the victims—COVID survivors, families and friends of the residents—but also for others. Like the EJI complex, like the Japanese American memorial, a monument to the residents would develop the education of the heart, unwinding prejudices from within.

Such a national emotional reeducation develops unevenly. Some people become (per Emily Dickinson) Vital Kinsmen. Not everyone, however, will visit a victims' monument with quiet reverence. In our divided nation—whose population includes "hoaxers," anti-vaxxers, dementists, and garden-variety ageists—some may scoff at the idea of a monument for nursing-facility residents, those losers?! As the COVID Era went on, I began to observe "evasive memory," as described by Larry L. Langer, the renowned author of *Using and Abusing the Holocaust*. False witnessing in the Holocaust context came from people denying their documented complicity with organized murder.

The Eldercide is a congeries of wrongs and crimes, not all attested in documents; it involves many perpetrators, local and national. Refusing to confront the reasons why so many died needlessly may seem another tempting return to the Before Time.

People who never intend to visit may—merely by learning of the memorial's existence—be forced to acknowledge, at a minimum, that a group powerful enough to build an approved, complex, and costly monument holds the victims in high esteem.

Some of the grief-stricken families may be confused about whether the people they lost would have died "anyway," as the public seems to believe. Visitors to a Monument to the Victims of the Eldercide may feel shock and outrage at learning that beyond the tragic singular event that bereaved their family lay disdain, neglect, malfeasance, ignorance, or corruption on a large scale—that there was, in fact, an eldercide. Some visitors who trusted authorities (in church services or at political rallies, events brazenly held without masks) may find appropriate redirections for their anger. At the Democratic National Convention in 2020, Kristin Urquisa rebuked the Republican lies, because her father's "only preexisting condition" was "trusting Donald Trump, and for that he paid with his life."

The millions who are grieving must now do so separately, standing stock still beside an empty chair at the table. They cannot heal fully until a monument, or, better, a transformation of public policy, proves that the United States recognizes that their losses are national losses. In the midst of death, we are joined in solidarity.

"WE ARE STILL WITH YOU"

The visionary next step is to seek out artists and architects who can turn our best knowledge of causes and villains, our worthiest feelings, into a durable witness that rises up visibly and permanently from the earth. Such a monument will be as perpetual as terrestrial materials can be. Ideally, it will be on the Mall. Like the grove that welcomed Oedipus, the Mall offers a special space in our culture for transcending narrow politics. It flourishes liminally between the secular and the revered. Here, if anywhere, a transvaluation can occur that would be uniformly honored.

Every detail should be designed with the aim of restoring honor to the victims and integrating the history of compound ageism and subordination into general knowledge of US life and culture.

The monument the country needs would be beautiful and dignified, soothing and unifying. Imagine something that moves visitors like Maya Lin's long, deep, dark Vietnam Veterans' memorial in Washington, DC, or the brilliantly colored, diverse AIDS quilts. This one, I suggest, should be a noble structure of rich somber colors, rare materials, and fine craftsmanship, expressing the abundant ways the individuals are remembered by those who loved them. I imagine precious insets like those that adorn the exquisite church of the Miracoli in Venice: jasper and porphyry, and marbles like Parian, Carrara, Swedish green, and rose Etowah from Georgia.

The monument would both symbolize and illuminate the lost residents' full lives and multiple relationships. Across the country, nursing homes could create a wall of photos of the COVID victims with their names and stories, which would help assuage the grief of local survivors and caregivers. In Washington, the shrine could borrow ideas from the Museum of Memory and Human Rights in Santiago, Chile. That museum has a wall fifty feet high, covered with photographs of those who were savagely executed by the military government during the years of dictator Augusto Pinochet. Ariel Dorfman, a Chilean writer, came to the Museum for his own act of commemoration. He describes visitors viewing the photographs from a balcony overlooking the lofty wall: "A small digital screen . . . allows a particular victim's name to be typed in so that the person's photograph lights up on the wall." Along the inner rim of the balcony, a shrine of candles burns perpetually.

Wherever mourning occurs, being able to read or touch the names is requisite. The National Eldercide Memorial for Nursing-Facility Residents Who Died of COVID must carry as many names as can be ascertained and their dates of birth and death, like the walls of a vast mausoleum. Wall plaques would explain that these people did not need to die, that they wanted to live, and that many others did survive. For some fortunate visitors who had bequeathed audio- or videotapes to the archive, typing in the name of a loved one on the digital screen could produce the poignant look and sound of life. In a country that sometimes willed them gone and forgets their absence and their existence, their own photos, words, and voices would evoke their *presence*. To Ariel Dorfman, the Chilean shrine "enacts the message that a museum dedicated to memory is designed to convey: remembering the dead is a way of keeping them somehow alive, and not so alone."

ONLY REMEMBER!

A memorial for all 1,100,000 US COVID victims is not likely, certainly not soon. But were it to be realized, that decision would entail a grave historical injustice and public health loss. It would bury the hundreds of thousands of stigmatized residents a second time, amid the mass of a more highly valued group. Only a monument focused on nursing-facility victims could frame the Eldercide properly, so that it may never happen again. Ideally it would accompany and mark an end to the residents' continuing plight.

The monument—a museum and library—would display the system that produced the Eldercide as its original sin and cause. One installation, at the end of a long corridor, would allow visitors to peep into an exact replica of a typical facility space: 8 by 12 feet square, furnished with a single bed, bureau, armchair, a walker, and some of the sparse personal mementos described in the prologue. Here, in situ, would be a place to listen to actors reading the residents' rare testimonies of their year of living dangerously in lockdown.

Their published memories would appear on the shelves of the library. An archive of writing and podcasts and TV news stories would be polyphonic, collecting the voices of family members who suffered losses, progressive nursing-home advocates, medical researchers, historians, ethicists, psychologists, anthropologists, gerontologists and age critics, and poets. Its genres would go from lament to analysis to jeremiad to policy paper—as this book does. Inside the bookstore, anti-ageist materials would be available for sale inexpensively, including editorial cartoons (like the one that opens chapter 2) and posters. One in my collection shows the WeCare Wall in Brooklyn in March 2021, for fifteen thousand lost residents.

Some texts might record confessions. Like retired military repenting wartime decisions, retired owners of the nursing and veterans' facilities industry, stockholders, and politicians might publicly apologize for diversions of CMS funds. Those pressured into moral injury would testify. Those who, with more agency, put lethal decision-making into hospital guidelines, or made the decisions in hospital ICUs or doctors' offices, might also be moved to do so. (In July 2021, Ezekiel Emanuel co-wrote an article about mandating vaccinations for all LTC workers, which ends on a possibly repentant note: "This is the logical fulfillment of the ethical commitment of all health care workers to put patients as well as residents of long-term care facilities first." This article appeared in *Annals of Internal Medicine,* not in one of the major media that had published Emanuel's sensational duty-to-die essay.)

The monument would consolidate in one place the narrative of the failed public health system, with administration after administration, state after state, corrupted by private corporate interests and deformed by US ideologies: neoliberal market forces, individual self-reliance, and state capture, all entangled in the cult of youth and the fear of growing old in such a society. The initiative might inspire books and documentaries that further reveal the social escalations of contempt and aversion toward indigent old people—everything that was festering in the body politic before 2020 and went hugely wrong in the COVID Era.

Initiating a memorial—answering the opponents—getting the memorial funded; admiring it as a new physical and symbolic landmark in the nation's capital; and recounting the quest as other monumental monument stories have been recounted, with admiration for heroic obstinacy, would also *teach.* Brian Stevenson said about the Lynching Memorial, "We want this place to inspire and motivate people to no longer be silent about this history." The visitors to the Residents' Memorial might leave with a determination to speak truth more urgently when it comes to confronting our history of violent exclusions based on age, race, class, abilities, and gender. Visitors could try to turn "ageist" and "ableist" into epithets as powerful as "racist."

Vowing "Never again" is the impetus for overlapping missions that constitute the Eldercide Project. #OldLivesMatter is the slogan that can help our society once again think of all older adults as individuals with an equal right to life, wherever they reside, whatever their physical or cognitive or economic conditions. Working toward a memorial would support the extraordinary nursing-facility transformation movement, described next. Arguing for a memorial to the dead of the Eldercide doesn't assume that achieving a monument would mark the end of the work. It might propel the real work of change.

RECKONINGS

And moral debts need to be paid.
Apologies, commemorations, and plans go only so far.

SHENNETTE GARRETT-SCOTT

THE TWO FRIENDS

VISITING VERA: "I NEVER THOUGHT I WOULD END UP LIKE THIS"

I was a child when I came to love Vera in the simple way affectionate children can wholly trust certain people and take them for granted as protectors. Summertimes, my mother mainly hung out with two sisters-in-law and welcomed Vera as a close friend. The four women drove their children to Rockaway Beach to play together while they sat in a tight circle talking childbirth, hapless husbands, beautiful cheap purchases. Aunt Vera always brought good things to eat. She would hand out cold watermelon and say "Scram," with her fabulous deep gurgling laugh.

Vera Curtisz Feldmann and Betty stayed friends forever. Like my mother, Vera became a public school teacher. Over thirty-two years, she must have taught nine hundred children to read. Whenever I visited Vera's daughter in a distant state, I would visit Vera. First in her immaculate two-bedroom apartment, stocked with tchotchkes; later in her nursing facility. I called her just to catch up on family gossip and hear her laugh. Her laugh was swooping, whooping, welcoming—it made you feel as if *you* were the one to make her day. She kept her wavy hair its forever color, a fiery auburn.

If I had some trepidation about crossing the threshold where Vera lived after a stroke, it was not from squeamish fear of disabled people. It was *my fabulous Aunt Vera* I came to see, a petite woman in her nineties, considered charming all her life. Her daughter, whom I will call Rose, had told me Vera wasn't so well, nor was she happy. I expected she would not be too different from the funny, generous woman I had admired back when I was overhearing those half-naked women telling secrets. Perhaps all the lost and the living souls in the facilities speak to me because of my long-ago admiration for Vera, and for my parents, aunts and uncles, and grandparents in their old age. Just as those blue sunlit salty days of our past remain in permanent communication, now that I too am old, with my heart.

My last visit to Vera took place about fifteen years ago. Later, I asked Rose what had impoverished her mother. Rose agreed to let me tell intimate financial facts because she feels the systemic harms need to be understood.

"A GREAT COMFORTER"

In Plato's *Republic,* Socrates says to Cephalus, "Old age sits lightly upon you, not because of your happy disposition, but because you are rich, and wealth is known to be a great comforter."

Vera, widowed, cannot be scorned for impecuniousness. Vera had joined the middle class as soon as she started teaching. Like my mother, she worked her way up from low-income, first-American-born-generation origins. These admirable forebears did the most valuable work then available to women. Vera and her husband lived for decades in a modest suburban house they had paid off. When her husband began to show he was cognitively impaired, they moved near their adult offspring. She was only seventy-five. Her husband spent some hours each day in a day facility, which was costly. She was his primary caregiver, exhaustingly. Sometimes on the phone I could hear him bellowing in the background.

Vera and her ailing husband used up the house-sale money. After he died, she lived in good health until she was eighty-nine, when a stroke ended her independence. The rental apartment took her entire income; there was nothing extra to enable her to live there with aides—her first choice. When the level of care she needed determined the move to the nursing facility, she said, "I worked so hard all my life. I never thought I would end up like this."

Vera received about $3,000 a month from her pension and Social Security. In her nineties, she was hospitalized for pneumonia. Rose explained what happened next:

> After 100 free days of rehab, the nursing home she was in charged $245.00 per day, i.e., approximately $7,350 per month! . . . So we had to get Medicaid to cover the difference between her $3,000 per month and the nursing home cost. To get Medicaid, you must give all your assets to the nursing home and all your income as you receive it.

To wind up in a place that values you, dollar-wise, at about two-thirds of what you had been worth when you were there on Medicare for a hundred days, *while you are still paying everything you have*—that goes beyond irony, beyond the loud laugh of despair. Vera had been a teacher, an *authority*. The hybrid system that Congress devised feels like an ageist joke on disability and old age.

Vera greeted me in her half room. She apologized, saying the space was not as clean as she had kept her own home. It was tidy. I knew the aides didn't talk to her; assistance was impersonal; the food was mediocre. The building was well-lit and neat, but the facility lacked amenities. Later, macular degeneration prevented Vera from watching TV. Her sister moved. Vera was bored; she was sometimes unhappy.

Both she and my mother had delightful dispositions, but "happiness in old age" is not a choice everyone can make. One keyword is *money*: for the Americans who lack it, for the nursing corporations that collect it. Middle-class people never think financial ruin and private humiliation could happen to them. Or maybe that is all they think about, with aversion.

THE RUIN OF WANT

Vera's story of "ending up" on Medicaid is typical. An official sensitively explains: "When expensive risks transpire during a phase when we can't work and earn, we can quickly become financially devastated. Long-term care is one of these risks." Costs for dealing with ill health or disability sneak up on those formerly safely lodged in the middle class, like Vera. Studies estimate that between 10 percent and 25 percent of all nursing-home residents who start off paying out of pocket—middle-class people—eventually spend down their assets to obtain Medicaid eligibility. People are pauperized.

Parents and grandparents who are impoverished may be loved and respected. The obvious ruin of want, however—hunger; inability to pay for rent, heat, and medications; possible eviction—digs deep into the soul. Falling lower than your children, so low that you can't help them out in their need as you would like, and they know you can't—that is another indignity.

Nursing facilities are full of people like Vera in all the embraceable human ways who have been "bruised by misfortune." When a Mrs. Smith took the step from the eighth floor to the basement, she said, "That's the longest step I ever took." People with rich temperaments have survived other calamities. They may support one another's dignity. But once admitted to a facility on degrading Medicaid, everyone confronts age segregation and the stigma of dependency.

It must be hard to maintain a subjective sense of your value when that value is disregarded in everyday reality. In institutions that pay lower than living wages, negligent treatment occurs and premature, *extra* deaths follow. Outside of the rare well-run places, the risk is high of being in mortal danger. The Eldercide continues.

A catastrophe that captures over a million people a year cannot be laid to individual fault. One main cause of no-fault poverty is income inequality. Elites have had the power to keep wages low and magnify their own tax and wealth privileges. The "retirement-income crisis" has been known for decades and lamented impotently:

> After three decades with *no growth* in the aggregate income of the bottom 90 percent of Americans, a new report by the National Institute on Retirement Security [2017] finds that . . . the typical household nearing retirement [has been able to accumulate] only $14,500 in retirement savings.

If Vera had had $14,500 in savings, just holding onto her bed would have spent it down in months.

BETTY: DOWN FROM THE PENTHOUSE

Vera's friend Betty—my mother—hadn't wanted to leave her home either. Only after recovering from two agonizing falls, when she was ninety-one, did she agree to move near us. Unlike Vera, she *liked* the idea of congregate living. We toured three communities; she chose one. The communal dining room looked out on a garden. This non-profit charged a monthly fee like a condo. The small living room that I called her "jewel box" displayed some art and furniture from the Florida high-rise she had called home for thirty years. Betty possessed a nice union-negotiated pension after twenty-five years of teaching first graders, on top of her Social Security—just like Vera. The main difference was that she had not had an ailing husband. She was able to save. And a divorce settlement gave her the condo.

Until she had to leave it. Even if you've chosen your surroundings, it can take years to get over making the big move that one expects to be final. Mostly, my mother's demeanor was as calm as her blood pressure. Occasionally, though, she referred to those losses. "I had a high view of the ocean," she would remind me. "Yes," I chimed in, "so high the pelicans flew *beneath* the balcony!"

Betty stayed healthy (all those daily walks on the beach). Her increasing blindness and memory loss, however, led us to hire aides. Savings allowed her to have "boughten friendship at her side," as Robert

Frost wrote, practically. From a bio I wrote, her pleasant, chatty companions learned her personal and professional backstory. She treated these women—an unmarried white former waitress, a South American immigrant mother, a Nigerian Christian—like younger friends, boosting their self-esteem as a gracious older woman can. After she died, her aides gave me a smooth, palm-sized stone with five words hand-painted on it: "Betty Morganroth, teacher and inspiration." She died in her own bed, without pain. I had been kneeling beside her, stroking her soft unconscious hand and whispering, shortly before she took her last breaths.

In their good years, Betty and Vera had met, fondly and energetically conversing. Both died before COVID, thank heaven: my mother in 2010, aged ninety-six; Vera in 2011, aged ninety-five.

RISKS

If the two friends had lived during the pandemic, who would have been most at risk? Betty had a door she could lock, well-paid aides she could trust to protect her health and their own. The nurse on site was an infection preventionist. As I reported, her place—a small, nonprofit, stand-alone facility—had had *no* COVID illnesses when I checked in January 2021.

Our dear Vera had easily survived a hospitalization for pneumonia; would she have survived COVID conditions? This thought—that she might have been neglected in an understaffed place, had she been alive in 2020—is too painful to imagine. No one should be nakedly exposed to death because, after a long rich life, they need a little help with the mundane routines of daily life.

AND CRUEL AND LETHAL

"U.S. nursing home care is ineffective, inefficient, inequitable, fragmented, and unsustainable." It's worth repeating that takeaway of the landmark 2022 report from the National Academies of Science, Engineering and Medicine, with my additions, "cruel and lethal." Allowing for exceptions, nursing facilities "embody the worst aspects of the privatization that so many of our elected officials have championed," Laura Katz Olson, a political scientist, concluded in *The Politics of Medicaid*. Dr. Marc Cohen, co-director of a LeadingAge Center, agrees. "The private market has suffered failure by all standards," he writes. The answer is comprehensive reform—really, transformation.

Anger at the industry and the government had been growing in the Before Time. LeadingAge, which represents approximately two thousand nonprofit nursing homes in thirty-eight states, some a century old, dared tell Senators Charles Grassley and Ron Wyden that continuing as-is was "insanity." That letter was sent in December 2019. Months later, the pandemic proved them right. Disgust grew at the catastrophe of the Eldercide. Everyone who cared enough already knew exactly what was wrong. At the Senate Finance Committee's 2021 virtual hearing on "A National Tragedy: COVID-19 in the Nation's Nursing Homes," Senator Wyden impatiently declared, "You could fill a library with the watchdog reports calling public attention to these issues."

EVERYONE KNOWS WHAT NEEDS TO BE DONE

How can a future Vera—say, perhaps half of the Gen Z children who will live to be one hundred and not have means—be well protected? The COVID Era is not over; the virus that will cause the next pandemic is foretold. What reforms are needed to keep the luckless from ending up abandoned in potential "death houses"? The nation is responsible for assuring that an eldercide can never happen again. "Reckonings" should mean the government doing everything to make sure older adults like Vera, trapped at the bottom, age either "in place" or in a place they can inhabit comfortably.

What Vera wanted—what I dare say everyone wants who gives two seconds of thought to living into old age and needing assistance they cannot afford—is long-term care adapted to basic human needs and desires. "Safety." "Quality" care. Ideally, care provided in her original community. Transportation to libraries and medical appointments.

If it must be in a congregate facility, a room and private bath. Good food. Privacy *and* social life, both. Aides who receive decent salaries and respect, reasons to stay in the job; time to do their best for each resident; and training. Good programming: art and music. Outdoor space. Some creature comforts. Respect. Respect for elder rights. Competent administration: rapid responses to complaints. No theft, no abuse, no fraud.

The future of old age must not depend either on private "wealth" or on pauperizing "welfare." Policy change—helping people stay out of institutions and transforming the remaining facilities in the failed federal-state system of Medicare and Medicaid—was long overdue. Yet nothing happened in 2021.

2022: THE YEAR OF TRANSFORMATIONAL CHANGE?

The year 2022 opened with great expectations. In February 2022, during his second State of the Union address, President Biden devoted a few earnest minutes to the residents' fates. "As Wall Street firms take over more nursing homes, quality in those homes has gone down and costs have gone up. That ends on my watch," he boldly declared. To have "nursing homes" and the takeovers of "Wall Street" mentioned together in a presidential speech, even without a plan to end private-equity investment or improve residents' quality of life, was extraordinary.

In 2022, however, remedial bills sat idly in a divided Congress. Gridlock benefits the status quo. New guidelines for closing facilities that put residents in jeopardy applied to fewer than 0.5 percent of the total number, the worst of the worst, already singled out for violations. Few midterm political races bothered to mention grim facilities or resident deaths. Representative James E. Clyburn's Select Subcommittee on the Coronavirus Crisis dedicated only one session to the 20 percent of Americans who died under CMS's aegis. Unlike Bennie Thompson's and Liz Cheney's televised January 6 sessions, Clyburn's exposé received little notice. Deprived of a laser-like public focus on the Eldercide, Biden seemed stymied.

A NATIONAL SOLUTION IS POSSIBLE

Growing old in the United States is like standing on a mountaintop in the path of a predicted hurricane. Long-term care (LTC) is a national problem by no means limited to people like Vera. These are the hard facts: by 2030 a fifth of Americans will be over sixty-five; about 70 percent will need short- or long-term care, at home or in assisted living or in a skilled facility. The number of aged poor people has increased since the mid-1970s. If nothing is done, a full half of people over sixty-five will be unable to afford the basics—housing as well as food and medical care—let alone be able to pay for private care like my mother's.

As people grow older, many learn with terror that the safety net for their old age is full of holes, shredding. Fear of aging into old age and being abandoned is another feature of the neoliberal market economy surrounding us. It invades inner life, adding economic anxiety to the psychological assaults of ageism.

Millions need a federal LTC benefit. A federal program with pooled benefits, like Social Security, would be the simplest, most popular, and most effective answer. LTC insurance eliminates the cruel neoliberal charge, laid freely on people with cognitive impairments, incurable cancer, disabilities, or chronic illnesses—if they have no money—of being an expensive "burden." The US doesn't have such a program or a strategy to get one. LTC insurance was originally part of President Obama's Affordable Care Act. To make the rest of the bill passable, the CLASS Act (Community Living Assistance Services and Supports) was dropped. More than 260,000 are still enrolled in the single existing Federal LTC Insurance Program—mainly federal and Postal Service employees and uniformed service members. The rest of us confront the private insurance market for long-term care, where premiums are high and rising.

The national failure to act draws attention to the state of Washington, the first and as of 2023 the only state to establish its own all-embracing LTC insurance pool. Ben Veghte, who is entrusted with the WA Cares Fund, explained the principles and the method. "Insurance is just a smart way rich, middle class, and lower income individuals all protect ourselves against risks through risk pooling." Like Social Security, this LTC program is not welfare but a "defined contributory insurance program sponsored by the government."

Everyone in the state now must either have bought private LTC insurance or joined the public pool through a small payroll deduction. Beginning in 2026, each resident who has paid in can receive up to $36,500. Based on the Genworth Cost of Care, that amount could pay for up to twenty hours of home care every week for a year. Not opulent, but time to exhale after a catastrophe.

Some people earn too little to make any contributions. There is a solution: lifting the class and status of those millions who are on the cusp. "Targeted income" means disbursements to the neediest. As long as the trillion-dollar government programs lasted, in 2020–2021, they ended a massive amount of hunger and child poverty. The practice is effective. "Lo and behold, if you give people money, they are less poor," said Elaine Waxman, an economist and senior fellow at the Urban Institute.

Conservatives jibe at "handouts" to disabled and chronically ill paupers, having driven Emersonian self-reliance to grotesque extremes of meanness. Establishing an income floor for LTC would undermine "burden" discourses. Endowing people with an independent and respectable old age would weaken sexism, ageism, ableism, dementism, and classism. Being assured of that floor enables a person standing respectably on it to achieve other states of being that she has reason to desire, as Amartya Sen, the economist who discovered female "extra deaths," explained. John Rawls's *A Theory of Justice* encouraged readers to reconceive society as if they might find themselves on the bottom. Until I wrote this book, I didn't know how many bottoms there were, or where that deep basement could be found.

After the Eldercide and the million other COVID deaths, a national and portable LTC insurance program should have been inevitable. Given the strife of forces, it is barely on the national radar.

STATE BY STATE
MONEY FOLLOWS THE PERSON

The next-best, or least-bad, options go, as ever, state by state. "Medicaid is firmly anchored in the states, even more so as a result of the ongoing devolution of power since 1980," Laura Katz Olson explains. Unfortunately, "localities have a glaring inability to lead the way" because of fiscal constraints: "virtually all [the states] require balanced budgets." Our social contract thus depends on fifty crazy-quilt exhibits of uneven interest in impoverished old folks and their safety, well-being, health, and housing.

Money Follows the Person (MFP) is a national program: still "welfare"—but the novelty is that it helps eligible persons move out of hospitals or institutions into their own homes or "the least restrictive setting possible," as the law requires. Bill Henning told me that his private nonprofit, the Boston Center for Independent Living, was one of the fiscal conduits and provided the counselors needed in today's overheated real estate market. The money went for essentials:

First and last month's rent. Support in housing search. Furniture. Support for extra services during a transition. Food for a month. Moving costs. Lots of critical things, and it worked, the number of transitions increased a lot.

Caregivers visit MFP participants at their own homes. Mike Batista, an AARP Montana director, says, "There is a dignity that comes with aging in the home one's spent their entire adult life paying for." It's where helpful neighbors and familiar streets are found. In Montana there's a waiting list two hundred people long for the services. (Vera had sold her last valuable asset, her house. In her state, she might have languished at the bottom of a waiting list.) When a 2022 bill made MFP 100 percent federally funded, only twenty states took advantage of it. In Massachusetts, MFP returned in 2023, for four years, for a minuscule number of people: only up to six hundred a year. The number still living in the facilities was down to thirty-one thousand in 2022. Of these, 21,000 are on Medicaid; many wish to live elsewhere.

The Center for Public Representation, a national public-interest law firm, filed a class action lawsuit, now known as *Marsters v. Healey*, that sought to compel Massachusetts

> to expand its existing residential programs so that people with disabilities in nursing facilities [including medical conditions, physical disabilities, and mental illness] can . . . have meaningful options to live successfully in the community.

In April 2024 CPR won a quicker settlement than anyone had imagined, which slowly, over eight years, will give up to 2,400 such residents the chance to get out. During the Eldercide, people who needed post-acute care and anxious others found alternatives: occupancy of nursing facilities went down from 81 percent before COVID to 68 percent in 2022. A state's funding ratio still could remain unbalanced toward institutional rather than home-based care. The industry is doing fine financially; it is slated to grow faster than inflation as the so-called Boomers grow older. State legislators' bias toward keeping needy people in a privatized market confers unfair power on the chains: One weapon against regulation is threatening to close facilities. Threats scare honest legislators, conscientious departments of health, and CMS. And the bias denies the public's deep desire to age in place: 88 percent of people over sixty-five would prefer to do so.

LET NO ONE DIE UNDER A BRIDGE

Even if every state funded Money Follows the Person and found housing to deinstitutionalize residents who were eligible and wanted to move (a utopia) the nation would still need some minimal number of skilled nursing facilities. Low-income and even middle-income families are rarely capable of providing 24/7 care at home for members with multiple chronic or terminal illnesses or disabilities. Some people don't have families. Some will become homeless. A county executive in Pennsylvania, Lamont McClure, knows where the bottom is. "There are 400 people in the county every year who have nowhere else to go," McClure said, "and as long as I'm here, they're not going to die under bridges."

In 2020 Dr. David Gifford, a geriatrician, described the nation's facilities with exuberant practicality as

> an incredible asset in the health care delivery system. There are about 3200 counties, and there's a nursing home in almost every county in the country. And in many counties, they are the largest health care delivery system in that county. And . . . you have a physical building, you have staff, you have transportation vehicles there.

Investors had cottoned on. Right after the start of the pandemic, when buyers might have shied away from the contamination of "death houses," "a continued frenzy of transactions" found large private companies buying them up. Real estate broker Josh Jandris understood the allure: "The best opportunity when buying an asset is . . . buying from a not-for-profit seller, because the dynamics are in your favor. You have really strong occupancy, you typically have a very good reputation, you have high revenue . . . what everybody wants."

The value of these "assets"—as well as the need to eliminate the ongoing evildoers—suggests to serious planners that the entire failed hybrid system is ripe for nationalization as a public authority.

A NATIONAL SOLUTION II

A secretary of elder *and* disability affairs could head the new public authority, sit in the cabinet, and report to the president. It's efficient to reconfigure a program that serves overlapping populations. The secretary would be a renowned public servant with high-level expertise rather than partisan political sway. The office would need to possess credibility and independence—and a secure revenue stream.

The supreme benefit of a federal department is that it would prevent the ongoing Eldercide. It would put 1.2 million current residents in the spotlight, out from under HHS and CMS, where they so easily get lost. Twenty-five separate agencies now regulate aging services alone, without including others for people with disabilities.

In lieu of the fifty-state mishmash, this new department would avoid the fluctuations of state budgets—the instinct at budget-balancing time to, say, keep the Personal Needs Allowance stingy. It would expand successful programs kept spotty by grudging states. It would provide sufficient funding and oversight of the survey process. Ongoing failures to take responsibility operationalize abandonment.

The authority could close demoralizing, anachronistic buildings built on the old hospital long-corridor model and, with help from Housing and Urban Development and income from sales of unneeded assets, replace them with small houses that integrate justly paid aides into the residents' daily lives. Small homes offering skilled care and a cook—"community homes"—house ten to twelve people. The aides in the Green Houses—called shahbazim—read to them, walk and play games with them, and help them make decisions for themselves. Employees tend to stay. Residents' better health and higher satisfaction lower costs and improve ratings.

Government ownership would prevent sudden closures, common whenever private investors buy only to flip, or when they drive a facility into bankruptcy. Displaced residents must all too quickly scatter, find a more distant facility, shelter with their unprepared families, or, indeed, end up homeless, under bridges.

A public authority would ipso facto eliminate private equity and the industry's lobby, with its history of derailing improvements. In a "surreal lawsuit," when New York nursing-home owners were given a profit maximum, they sued: it turned out they make nearly a billion dollars a year understaffing homes and shortchanging patients; they want to prove that the state's clawing some of it back is an illegal "taking."

Behind the sidelining of urgent bills, the knuckling under to the industry, Laura Katz Olson writes, there is often a seductive lobbyist talking into the ear of legislators, "crying wolf" about money and "conflating their [business] needs with those of Medicaid recipients."

A celebrated neurologist told me he had discovered, when serving on a committee in Ohio, that some legislators traded stocks or had ownership positions in the facilities they were regulating. Nationalization would bring democratic control to this warped and corrupting system.

Nationalization would also mean intelligent planning (say, for where new facilities need to be located). No accountancy scams or tax evasion. No need for a sketchy profit ceiling. No evasion of unionizing. No evictions of people with more severe disabilities or Alzheimer's. No avoiding low-income or rural regions. The new system could make civil servants out of medical directors, nurses, aides, and managers, with a corresponding rise in their sense of professional responsibility.

Finally, nationalization would eliminate the element of state capture. Conservatives have long attempted to "destroy the New Deal project" of safety nets and instead subject programs like Medicaid "to a neoliberal, free-market model." Martha Patterson-Cohen, a gerontologist, explains why a degree of state capture appears permanent. "Neoliberalism is a political philosophy resulting in state policy that supports private interests. It has become the power tool of capitalists to prop up an economic system which ignores society, demands individualism, and justifies this destructive system by convincing people that this is 'freedom.'"

Like national LTC insurance, no one believes that nationalizing care for those who need it, under whatever euphemism, is in the cards. But it's always a good time to excite public enthusiasm with bold imaginings.

IN ONE STATE

WHAT WOULD A GEN Z VERA NEED?

WHAT WILL SHE GET?

Meanwhile, incremental "reform" of facilities occurs unevenly, state by state. A state holds the right and powers to specify the services owners produce. Massachusetts is a progressive state. It is one of the richest states in the country, in terms of income per capita and similar measures. By the end of the legislative session in 2023, what was Massachusetts able to accomplish for a Vera of today or any future indigent Gen Z Vera, and in what did it fail?

Vera's top desire was a private room with her own bath, after the *small-house* model. Some people prefer a companion; otherwise, the arguments for single rooms, for safety, privacy, and self-esteem, are strong. Lawmakers passed a bond issue ($400 million) to give veterans in the Holyoke Soldiers Home, which had received stinging publicity, single rooms in a renovated facility with fresh amenities. For nursing-home residents, there was no bond issue. The best bill the legislators could pass mandated no more than *two* people to a room. Many owners of facilities (two-thirds with low ratings) protested even that, although the system has thousands of empty beds. In 2023 the owners took the issue to court.

Safety is the supreme requirement. The word "safety" may sound vague, but nothing is more basic than appropriate staffing. It means *keeping people alive.* A thorough 2001 report to Congress included the effects of understaffing. A resident with quadriplegia who was ventilator dependent told inspectors he asked for help at night when he needed suctioning: "Two minutes not being able to breathe is scary. . . . I timed them [staff] one night and it took them 28 minutes to answer my call light."

Extra staff minutes a day may seem too few to fuss about, but they make the difference between life and death, every day. A Connecticut study found that even a twenty-minute increase in care offered by staff may translate into 22 percent fewer deaths in those facilities. "In the often-contentious world of nursing home policy . . . [the need for adequate staff numbers is] one thing everyone agrees on," Professor Konetzka told the Senate hearing on "A National Tragedy." "Even perfect infection-control procedures will not improve safety of nursing-home residents without the staff to implement them."

For the residents personally, at a minimum, appropriate staffing means getting meds and food on time; receiving frequent help with bathing; not being drugged; having an aide who has time to speak to you. Such modest desires are not beyond good government; in fact, facilities are tasked, in an idealistic way, with enabling residents' "goals, preferences and values" Attentive care necessitates training. CMS had once obliged nurse aides to undergo at least seventy-five hours of it. Come COVID, CMS waived the requirement. Then they restored it. Massachusetts was one of seventeen states that asked to be kept on the lower standard. What adherence to a care plan can there be if your state prefers picayune training requirements? Massachusetts also rates badly for inflicting antipsychotics on inmates—oversedation is another common result of inadequate staffing—but its hundreds of facilities received zero harm citations for drug overuse.

The leader of Moving Forward, Alice Bonner, who served two years as director of the Division of Nursing Homes in CMS under Obama, believes surveillance is key to ensuring safety. Inspectors, with unfettered access and authority to issue citations, are lacking. Federal funding has been stagnant since 2015. Massachusetts is chronically listed in the bottom 10 percent of states, late in holding inspections and late in resolving complaints. The Department of Public Health (DPH) has three thousand employees across a patchwork of agencies responsible for nursing facilities: for example, licenses, funding, ombudsman— but not enough inspectors. Eighty-two nursing-home inspectors were shouldering the highest caseload of any state in New England. They are supposed to drop in at intervals of no more than fifteen months— shorter intervals would be safer—but in 2023 thirty-two homes hadn't had a recertification survey since 2019. Those who call DPH a failed agency point to the Division of Health Care Facility Licensure and Certification, where latent powers sleep.

"Safety" for residents also requires competitive wages and benefits for aides. The grim turnover rate in nursing homes in the Before Time should alone have indicted low pay for lethal risk to residents. If the federal minimum wage had been even 10 percent higher, Krista Ruffini, an economist at Georgetown University, estimates there would have been fifteen thousand fewer resident deaths in the short months between February and mid-May 2020, possibly the deadliest part of that terrifying year.

In Massachusetts, "a staggering 1 in 5 of all the people living in senior care sites before the pandemic" died of COVID in the first year. Taking responsibility, Massachusetts became the first state to mandate that 75 percent of owners' revenues go to patient-facing care (defined here as nursing, dietary care, restorative therapy, and social work). Reformers suggest that revenue might in fact cover *true costs* if they could only be ascertained. Is that mandate working? No consolidated audit has been done, but at the latest self-report (2022), almost a third of state facilities admitted to spending less than required.

"MAY YOUR HANDS BE STRONG" (HEBREW PRAYER)

The people striving for reform are indefatigable and resolute. Together they represent thousands of years of research and intense experiences. Almost everyone became radicalized by the accelerated horrors of institutional care in spring 2020. One economist told me she became "obsessed." Assemblyman Ron Kim of Queens, a passionate advocate, whose uncle died in a nursing facility in 2020, called the nationwide catastrophe "a mass murder." Something happened to which advocates cannot reconcile themselves. They do not forget.

In my state, a broad coalition (with experience in disability, elder and veterans' affairs, home care, nursing facilities, mental health, Alzheimer's, ethics, medicine, law, and housing) came together, amazingly, amid the pandemic chaos of 2020. As soon as I discovered Dignity Alliance Massachusetts, I read their cogent position papers; I joined their meticulously well-organized biweekly Zoom meetings. Organizations that advocate on behalf of the poor are scarce. I came to admire the group for their pooled knowledge, total sincerity, egalitarianism, ability to lighten up and keep going, collective hope, and relentless activism.

Paul Lanzikos is the steady co-chair of the Zoom meetings. A former head of Elder Affairs when it had the governor's ear, he produces forward motion: agendas, the alliance's informative website, the weekly *Dignity Digest* that attracts a thousand readers. Bill Henning, also part of the alliance, with a wry look on his lean face, radiates irony and good sense from the Boston Center for Independent Living.

Dick Moore, former state senator and chair of the Joint Legislative Committee on Health Care Financing, a calm humorist, provides expertise to turn the alliance's endorsements into legislative acts. Arlene Germain, she of the curly white hair, ready smile, and scrupulous accuracy, supplies the learned footnotes. With others, Germain had originally run family-led councils in loved ones' facilities. What they observed led them to found Massachusetts Advocates for Nursing Home Reform (MANHR). For twenty years, MANHR was the *only* such group. Then Dignity opened a bigger umbrella.

Dignity folks are pragmatic. They plan concretely. (In 2022 members interviewed all candidates for statewide offices, after asking them to put their plans for the facilities in writing. Members are trusted to be wonky; they meet and speak frankly to the new officials the Maura Healey administration brought in.) Doggedness, not passion, is a requisite for activism. Most of all, in an NGO without funding, these volunteers are disinterested.

In 2022, an election year, when reform was supposed to occur all over America, not much happened. In October, tireless New York State representative Ron Kim told Gray Panthers NYC bluntly, "We are failing."

2023

The next year, in Massachusetts, some progress was made but not in staffing. Howls from the lobby prevented the 3.58-hour state standard from rising even to 4.1, according to Dick Moore, former state senator. It had been three years since the pandemic began. If your mother had an untreated wound on her heel or got a shower only every few weeks, would you want to wait three *days* for a remedy, let alone three *years*?

Many items that Dignity advocated passed. The legislature had a historically high amount of money to dole out, $56 billion. It earmarked 0.2 percent of that amount, almost a fifth of all additional monies allocated to nursing homes, to support wages and training for direct-care staff. $14,300,000 went for investments in home-health nursing rates, to bolster that workforce.

One form of resident dumping needed to be stymied: finding that you cannot get back into your half room after a hospital stay or a visit outside. So: "No nursing home shall reassign a patient's bed during a [reimbursable] leave of absence." That assurance had been long withheld; in 2024 it may pass. There's an overlooked regulation that closing a facility requires giving residents at least three months' notice; this regulation may now get enforced. A sum of $500,000 was allocated to study LTC funding programs. Using her independent power, the new attorney general, Andrea Campbell, opened an Office of Elder Justice and staffed it.

Promising, yes, but few in the know consider these outcomes "transformational." What was forgotten? Converting double into single rooms. Mandating that 90 percent of revenue go to patient-facing care. Improving staffing ratios for people with traumatic brain injuries or who are dangers to others. LTC workforce training and career paths, to reduce turnover. Requiring CNAs to get 120 hours of training instead of seventy-five. Raising the Personal Needs Allowance, still flat at $78.20 a month when, after decades of inflation, it should be at least $160. Air conditioning, as New England's burning summers heat up the residents' tiny spaces and endanger their lives.

Massachusetts's appalling Eldercide in 2020 and the current issues belie the state's reputation for progressivism, its admired medical and surgical care, and the relative wealth of its citizens. Its long, painful record of underserving residents may derive from executive unwillingness to enforce regulations, donations from nursing-home executives (Governor Baker received $52,510 and House Speaker Robert DeLeo $47,170 in the year before May 2020, according to the Office of Campaign and Political Finance), legislative lethargy, and a Department of Public Health that has been lax and uncoordinated.

For 2024, the $56 billion surge in revenue resulted from a bonanza of tax dollars, CARES and American Rescue Plan money, and the first tranche of the state's "Millionaires' Tax." Governor Healey's windfall achieved free school lunches for children and made community college free for people over twenty-five; a billion and a half dollars (in surplus) went into the Rainy-Day Fund. Pride over popular accomplishments keeps blinders on for low-priority people. Compound ageism makes failures expectable and sidelines reformers. When the session's legislative opportunities had ended, one leader of the nursing-facility transformation movement told me bluntly, "We got crumbs."

A TITANIC DOMESTIC WAR

On September 1, 2023, the Biden White House boldly acknowledged the pitiful situation, saying, "The nursing home industry receives nearly $100 billion annually from American taxpayers, yet too many nursing homes chronically understaff their facilities—resulting in poor, sub-standard care that endangers residents." In this way the Eldercide— even if no one named it as such—became a "publicly known fact," a gash in the entrenched system's polished surfaces. Even so, James Butler, a media expert, warns, "The road from publicly known fact to political consequence is even less travelled."

Biden's State of the Union speech had raised hopes about the most crucial safety issue—staffing. Congress has never set a national staffing floor. The last relevant gesture took place in 2001, when a Congressional commission was followed by CMS merely *preferring*, rather than requiring, 4.1 hours of staffing per person per day, below which quality of care would be compromised. Advocates, having watched twenty years of government inaction, were braced for disappointment. The for-profit lobby often lavishly lays out over $100 million a year. In 2021, only 6 percent of US nursing homes achieved 4.1 hours per person. Inspectors rarely cite any facility for "insufficient staffing": that charge accounted for just 1 percent of citations in 2018–2020. Meanwhile, the meaningful minimum number of hours per person per day that wise heads suggest is in fact now 4.55—actual contact time, adjusted for case mix and including nights and weekends.

On September 1, 2023, with Biden's confident, soothing imprimatur—"We're ending the abuse today," he wrote in *USA Today*—his CMS finally announced a standard: 3.0 hours. The for-profits were livid at being regulated at all. Their allies threatened that the extra expense of direct-contact salaries would cause many places to close: "Hundreds of thousands of vulnerable residents . . . could be forced out." Some advocates and organizations politely said Biden's three hours were "a start." The forthright position of Dignity Alliance Massachusetts was that the proposed rule "does not go far enough to protect nursing home residents and nursing home staff." They argued plausibly to CMS that "these additional staffing requirements are financially feasible, since the costs would be less than five percent of the more than $100 billion that nursing homes receive from Medicare and Medicaid annually." When the Biden administration announced the final number of care hours per person in April 2024, the rule had been adjusted *up*, amazingly, to 3.48 hours. It will take years to go into effect. Some reformers were still aghast that the per-person care level would remain, as experts had said about the 3.0 standard, "dangerously inadequate."

Is it likely that 2024 will mark the start of an Era of Nursing Home Reform? As of the latest information, nearly three-quarters, or 260 of Massachusetts facilities, fell below the state's slightly higher 3.58 standard. The state seems unable to compel the mandate. Seventy-two facilities (20 percent) even fell below Biden's original three-hour standard. To discover if the historic 3.48 rule will provide any improvement for you and your loved ones, consult a readable map that shows your state's minimum staffing level, if any. Mississippi, Vermont, and others have had no minimum. Whether in old age or disability you are likely to be abused or comforted, live or die, should not depend on whether your state has the will to enforce the new national mandate, hire enough surveyors to uncover wrongs, and follow the *Marsters* settlement in helping low-income older people and people with disabilities remain in or return to their own communities.

SAD CEMETERIES

In the years since 2020–2021, as the mortality counting dwindled and then entirely disappeared, the residents faded out of public notice. Media attention had wandered away, like sheep without a shepherd.

The residents were still dying or enduring long COVID or PTSD, but as a group they were no longer *linked* to dying or *seen* as suffering.

The years of fear, psychic abandonment, and distraction traumatized many Americans and atomized us. Creating a warmer social embrace of currently imperiled residents requires that we not shun them because their helplessness reminds us of our own, the frightening state of childlike weakness into which the pandemic threw every sentient person on the globe. Recovery seems uneven and slow. People want to "move on." Even good souls may look away from misery, humiliation, and squalor they cannot alleviate through public policy.

Some sorrows never find their fit audience. Some shames never create a meaningful monument. Marguerite Yourcenar, in a novel narrated by a grieving man, wrote, "Memory for most people is an abandoned graveyard. There rest the dead they did not cherish enough. Anyone prolonging their grief insults the forgetful, who wish to abandon those sad cemeteries."

Apathy, corruption, and ideology might not carry the day without the backstop of compound ageism. If a society like ours cannot provide security and comfort to a mere million people on the bottom, it has little hope of curing compound ageism, the most acceptable and unnoticed of our social plagues.

IF NOT NOW, WHEN?

[After] institutional failure to act in the face of spectacular . . . violence[, here are] the characteristic patterns of response: eventual acknowledgment, but only after a long delay; a call for action, but later, not now, at some point when the timing is better; reform, but in a way that advertises good intentions while protecting established interests; hope that the most recent scandal will not be repeated, so that the exclamation "this is not [on] us" may actually possess some truth.

CHRISTOPHER BROWN

This portrait of guilty pious governments, by Christopher Brown, a professor of history, fits the story of the Eldercide. The unconscionable mortality of the residents—now said to amount to two hundred thousand dead—constituted "spectacular violence." The institutional failures include Trump's delays, denials, and lies; CMS's dry, bland equivocations about oversight; the Republican drive to stabilize the economy by plowing under the bones of older adults; the granting of immunity from prosecution to thousands of facilities that had been unscrupulously dilatory about safety; ageist medical triage around DNRs and ventilators. All too apt, then, the first sentence of Louise Erdrich's summary at the end of her historical novel *The Night Watchman*, about a Congressional attempt to end promises made to Native Americans: "Lastly, if you should ever doubt that a series of dry words in a government document can shatter spirits and demolish lives, let this book erase that doubt."

A titanic political war over assisting the neediest roils our democracy on many issues. In this case, on one side are the brute facts: the COVID catastrophe in the nursing facilities and the endless everyday failures of care that produce a devastating but scarcely visible eldercide, year in and year out. On the other side: a rich major industry tenaciously wooing legislators. The industry quickly found members of Congress to oppose the new staffing standard. The top experts at NASEM grasped that the ultimate issue was power. They wrote, "The pandemic has indeed 'lifted the veil' on US nursing homes. The big question is whether the country has the will to do anything about it." Every visionary of good will who is trying to foil the plunderers, up to and including this president, has until now fallen back onto what some call *compromise*, which amounts once again to "tinkering with small ways to make incremental improvements."

In the short term, the hidden maltreatment of eldercide continues in many places, *business as usual*. Anyone can predict a desperate fate for many. Tragically lost.

SPARKS

Yet the COVID Eldercide pricked consciences. All the hearings—Representative Doggett's in 2020, Senator Ron Wyden's on "A National

Tragedy" in 2021, Representative James Clyburn's in 2022, Senator Bob
Casey's "Uninspected and Neglected" in 2023—and the NASEM report may have provided Biden with humane backup. Given the chance,
Democratic political leaders may push harder. Senator Elizabeth Warren, at a hearing in 2024, spoke for reformers when she said, "During
the pandemic, private-equity-owned nursing homes had a 40 percent higher Covid mortality rate than other nursing homes. I'll say
it bluntly: turning private equity loose in our health care system kills
people." "What was immoral will be illegal," Senator Ed Markey foretold, of his newly proposed Health over Wealth Act.

Collective memory is tricky. Inside, we the people may hoard burning shame or clamor for reparation. In the deepest ash lie the sparks
of the fiercest fire. In the AIDS crisis of the Reagan 1980s, ACT UP's
broad coalition raged into effectiveness because it showed firsthand
how abandonment by the state could kill. Now, alas, because of the
Eldercide, we have the same kind of evidence. The voices this book
presents may be heard. The living, like the dead, are saying, *Can you
give me back my old age?* Our society may recognize that odious conditions and unnecessary deaths are unnatural; their sociopolitical, financial, and discursive agents can be opposed, and some could be
brought to judgment.

The time is right for Erdrich's final audacity in *The Night Watchman*:
"Conversely, if you should be of the conviction that we are powerless
to change those dry words, let this book [about a tribe's successful re-
sistance] give you heart."

A valiant civic constituency has girded up. Against the documents
that betrayed the residents are other watchdog documents (hundreds
cited in the endnotes) that tirelessly educate and promote remedies.
After canvassing the members, Dignity Alliance Massachusetts wrote
up a 2025 budget for Governor Healey based on still-outstanding
needs. When advocates appear to lose ground, they do not lose heart.
Name any similar group—the eight hundred allies of Moving Forward
or the thousands of Marked by COVID, the National Consumer Voice
for Quality Long-Term Care, the National Center for Medicare Advocacy, the Long Term Care Community Coalition, Elder Justice Coa-

lition, AARP, Justice in Aging—and you will find them busy creating the genuine solidarity that has eluded Congress so far. The election of 2024 could open another opportunity to renovate nursing facilities and invent long-term care, perhaps only state by state, perhaps nationwide.

Even more conclusively than before COVID, the current 1,200,000 residents stand in for all the rest of us. Supporting them strengthens our campaigns against the escalating issues of *simple* ageism—the kind that millions now growing older may well face in "aging America."

The war against simple ageism is only in its first decades of vital resistance. Social justice movements take decades to succeed, if they do. Some groups win a right (like abortion, or pre-clearance for voting) and then lose it. Age-justice and disability-justice activists, like others, however, possess mysterious ethical and emotional sources. Memory goes on raging inside them. The war almost always goes on.

Goodness can be defined as listening to suffering, defying frustration, and making the wisest next strategic moves as efficiently as possible. Let us take heart from the grieving and aggrieved relatives and friends who cry for action; from the growing number of agewise younger activists and the countless ally organizations around the globe who take up the anti-ageist cause; and especially from the undaunted reformers, dug in for the long term to pursue age justice. Ever growing in numbers, they fight on, reminding us tirelessly that older people have an equal right to live. We find ourselves churning toward a vast, slow, thorough, blessed transformation of human consciousness. The great wave of true caring moves ahead.

April 2024

UNDERCOUNTING THE DEATHS OF RESIDENTS

One final word of warning . . . figures have limitations. . . . There can be no statistics unless someone has first done the counting. . . . All statistics are answers to specific and extremely narrow questions and if they are used to answer other questions, whether in their crude form or after more or less sophisticated manipulation, they must be used with extreme caution.

E. J. HOBSBAWM, *Industry and Empire*

"The true toll of COVID-19 on nursing home residents may never be known . . . [A]lthough current measures of COVID-19 prevalence and mortality reflect a devastating public health crisis for the nursing home population, it is likely that even more lives were impacted," Dr. Elizabeth White of the Brown University School of Public Health concluded in a *JAMA* article in September 2021, commenting on the absence of complete and reliable data.

Any estimates of the COVID dead in the nursing facilities are unquestionably undercounts. I use 112,300 for the first year, 2020. The federal underreporting of residents' deaths in that year is estimated to have lost at least 16,000 people. The toll would then be not 112,300 but 128,300. Another estimate, from only thirty-nine states, up to May 28, 2020, adds 40,000 more, or 152,000 resident deaths in just 2020.

No one can know the true totals, for many reasons. The overriding one seems to be that the public is not meant to know what went on in the spring of 2020. The earliest and most significant cause of the failure is that from January 2020 until May 24, 2020, the Centers for Medicaid and Medicare Services (CMS) was not requiring statistics from the facilities. These were the same months when CMS investigations had partially ceased. This lapse of months in data collection was not corrected. "Retroactive reporting is not mandatory, and the accuracy of reporting at the state level is unknown," was the caution on the AARP Nursing Home Dashboard in 2021.

Representative James Clyburn's House Select Subcommittee on the Coronavirus Crisis, having tried to obtain accurate counts of cases and deaths directly, from only five of the largest chains (including Life Care), concluded that the chains' "use of convoluted corporate structures may have helped to obscure profits and avoid legal and regulatory accountability." The way that CMS asked for infections and deaths made it harder to attribute responsibility because it allowed data to appear "under names and corporate structures that can obscure common ownership."

CDC's National Center for Health Statistics is supposed to capture all deaths from all causes across the nation in their Vital Statistics System. In Massachusetts, cities record death certificates and send them to the Registry of Vital Statistics. States register all death certificates.

States had different rules for reporting COVID-19 deaths. Often the counts were not uniformly disaggregated by race or gender. Some states did not ask the owners of facilities they allegedly monitored how many residents had died in their location. Some health departments reported the number of COVID deaths in nursing homes but not in a format easy to understand. (Other state reports of COVID data obfuscated the residents' deaths, a central concern of this book, by sometimes including deaths of staff and/or all people in assisted living and other elder housing: These locations are not under government control.) Some news sources also reported such inclusive, confounding data. As long as counting continued, this practice blurred the residents' death counts. It had the effect of diminishing the gravity of nursing-facility mortality and hiding the responsibility of the owners.

Lack of transparency is a long-term problem. Incomparability of data crucially weakens public health policy.

Some states—notoriously New York and Massachusetts—found ways to fudge the count of residents' deaths to make the toll seem less horrifying. As of September 2020, the *Boston Globe* reported that 66 percent of the state's 9,160 COVID deaths had been residents of LTC facilities—a worse record than that of most states.

Massachusetts then changed the way it counted this data. "On April 14 [2021], Massachusetts had one of the highest reported nursing home COVID-19 death rates in the country, with 9,018 [*sic*] dead. The next day, it plummeted 39 percent to 5,502, according to the official state count," Kay Lazar reported for the *Boston Globe* in a story that exposed the change and raised serious questions. Under the headline "How the Baker Administration Ill Serves Those in Elder Care," the drastic drop was also reported by GBH News. As of November 10, 2022, Massachusetts reported cumulative deaths in nursing homes as 6,223 (2,509 men and 3,338 women), with staff deaths at 24. With total state deaths reported as 20,697, nursing-facility deaths still stood at an extraordinary 30 percent. Soon after, counting them stopped.

States sometimes presented readers with huge, unwieldy data sets. The Massachusetts Department of Health did a preposterously opaque and frustrating job of reporting the COVID mortality. In 2020, the legislature forced on it the reporting system known as "Chapter 93." As of December 2021, this spreadsheet listed every nursing home in the state, but the number of deaths in each was often presented within a 1 to 4 range. There was no way to determine actual COVID deaths even approximately.

Different states defined deaths of people in long-term care differently. The COVID tracker from *Atlantic.org* reported in September 2020 that "New York, for example, reports LTC deaths only when they occur in a facility, not when an LTC resident is transported to the hospital and dies there." Further contributing to the underestimation of LTCF deaths is that in March and part of April 2020, while testing for COVID was largely unavailable, COVID deaths were counted as such only if backed by a positive test. The *Atlantic* noted that if states all used consistent reporting rules, "the official death count in LTCs would likely be substantially higher."

Counting deaths in a consistent way nationally was also obstructed by a technological problem. Each state health department buys its own computer tracking systems, and it makes its data decisions without any coordination. Many states end up with databases that do not connect easily to their other systems or to the CDC. So data does not "flow"; instead, it's been described as a series of manual hops, skips, and jumps through disjointed systems. This fact demonstrates the fifty-state "crazy quilt" described earlier.

Absence of data weakens activism. On March 7, 2021, the *Atlantic's* Covid Tracking Project closed down. The *Boston Globe* stopped reporting the death toll in Massachusetts nursing homes in 2021. AARP provided resident mortality data state by state, updated monthly, into 2022. On December 4, 2023, the Massachusetts legislature repealed Chapter 93 reporting.

Is it right to blame the media, as I do, for overemphasizing the astonishing totals in nursing-home mortality and point out, as I do, the error of government agencies as well, in making residents and then people fifty and over seem uniquely compromised? Defenders can argue that in the COVID Era, data *was* the story. The story of mortality, however unreliable, was gripping and staggering. The rapidly rising totals of resident deaths in the spring of 2020 certainly caught my attention, and they led many besides me to wonder why so many were dying and, perhaps, who was responsible. *Why* and *who* are the first "upstream" questions.

I do mention one other benefit of the media focus on sensational data. By alarming the public week after week, month after month, the press presumably put pressure on a slack government and on unprepared facilities to develop a reliable test, do more testing, and get usable PPE to the facilities. If such pressure was the intent, the intent was honorable and left a record of government failure.

My counterargument, probably clear long before this, is that by ignoring the data that this book makes much of—the huge percentage of survivors and the likelihood that most deaths were premature—and by failing to collect the oral histories of the survivors (many brave and resilient, some desperate, some rationally complaining), the media reinforced the image of frailty and attached it to all older adults. Thus, they abetted the sense that medical care for the older population is futile, and they amply contributed to the heightened ageisms of the ongoing COVID Era.

Moreover, insofar as the media discontinued the nursing-home story at a time when legislators were considering doing something to fix it, journalism abetted forgetfulness and continued the lethal neglect of the main issues.

ACKNOWLEDGMENTS

I thank Tim Hartman, the artist whose cartoon illuminates not just chapter 2 but the entire section "Instead," who graciously revised the work and gave permission for its use.

My indefatigable first-stage editors, David Gullette, Connie Wilson Higginson, and Andrea Petersen, see new work before anyone else and help me avoid pitfalls. Connie provided line edits with her sharp precision tools. Andrea offered big-picture notes and searching queries. David reads with his fine ear for tone, nuance, grammar—everything. Vega Gullette valuably helped at the proof stage.

Many short-form editors recognized the importance of the topic early. Boris Dralyuk of the *Los Angeles Review of Books* published my articles on "Ageism in America," as he called the series, in 2020. *Tikkun*, led by Rabbi Michael Lerner, published my earliest piece of fact-based outrage in April 2020. A section about Biden's failure to mention residents in his commemorations was originally published on WBUR's *Cognoscenti*, thanks to my editor, Cloe Axelson. On December 7, 2020, thanks to editor Rich Eisenberg, *Next Avenue* published my piece "Why We Need a COVID-19 Memorial to Those Who Died in Long-Term Care Facilities." In early 2021, *Dissent* first published an article about failures in the history of nursing facilities, which was then reprinted by the American Society on Aging and in *The Long Year:*

A 2020 Reader (Columbia University Press, 2022), edited by Thomas J. Sugrue and Caitlin Zaloom. *Theory, Culture and Society* 35, no. 7–8 (December 2018) published a first version of chapter 8 under the title "Against 'Aging': How to Talk about Growing Older." My thanks to editor Mike Featherstone, a leader in studying ageism along with our mutual friend, the late Mike Hepworth.

My Brandeis Social Issues group was crucial to the development of the book, starting in January 2021, when Helen Berger, Jan Friedman, Selina Gallo-Cruz, Ruth Nemzoff, Robin Robinson, and Phoebe Schnitzer gave me feedback on a trade book proposal. With important additions over time—Edie Cheers, Ama Saran, Mei-Ling Ellerman, Shane Snowdon—the group then read chapter after chapter. I have never before had the luck of having a book read by a whole group with such varied disciplinary backgrounds and interests.

In casual conversation and in an interview, Derrick Jackson provided important ideas. He and Michelle Holmes believed in the mission and saw its deep connections to anti-racism. Dr. Holmes's activism also influenced my thinking about the 2020 triage guidelines and about many puzzling theory intersections.

Marlene Goldman read the prologue and chapter 1 at an early stage and said the sentences were like "sledgehammers," which encouraged me with the writing. Ruth Ray Karpen's reading of the prologue delicately led me to better expression. The emails of Andy Wengraf, one of my high school friends, provided pithy, usable commentaries and articulated his political wisdom.

Harry (Rick) Moody wrote me and forwarded relevant materials as a philosopher and sage, a gerontologist, a director of the Institute for Positive Aging at the International Longevity Center (New York) and friend of Robert Butler's, and as a general upbeat encourager. Paul Kleyman, of Generations Beat Online, let me pick his brain about the media, and he also cheered me on.

Ian (Matt) Nelson, research scholar at the Scripps Gerontology Center, Miami University of Ohio, gave generous help explaining the data; he and Jane Straker, director of research at Scripps, found the exact data points I needed amid the welter of problematic compilations.

Any mistakes are my own. Corinne Field asked a historian's pertinent, improving questions about gerontology and age studies.

My Brandeis interns, Vishni Samaraweera (spring and fall 2021 and fall 2022) and Allison Sukay (spring 2021) did important research. Vishni found some of the missing voices and provided the data proving how hard they were to find. Allison worked on the section of the COVID monument chapter that deals with the Equal Justice Institute. Sophia Koolpe and Ishaan Bhatia, also Brandeis students, provided important help in spring 2022. Vishni returned (fall 2022) for the hard detail and finish work of endnotes and bibliography. Wenli Cai patiently put the online bibliography into final shape (spring 2024).

Grant Ujifusa graciously answered all my questions about his roles in providing our capital with the memorial to the Japanese American internees and troops. Larry Langer, an eminence in Holocaust studies, answered questions about Holocaust writing. A distinguished physician, Phil Stubblefield, read the chapter on medical ageism. Scholars from numerous disciplines, nurses and physicians, leaders of reform groups, and social workers in nursing facilities responded to my queries with alacrity, truth, and positive energy.

More people than I can name became allies—providing not only materials but also encouragement: among them, memorably, Ashton Applewhite, Charlene Harrington, and Sheila Serio Lindenbaum. Dignity Alliance Massachusetts has been an invaluable resource. Arlene Germain read an early draft of the epilogue and provided data time and time again with great patience. She, Richard Moore, and Paul Lanzikos helped with insider wisdom.

Beth Vesel, an NYC agent, led me through writing a proper trade proposal and had faith in the importance of the book.

My University of Chicago editors, first Mary Al-Sayed and then Dylan Joseph Montanari, appreciated the mission of the book. Dylan guided me adroitly through the final stages of the approval process and gave good notes on the MS. Fabiola Enríquez Flores's concern for details matched my own. Jessica Wilson, a meticulous copy editor, made sure all the (hidden) endnotes would be useful. Brian Chartier, the book's designer, took my concept for the cover, a collage of faces, and made of it a powerful voice for the voiceless. Sean Gullette added a brilliant tweak to the interior design. The UCP publicity and marketing team further helped shepherd the book into the world. At the last minute, updates could be added thanks to the flexibility of the production team, especially Stephen Twilley and Sabrina Szos.

My thinking about certain concepts and about argumentation, and my search for a style adequate to the pain of the losses, the horror of the events, and the ironies of the responses, were aided, over the years of research and writing, by reading the work of Bryan Stevenson and Isabel Wilkerson, and by rereading the work of Hannah Arendt, James Baldwin, Vasily Grossman, George Orwell, Rebecca West, Edward Said, and Leo Tolstoy.

NOTES

The complete bibliography for this book appears online, at https://
press.uchicago.edu/sites/gullette/index.html.

DEDICATION

"ASKS ME NOT TO LET HIM DIE ALONE" Emmanuel Levinas, quoted in Judith Butler, *Precarious Life: The Powers of Mourning and Violence* (New York: Verso,
2004), 131.

PROLOGUE

"THINKING ABOUT THIS EVERY SINGLE DAY" Chris Kocher, "Healing Hearts—
Moving Forward from COVID-19 Loss," Gray Panthers webinar, Transformation Tuesday, December 14, 2021, organized by Jack Kupferman, https://www.youtube.com
/watch?v=USfd-FKEHg4&t=28s, at 30:00.

"WATCHING AN ENTIRE LIBRARY BURN" Virginia Hedrick, Zoom panel, California Consortium for Urban Indian Health (CUIH.org), February 12, 2021.

"A SYMBOL . . . OF NATIONAL COHERENCE AND INCLUSIVENESS" Simon
Biggs, quoted in Rüdiger Kunow, *Material Bodies: Biology and Culture in the United
States* (Heidelberg: Universitätsverlag Winter, 2018), 248.

50 PERCENT OR MORE OF DEATHS WERE OF RESIDENTS Rossana Lau-Ng,
Lisa B. Caruso, and Thomas T. Perls, "COVID-19 Deaths in Long-Term Care Facilities," *Journal of the American Geriatrics Society* 68 (2020): 1895–98.

1,700 HAD DIED Beth Schwartzapfel, Katie Park, and Andrew DeMillo, "1 in 5
Prisoners in the US Has Had COVID-19, 1,700 Have Died," *ABC News*, December 18,
2020.

AT LEAST 112,300 Blake Ellis and Melanie Hicken, "Government Action Took

Months as Nursing Home Employees Died," CNN, February 18, 2021. This figure of 112,300 was retrieved with help from Ian Matt Nelson, Research Scholar at Scripps Gerontology Center, Miami University of Ohio, Oxford, Ohio; see also "AARP Nursing Home COVID-19 Dashboard Fact Sheets," AARP Public Policy Institute, updated September 14, 2023, https://www.aarp.org/ppi/issues/caregiving/info-2020/nursing-home-covid-states.html.

ALL TRUE COUNTS OF THE 2020 COVID TOLL UNCERTAIN The Centers for Medicare and Medicaid did not ask for data from nursing facilities through the early months of 2020, which may have been the most deadly period. See the appendix.

"CASES ARE SO PROFOUNDLY CONCENTRATED" Mark S. Lachs, "COVID-19 and Aging, a Tale of Two Pandemics," *Nature Aging* 1 (January 14, 2021): 8–9.

"UNDERVALUED LIVES ARE LEFT UNDERPROTECTED" Howard Steven Friedman, quoted in Cass R. Sunstein, "What Price Is Right?" *New York Review of Books*, June 10, 2021.

"OFFERED FOR OUR ADMIRATION" Simone Weil, "The Iliad, or the Poem of Force," trans. Mary McCarthy, *Politics* (November 1945).

"SAID GOODBYE TO FIVE CLIENTS . . ." Elliot Kukla, "Where's the Vaccine for Ableism?" *New York Times*, February 4, 2021, https://www.nytimes.com/2021/02/04/opinion/covid-vaccine-ableism.html.

MOST WERE WHITE Priya Chidambaram, Tricia Neuman, and Rachel Garfield, "Racial and Ethnic Disparities in COVID-19 Cases and Deaths in Nursing Homes," *KFF.org*, October 27, 2020. CMS did not require nursing facilities to report race or ethnicity for COVID cases and deaths, making it difficult to document the full scope of the pandemic on residents of color.

IN 2016, 12 PERCENT OF THE CENTENARIANS WERE AFRICAN AMERICAN Administration for Community Living, US Department of Health and Human Services (hereafter HHS), *Profile of African Americans Age 65 and Over: 2017* (Washington, DC: Administration for Community Living, 2017).

AROUND 16 PERCENT WERE *YOUNGER* THAN SIXTY-FIVE Elaine K. Howley, "Nursing Home Facts and Statistics," *US News*, November 2, 2020. (2015–2016 data from National Center for Health Statistics.)

"THE BEST THING ABOUT . . ." Ponch Hawkes, quoted in Brigid Delaney, "Reclaiming Women's Bodies from Shame: A Photographic Illumination of Ageing," *Guardian*, March 8, 2021.

"ALL AGING IS 'SUCCESSFUL'" Ashton Applewhite, *This Chair Rocks* (Los Angeles, CA: Networked Books, 2016).

A BROAD SPECTRUM OF COGNITIVE ABILITIES Patrick Kutschar and Martin Weichbold, "Interviewing Elderly in Nursing Homes—Respondent and Survey Characteristics as Predictors of Item Nonresponse," *Survey Methods: Insights from the Field*, January 24, 2019.

ONLY 4 PERCENT SUFFERED FROM DELUSIONS Katie Thomas, Robert Gebeloff, and Jessica Silver-Greenberg, "Phony Diagnoses Hide High Rates of Drugging at Nursing Homes," *New York Times*, September 11, 2021.

CARDIAC DISEASE . . . IS THE MAIN ILLNESS RESIDENTS ARRIVE WITH "Cardiovascular Diseases Affect Nearly Half of American Adults, Statistics Show," *American Heart Association News*, January 31, 2019.

ON THE WALL OF ONE WARD-LIKE ROOM HANG . . . J. van Hoof, M. L. Janssen, C. M. C. Heesakkers, W. van Kersbergen, L. E. J. Severijns, and L. A. G. Willems, "The Importance of Personal Possessions for the Development of a Sense of Home of Nursing Home Residents," *Journal of Housing for the Elderly* 30, no. 1 (2016): 35–51. The objects I describe are mentioned in this article or in other articles or are visible in Web photos. One is invented.

"WANTING PLEASURE" Ashton Applewhite, in Sue Jaye Johnson, "The Pleasure Report," Substack newsletter, February 19, 2021.

MORE LIKELY TO FIND THEMSELVES IN A FACILITY Movement Advancement Project (MAP), "LGBT Older People and COVID-19: Addressing Higher Risk, Social Isolation, and Discrimination," issue brief, May 2020, https://www.lgbtmap.org/file /2020%20LGBTQ%20Older%20Adults%20COVID.pdf.

THE PBS DOCUMENTARY *SENIOR PROM* Luisa Conlon, dir., *Senior Prom* (Los Angeles, CA: JPC Films LLC and LC Productions LLC, 2021), premiered June 1, 2021, on the PBS show *Independent Lens*.

"THE SLOWEST-MOVING OF THE STIGMAS" Michael Bérubé, "Term Paper," *Profession* (November 2010): 115.

"TREAT US WITH PATIENCE, NOT HOSTILITY" Quoted in Susan McFadden, *Dementia-Friendly Communities* (London: Jessica Kingsley Publishers, 2020).

SANG IN CHORUSES Theresa A. Allison and Alexander K. Smith, "'Now I Write Songs': Growth and Reciprocity after Long-Term Nursing Home Placement," *Gerontologist* 60, no. 1 (February 2020): 135–44.

"A LOT OF COMFORT IN THAT" Allison Williams, "CNA Margaret Ditto Cares for Nursing Home Residents in Sickness and in Health," *SeattleMet*, March 30, 2021.

CNAS DO 90 PERCENT OF THE DAILY HANDS-ON WORK Emily Paulin, "Inside the 'Staffing Apocalypse' Devastating U.S. Nursing Homes," *AARP*, June 9, 2022.

MANY PERMANENT RESIDENTS WERE WELL ENOUGH . . . Meg Coffin, CEO, Center for Living and Working Inc., letter to the editor, *Boston Globe*, July 12, 2021.

SKILLED, RESPECTFUL CARE "Skilled Nursing Care: Case Studies," Hillsboro House, accessed February 2, 2024, https://hillsborohouse.org/about/skilled-nursing -care-case-studies/.

PSYCHOSOCIAL JOYS OF GROWING OLDER Louise Aronson, *Elderhood: Redefining Aging, Transforming Medicine, Reimagining Life* (New York: Bloomsbury, 2019), 255–56.

BIG MOVE Anne Marbury Wyatt-Brown, Ruth Ray Karpen, and Helen Q. Kivnick, *The Big Move: Life Between the Turning Points* (Bloomington: University of Indiana Press, 2016).

LEAVE THEIR PETS Tom Snee, "Animals and the Elderly: Law Professor Aims to Allow Nursing Home Residents to Have Pets," *Iowa Now*, June 11, 2012.

THERAPY . . . IS OFTEN UNAVAILABLE Margaret Morganroth Gullette, "Preventing American Eldercide: From Lethal Jeopardy toward Safety and Well-Being?" *Women and Therapy*, forthcoming 2024.

AN OUTRAGED DIATRIBE ON *LAST WEEK TONIGHT* John Oliver, "Long-Term Care: Last Week Tonight with John Oliver," aired April 12, 2021, on HBO, available at https://www.youtube.com/watch?v=2xlol-SNQRU.

IT'S A TREMENDOUS LUXURY Heather Davila, Weiwen Ng, Odichinma Akosionu, Mai See Thao, Tricia Skarphol, Beth A. Virnig, Roland J. Thorpe, and Tetyana P. Shippee, "Why Men Fare Worse: A Mixed-Methods Study Examining Gender Differences in Nursing Home Resident Quality of Life," *Gerontologist* 62, no. 9 (October 19, 2022): 1347–58.

FEEL SURPLUS Audre Lorde, "Age, Race, Class and Sex: Women Redefining Difference," paper delivered at the Copeland Colloquium, April 1980, Amherst College, Amherst, MA, reprinted in *Sister Outsider* (Berkeley, CA: Crossing Press, 1984).

WOULD "RATHER DIE" Thomas J. Mattimore, Neil S. Wenger, Norman A. Desbiens, Joan M. Teno, Mary Beth Hamel, Honghu Liu, Robert Califf, Alfred F. Connors Jr., Joanne Lynn, and Robert K. Oye, "Surrogate and Physician Understanding of Patients' Preferences for Living Permanently in a Nursing Home," *Journal of the American Geriatrics Society*, April 27, 2015.

"EVERYONE HAS HAD TO FIND SATISFACTIONS . . ." John Leland, "Notes from the End of a Very Long Life," *New York Times*, January 9, 2022.

"KEY CONSTITUENTS" A. N. Rahman and J. F. Shnelle, "The Nursing Home Culture-Change Movement: Recent Past, Present, and Future Directions for Research," *Gerontologist* 48 (2008): 142–48.

VALUED AT OVER $141 BILLION "Nursing Care Facilities in the US," *Ibis World*, August 30, 2022. The hospice industry was valued at $22 billion.

"EVERY DAY IS PRECIOUS" Marshall Keely, "Nursing Home Celebrates 6th Resident Reaching 100," *WNEP*, July 28, 2021.

"TEARS IN THE EYES?" Tyler Job, "La Crosse Healthcare Workers and Nursing Home Residents Talk about Experience after Getting COVID Vaccine," *News8oo*, January 21, 2021.

"NOBODY WANTS TO [DIE]" Allison Latos, "9 Investigates: Tracking COVID-19 Vaccines in Long-Term Care Facilities," *WSOC TV*, February 17, 2021.

"OLDER ADULTS DO NOT WANT TO STOP LIVING" Jasmine Travers, quoted in Amanda James, "Witnesses Recount 'Dire Conditions' in Nursing Homes during Covid-19 in Congressional Hearing," *MedCity News*, September 23, 2022.

CALCULATED AGEISM Anne E. Barrett, Cherish Michael, and Irene Padavic, "Calculated Ageism: Generational Sacrifice as a Response to the COVID-19 Pandemic," *Journals of Gerontology: Series B* 76, no. 4 (April 2021): e201–05. They looked at thousands of retweets and created a typology.

"*WHAT WAS I THINKING?*" Jane Miller, "At Home," *London Review of Books*, June 4, 2020.

"WHAT WE'VE SEEN ACROSS THE COUNTRY . . ." Ginger Christ, quoted in Alex

Kacik, "Beyond the Byline: How Residents' Stories Shape Our Coverage of the Vaccine Rollout," *Modern Healthcare*, February 5, 2021.

AN APPROACH SOME CRITICS CONSIDER TO BE OVERLY "MILITARISTIC" Danny R. George and Peter J. Whitehouse, "The War (on Terror) on Alzheimer's," *Dementia* 13, no. 1 (2014): 122.

A VENN DIAGRAM OF MULTIPLE OVERLAPPING OVALS Corinne Field helped me with this description via a series of emails, November 2021.

"IF IT HAPPENS TO A CHILD OR A DOG . . ." Tracey Pompey, quoted in Jayme Fraser and Nick Penzenstadler with Jeff Kelly Lowenstein, "Many Nursing Homes Are Poorly Staffed. How Do They Get Away with It?" *US News*, December 2, 2022.

"[THEY] ARE PART OF THE MAKE-UP OF MOST OF US . . ." George Orwell, "Notes on Nationalism," in *The Collected Essays, Journalism, and Letters of George Orwell Vol. III (1943–1945)*, ed. Sonia Orwell and Ian Angus (New York: Harcourt Brace Jovanovich, 1968), 380.

"WE DON'T HAVE TIME . . ." David Swanson, "Top Ten Things People Pretend They Don't Know," *Counterpunch*, January 11, 2022.

CHAPTER ONE

179,000 The toll of 163,128 nursing facility residents comes from "AARP Nursing Home COVID-19 Dashboard," AARP Public Policy Institute, updated May 18, 2023. Add sixteen thousand unreported deaths that occurred before May 24, 2020: Karen Shen, Lacey Loomer, Hannah Abrams, David C. Grabowski, and Ashvin Gandhi, "Estimates of COVID-19 Cases, Deaths among Nursing Home Residents Not Reported in Federal Data," *JAMA* 4, no. 9 (September 9, 2021): e2122885. See the appendix.

"SHE WASN'T AN AILING WOMAN" Marla Krohn, quoted in Janice Yu, "Family Members Express Concerns over COVID-19 Outbreak at Atlanta Nursing Home," *Fox5 Atlanta*, October 28, 2020, https://www.fox5atlanta.com/news/family-members-express-concerns-over-covid-19-outbreak-at-atlanta-nursing-home.

"WHEN PEOPLE TALK ABOUT DEATHS FROM COVID-19 . . ." Stephen J. Elledge, quoted in Joe Pinsker, "4 Numbers That Make the Pandemic's Massive Death Toll Sink In," *Atlantic.com*, January 5, 2021. See also Priya Amin, "People with Coronavirus Are Dying 10 Years Earlier Than They Would Have Naturally: Study," *ABC News*, May 10, 2020.

NOT ONE PERSON BECAME INFECTED Erica Carbajal, "Baltimore Nursing Home Has Had 0 COVID Cases," *Becker's Hospital Review*, January 22, 2022.

NURSING HOMES REMAIN HIGHLY SEGREGATED . . . Yue Lie, Xi Cen, Xueya Cai, and Helena Temkin-Greener, "Racial and Ethnic Disparities in COVID-19 Infections and Deaths across U.S. Nursing Homes," *Journal of the American Geriatric Society* 68, no. 11 (November 2020).

A FULL-TIME INFECTION-CONTROL SPECIALIST Maggie Flynn, "Keeping COVID at Bay," *Skilled Nursing News*, February 18, 2021.

QUICKLY REVEREND DEWITT BROUGHT IN MORE PERSONAL PROTECTIVE EQUIPMENT . . . Dan Rodricks, "How a West Baltimore Nursing Home Has Zero Covid-19 Infections," *Baltimore Sun*, June 18, 2020.

1,950 NURSING HOMES . . . HAD NO DEATHS AT ALL Michael L. Barnett, R. J. Waken, Jie Zheng, E. John Orav, Arnold M. Epstein, David C. Grabowski, and Karen E. Joynt Maddox, "Changes in Health and Quality of Life in US Skilled Nursing Facilities by COVID-19 Exposure Status in 2020," *JAMA* 328, no. 10 (September 13, 2022): 941–50.

DEATH RATE . . . WAS STATISTICALLY ZERO Sheryl Zimmerman, Carol Dumond-Stryker, Meera Tandan, John S. Preisser, Christopher J. Wretman, Abigail Howell, and Susan Ryan, "Nontraditional Small House Nursing Homes Have Fewer COVID-19 Cases and Deaths," *Journal of the American Medical Directors' Association* (Online: January 26, 2021).

"UNIONS GENERALLY DEMAND . . ." Maggie Flynn, "Unionized Nursing Homes Saw Lower COVID-19 Mortality Rates, Better PPE Access: Study," *Skilled Nursing News*, September 13, 2020.

"THREE TIMES AS LIKELY" President Joe Biden, "President Biden: Nursing Homes Are Putting Residents at Risk. We're Ending the Abuse Today," *USA Today*, September 1, 2023.

INCREASE NURSING-CARE TIME PER PATIENT Rachel M. Werner and Norma B. Coe, "Nursing Home Staffing Levels Did Not Change Significantly during COVID-19," *Health Affairs* 40, no. 5 (May 2021).

ONLY 11.7 PERCENT . . . WENT ON TO GET SYMPTOMS Sunil Parikh, Kevin O'Laughlin, Hanna Y. Ehrlich, Lauren Campbell, Adora Harizaj, Amanda Durante, and Vivian Leung, "Point Prevalence Testing of Residents for SARS-CoV-2 in a Subset of Connecticut Nursing Homes," *JAMA* 334, no. 11 (2020):1101–03.

NOT AGE ALONE Alessandra Marengoni, Alberto Zucchelli, Davide Liborio Vetrano, Andrea Armellini, Emanuele Botteri, Franco Nicosia, Giuseppe Romanelli, Eva Andrea Beindorf, Paola Giansiracusa, Emirena Garrafa, Luigi Ferrucci, Laura Fratiglioni, Roberto Bernabei, and Graziano Onder, "Beyond Chronological Age: Frailty and Multimorbidity Predict In-Hospital Mortality in Patients with Coronavirus Disease 2019," *Journals of Gerontology*, November 20, 2020.

"HOW DISPOSABLE THEY FEEL YOU ARE ONCE YOU BECOME A CERTAIN AGE" Judith E. Graham, "Seniors Decry Age Bias, Say They Feel Devalued When Interacting with Health Care Providers," CNN, October 17, 2021; Judith E. Graham, email to author, "Excellent Article about Medical Ageism," October 22, 2021.

MS. WOOD TOLD AARP David Hochman, "Four Months that Left 54,000 Dead from COVID in Long-Term Care," *AARP*, December 3, 2020.

"THE PASSION TO STRAIGHTEN THINGS OUT . . ." Hannah Arendt, in Hannah Arendt and Karl Jaspers, *Hannah Arendt / Karl Jaspers Correspondence, 1926–1969*, ed. Lotte Kohler and Hans Saner, trans. Robert and Rita Kimber (New York: Harcourt Brace Jovanovich, 1992), January 29, 1946.

THOSE RESPONSIBLE CALLED THE EVENTS A "NATURAL DISASTER," BUT

THERE IS NO SUCH THING Margaret Morganroth Gullette, "Katrina and the Politics of Later Life," in *There Is No Such Thing as a Natural Disaster*, ed. Chester Hartman and Gregory D. Squires (New York: Routledge, 2006), 104.

"INEFFECTIVE, INEFFICIENT, INEQUITABLE, FRAGMENTED, AND UNSUS-TAINABLE" David Grabowski, Marilyn Rantz, and Jasmine L. Travers, "Report: U.S. Nursing Home Care Is Ineffective, Inefficient, Inequitable, Fragmented, and Unsustainable," *STAT*, April 6, 2022. The volume *The National Imperative to Improve Nursing Home Quality* (Washington, DC: National Academies Press, 2022), a consensus study report by the National Academies of Sciences, Engineering, and Medicine, is known as the NASEM Report.

TURN ANY CREATURE . . . "INTO A THING" Simone Weil, "The Iliad, or the Poem of Force," trans. Mary McCarthy, *Politics* (November 1945): 322.

AS POLITICAL PHILOSOPHER DANIELLE ALLEN SHOWS Danielle Allen, *Democracy in the Time of Coronavirus* (Chicago: University of Chicago Press, 2022).

$18.20 PER WEEK "Paying for a Stay in a Nursing or Rest Home," Mass.gov, accessed December 6, 2023, https://www.mass.gov/info-details/paying-for-a-stay-in-a-nursing-or-rest-home#.

RESIDENTS CAN'T AFFORD Matt Sedensky, "In Nursing Homes, Impoverished Live Final Days on Pennies," *19 News Cleveland*, March 15, 2023.

"WORTH ABOUT TWO-THIRDS OF OTHER PEOPLE" Dr. James M. Perrin, "Structural Racism Infects How We Pay for Health Care," letter to the editor, *Boston Globe*, May 17, 2021: A9; American Council on Aging, "2020 Nursing Home Costs by State and Region," *Medicaid Planning Assistance*, January 14, 2021.

"NON-WHITE RESIDENTS EXPERIENCED MORE . . . DEATHS" Tamara R. Konetzka, "A National Tragedy: COVID-19 in the Nation's Nursing Homes," a virtual hearing before the United States Senate Finance Committee, March 17, 2021.

TRUMP HAD STOPPED TESTING Jeff Brady, "Federal Support Ends for Coronavirus Testing Sites as Pandemic Peak Nears," *NPR*, April 8, 2020.

AS WEST VIRGINIA'S GOVERNOR WAS FIRST TO DO Office of the Governor, Jim Justice, "COVID-19 UPDATE: West Virginia Becomes First State in Nation to Begin Testing All Nursing Home Residents and Staff for COVID-19," press release, April 20, 2020. On remedying government failures, see Allen, *Democracy in the Time of Coronavirus*, 87.

NONE DID Nina A. Kohn, "Nursing Homes, COVID-19, and the Consequences of Regulatory Failure," *Georgetown Law Journal Online*, April 26, 2021: 4, n14.

"COULD HAVE BEEN MANDATED" Elaine Ryan, email to author, "Re: A Query about Federal Billions That Went to Nursing Homes," August 10, 2021.

"NO STATE IS PROTECTING FRAIL ELDERS WELL" Mary Ellen Klas, "Why Are Coronavirus Deaths Doubling in Florida's Nursing Homes?" *Tampa Bay Times*, December 12, 2020.

BUDGETS SWING WILDLY DEPENDING ON THE BUSINESS CYCLE John R. Bowblis and Robert Applebaum, "How Does Medicaid Reimbursement Impact Nursing Home Quality?" *Health Services Research* 52, no. 5 (October 2017).

BUT THEY LEFT PEOPLE DEAD Reported speech, in Michael Lewis, *The Premonition* (New York: Norton, 2021), 42.

A DUTY TO . . . "PROMOTE . . . RIGHTS" "Nursing Home Residents' Rights," National Consumer Voice for Quality Long-Term Care, accessed February 4, 2024, https://theconsumervoice.org/uploads/files/long-term-care-recipient/CV _NHrights_factsheet_final.pdf.

ELDER JUSTICE ACT Laurinda Reynolds, "The COVID-19 Pandemic Exposes Limited Understanding of Ageism," *Journal of Aging and Social Policy* 32, nos. 4–5 (2020): 499–505.

CMS "IS RESPONSIBLE FOR ENSURING . . ." US Government Accountability Office, *COVID-19 in Nursing Homes: Most Homes Had Multiple Outbreaks and Weeks of Sustained Transmission from May 2020 through January 2021* (Washington, DC: Government Accountability Office, May 19, 2021).

A TIME "THAT WILL BE FOREVER BURNED INTO OUR MINDS . . ." Steve Annear, "Back in the Office, Back in Time," *Boston Globe*, July 21, 2021: A1.

"NO ONE SHOULD HAVE TO DIE ALONE . . ." *Frontline*, season 2021, episode 12, "The Virus That Shook the World," dir. James Bluemel, aired April 27, 2021, on PBS.

AN AARP STATE DIRECTOR FROM ARIZONA TESTIFIED Chorus Nylander, "AARP AZ Director Testifies before Judiciary Committee on Nursing-Home Immunity," *KVOA*, February 11, 2021.

"IN PRISON" Liz Seegert, "'I'm Very Lonely and Depressed'—Many Nursing Home Residents Say They Feel Like They Are in Prison," *Next Avenue*, October 12, 2020.

MARY MASON Mary Grimley Mason, "Locked In and the New Normal," *Disability Issues* 4, no. 2 (Spring 2020).

FEARED . . . "A DEATH TRAP" Mary Ann Thomas, "How a Trib Reporter Is Coping with Inability to Visit Mother during Coronavirus Uncertainty," *Tribune Review*, March 13, 2020.

"WE WERE REALLY LUCKY" Brynn Gringas and Theresa Waldrop, "Separated from Loved Ones for Months, Nursing Home Residents Face Even Lonelier Holidays during the Coronavirus Pandemic," CNN, November 26, 2020.

SHEILA LILES Colin Campbell, "For Maryland Nursing Homes, COVID Vaccines Bring . . . Sense of Hope and Normalcy," *Baltimore Sun*, March 5, 2021.

CHARLES MILLER Gringas and Waldrop, "Separated."

A REBEL SNEAKED INTO ANOTHER WING Sheldon Schwartz, "Adjusting to the New Realities," *Advocate* (Pennsylvania State Long-Term Care Ombudsman Program newsletter), July 2021: 2, https://ltcombudsman.org/uploads/files/support/July _2021_newsletter.pdf.

"THE MOST CALM PEOPLE" Eric Harvey, "Hebrew Home Comes Long Way since Covid," *Riverdale Press*, June 4, 2023.

"A MIXED EXPERIENCE" Tom Medlar, "Surviving Pandemic Pandemonium in Nursing Facilities," *Psychotherapy.net*, June 2, 2022.

"BED PAN" Hannah Catlett, "Senior Advocates and Lawmakers Respond to 19 News Nursing Home Investigation," *19 News*, February 19, 2020.

"DEATH IS EVERYWHERE" Chris Serres, "Deadly Toll Grows at Minnesota's New Hope Nursing Home," *Star Tribune*, May 1, 2020.

"NOT GIVEN A LOT OF TIME" Reed Abelson, "COVID Forces Families to Rethink Nursing Home Care," *Boston Globe*, May 9, 2021.

PATRICIA STAKED OUT THE PARKING LOT Patricia Sheppard, email to author, "Re: Lovely to See You . . ." March 17, 2021.

NURSING HOURS HAD FALLEN 20 PERCENT BELOW THE STATE AVERAGE Rebecca Ostriker, "Homey, Coveted, Costly—and Crushed by the Pandemic," *Boston Globe*, September 28, 2020.

"NO STIMULATION" Sarah Ravani, "The Pandemic Disrupted Many Bay Area Lives," *San Francisco Chronicle*, May 23, 2021.

"TRAPPED AND WAITING" Jack Healy, M. Richtel, and M. Baker, "Nursing Homes Becoming Islands of Isolation amid 'Shocking' Mortality Rate," *New York Times*, March 11, 2020.

"IT'S A VERY GRIM PICTURE" Dialynn Dwyer, "This Doctor Works in Several Local Nursing Homes," *Boston Globe*, March 23, 2021.

"THEY DO NOT SPEAK THEIR BIGGEST FEAR . . ." *New Day Saturday*, "House Passes Coronavirus Relief Bill," anchors Victor Blackwell and Christi Ruth Paul, aired March 14, 2020, on CNN Atlanta.

"THERE'S A LOT THAT WE DON'T KNOW ARE DEAD OR ALIVE" Louis Finlay, "Caregivers and Nursing Home Residents Hope for Answers Following News of Probe," *News10*, February 18, 2021.

"PETRIFIED" Jenna Carlesso and Dave Altimari, "The Clouds Are Starting to Open," *CT Mirror*, January 22, 2021.

"SHE SAID SHE WOULD KILL HERSELF" Christopher Collins, "A West Texas Nursing Home Sent Its COVID-Positive Residents Elsewhere. Now Two of Them Are Dead," *Texas Observer*, October 28, 2020.

"I COULD HAVE BEEN ONE OF THOSE THAT WAS STUCK" Briana Erickson, "'It's Really Getting Bad Here,'" *Las Vegas Review-Journal*, August 2, 2020.

YOU CAN HEAR HER PLEADING Erickson, "'It's Really Getting Bad Here.'"

"I CAN'T BREATHE" AARP, "The Behind-the-Scenes Fight against COVID in Nursing Homes," December 5, 2020, YouTube video, 17:17, from 12:55 to 13:36, https:// www.youtube.com/watch?v=WsgAWOxjrmo.

"NO OTHER REHAB CENTER WILL TAKE HIM" John Swaine and Maria Sacchetti, "As Washington Nursing Home Assumed It Faced Influenza Outbreak, Opportunities to Control Coronavirus Exposure Passed," *Washington Post*, March 17, 2020.

"I WANT SO BAD TO BE WITH HER . . ." Jennifer Roberts, "Horry County Family Tired of Waiting on McMaster to Lift Nursing Home Restrictions," *WMBF News*, July 31, 2020.

"LIKE REALLY SEE YOU" Alicia Lee, "With Nursing Homes on Lockdown, a

Woman Found a Special Way to Share the News of Her Engagement with Grandfather," CNN, March 19, 2020.

"HUG TENT" Liz Gelardi, "'Hug Tent' Allows Nursing Home Residents the Chance to Embrace Family," *Denver 7*, November 13, 2020.

"SNAPPED BACK TO BEING HER NORMAL JOVIAL SELF" Ravani, "Pandemic Disrupted Many Bay Area Lives."

"THEY DICKED AROUND WITH HIM" A true story. Patrick J. Doyle and Robert Rubinstein, "Person-Centered Dementia Care and the Cultural Matrix of Othering," *Gerontologist* 54, no. 6 (2014): 969, table 3. The rest of the conversation between sisters is fiction, setting the scene.

CARE HOME STORIES *Care Home Stories: Ageing, Disability, and Long-Term Residential Care*, Aging Studies vol. 14, ed. Sally Chivers and Ulla Kriebernegg (Bielefeld, Germany: Transcript Verlag, 2018).

CHRIS GILLEARD AND PAUL HIGGS Paul Higgs and Chris Gilleard, "Fourth Ageism: Real and Imaginary Old Age," special Issue: "Aging as a Unique Experience," *Societies* 11, no.1 (February 2021).

$30 MILLION Sidney Madden, Braeden Waddell, and Yanqi Xu, "Industry Lobbying Left Nursing Home Patients at Risk," *IRW* (Investigative Reporting Workshop), March 3, 2021.

UNABLE TO REQUIRE VACCINATIONS Centers for Medicare and Medicaid Services (hereafter CMS), "Biden-Harris Administration to Expand Vaccination Requirements for Health Care Settings," *CMS.gov*, press release, September 9, 2021, https://www.cms.gov/newsroom/press-releases/biden-harris-administration-expand-vaccination-requirements-health-care-settings.

"A VERY, VERY RADICAL THOUGHT" Kwame Anthony Appiah, interviewed by Chris Hayes, "Rethinking Identity with Kwame Anthony Appiah," *NBC News.com*, March 12, 2019.

CHAPTER TWO

HAZMAT SUITS Maria Sacchetti and John Swaine, "Wash. Nursing Home Faces $611,000 Fine over Lapses during Fatal Coronavirus Outbreak," *Washington Post*, April 2, 2020.

"AT LEAST ONE RESIDENT" CMS, "CMS Announces Findings at Kirkland Nursing Home and New Targeted Plan for Healthcare Facility Inspections in light of COVID-19," *CMS.gov*, press release, March 23, 2020, https://www.cms.gov/newsroom/press-releases/cms-announces-findings-kirkland-nursing-home-and-new-targeted-plan-healthcare-facility-inspections.

SEATTLE TIMES Asia Fields and Mary Hudetz, "Coronavirus Spread at Life Care Center of Kirkland for Weeks, while Response Stalled," *Seattle Times*, March 18, 2020.

"SHOW THEMSELVES MORE PLAINLY" Richard Ohmann, *Selling Culture: Magazines, Markets, and Class at the Turn of the Century* (London: Verso, 1996), 13.

0.6 PERCENT Avik Roy, "The Most Important Coronavirus Statistic: 42% Of U.S. Deaths Are from 0.6% of the Population," *Forbes*, May 26, 2020.

"MOST OF THE DEATHS ARE VERY OLD AMERICANS WITH CO-MORBIDITIES" Twitter took down Trump's tweets, including this one, quoted by Peter Baker, "Trump Embraces Fringe Theories on Protests and the Coronavirus," *New York Times*, August 30, 2020. See also Sonia Kruks, "Alterity and Intersectionality: Reflections on Old Age," *Hypatia* 37, no. 1 (Winter 2022): 196–209.

"NOTORIOUSLY SQUEAMISH" David Runciman, "Competition Is for Losers," *London Review of Books*, September 23, 2021: 18. In a sixteen-second clip, Trump is seen mocking the reporter in "Trump Mocks Reporter's Disability," uploaded to YouTube by the official CNN account on July 22, 2016, at https://www.youtube.com/watch?v=uNXgjnBpxGI.

PHOTOSHOPPED IMAGE David Smith, "The Age of the Elderly Candidate: How Two Septuagenarians Came to Be Running for President," *Guardian*, October 29, 2020. The tweet appeared at pic.twitter.com/wJN4zv0y8O(@realDonaldTrump), October 14, 2020; that account has since been closed.

STEREOTYPES TEND TO SURVIVE FACTS In fact, men were dying more than women, but early on it was hard to find data on nursing-home deaths by gender or race, even from the CDC. See Anushka Kalyanpur, Dannielle Thomas, Diana Wu, Laura Tashjian, May D. Sifuentes, and Rachel Hall, *Rapid Gender Analysis: COVID-19 in the United States* (Atlanta, GA: CARE USA, 2020), 6.

TWELVE OCCASIONS Calder Walton, "US Intelligence, the Coronavirus and the Age of Globalized Challenges," *CIGI Essay Series*, August 24, 2020.

"WE WERE VERY, VERY MUCH HINDERED" "Perspective Roundtable: Long-Term Care in the United States—Problems and Solutions," *New England Journal of Medicine*, May 19, 2022.

HAD THE WORST [PPE] Mark S. Lachs, "COVID-19 and Aging, a Tale of Two Pandemics," *Nature Aging* 1 (January 2021): 9.

"A LITTLE BIT OF A WEAK SPOT" Alex Spanko, "Trump Orders Formation of Nursing Home Quality, Safety Commission in Wake of COVID-19 Crisis," *Skilled Nursing News*, April 30, 2020.

JUSTICE IN AGING Eric Carlson, "Imbalanced Commission Report Does Not Do Enough to Make Nursing Homes Responsible for Resident Safety and Quality of Life," *Justice in Aging*, September 18, 2020.

PRAISED "THE ROBUST PUBLIC HEALTH ACTIONS" CMS, "Independent Nursing Home COVID-19 Commission Findings Validate Unprecedented Federal Response," *CMS.gov*, press release, September 16, 2020.

66 PERCENT OF STATE COVID DEATHS "Rate of COVID-19 Deaths among Nursing Home Residents in the United States as of September 27, 2020, by State," *Statista.com*, October 14, 2020.

VARIOUSLY ATTRIBUTED Charles F. Parker and Eric K. Stern, "The Trump Administration and the COVID-19 Crisis," *Public Administration*, March 29, 2022: part 3.

LULL HIMSELF Lisa Bortolotti and Kathleen Murphy-Hollies, "Exceptionalism at the Time of COVID-19: Where Nationalism Meets Irrationality," *Danish Yearbook of Philosophy* 55, no. 2 (January 17, 2022): 90–111.

"IT AFFECTS VIRTUALLY NOBODY" Timothy Bella, "'It Affects Virtually Nobody': Trump Incorrectly Claims Covid-19 Isn't a Risk for Young People," *Washington Post*, September 22, 2020.

SINGLE LARGEST DRIVER OF COVID MISINFORMATION Joan Conrow, "What Drove the COVID Misinformation 'Infodemic'?" *Cornell Alliance for Science*, October 1, 2020.

IF THE FIRST VICTIMS HAD BEEN *CHILDREN* Desmond O'Neill, "Protecting Our Longevity Dividend during Covid-19," *Irish Medical Journal* 113, no. 4 (2020): 50.

"WHATEVER NARRATIVE ABOUT IT CRYSTALLIZES FOR THEM" Cass R. Sunstein, "Once upon a Time There Was a Big Bubble," *New York Review of Books*, January 14, 2021: 30.

"MAKING UP PEOPLE" Ian Hacking, "Making Up People," *London Review of Books*, August 17, 2006.

"NOT JUST OLD, OLDER" Bob Woodward, *Rage* (New York: Simon and Schuster, 2020), 285; "PLAYING IT DOWN" xviii (March 19, 2020, interview); see also xix.

HE HAD KNOWN SINCE JANUARY 25 The head of HHS briefed Trump on January 25, 2020. See Andy Slavitt, *Preventable* (New York: St. Martin's, 2021), 12; German Lopez, "New Audio Proves It," *Vox*, September 9, 2020.

"TAKE YOUR HAT OFF TO THE YOUNG" Lauren Frias, "Trump Falsely Claims That for Young People COVID-19 'Affects Virtually Nobody,'" *Business Insider*, September 22, 2020.

"THOSE WHO WANTED TO PERSUADE" Nina A. Kohn, "The Pandemic Exposed a Painful Truth: America Doesn't Care about Old People," *Washington Post*, March 8, 2020.

CAMUS Quoted in Jacqueline Rose "Pointing the Finger," *London Review of Books*, May 7, 2020: 3.

"PROTECT AGAINST PUBLIC HEALTH EMERGENCIES" "Health Care," Patty Murray Working for Washington State, January 13, 2020, archived at https://web .archive.org/web/20200113063018/https://www.murray.senate.gov/public/index .cfm/mobile/healthcare.

"IN MY BACK YARD" Patty Murray, quoted in Lawrence Wright, "The Plague Year," *New Yorker*, January 4 and 11, 2021: 23.

WITHIN THE NEXT FOUR-WEEK SPAN Paige Cornwell, "'It Made the World around Us Stop,'" *Seattle Times*, August 28, 2020.

"THIS IS COMING TO YOU" Patty Murray, quoted in Wright, "Plague Year," 36. This account is slightly different from the one in Wright's book *The Plague Year: America in the Time of COVID* (New York: Knopf, 2021).

"YOU NEED TO PROTECT THEM" Liz Kowalczyk and Robert Weisman, "A Home to Die In," *Boston Globe*, September 27, 2020.

WHERE THEY WERE GOING Robert Weisman and Tim Logan, "Officials Are

Emptying Nursing Homes across Mass. to Create Coronavirus Recovery Centers," *Boston Globe*, March 28, 2020.

"THE MOST CHARITABLE INTERPRETATION" Roy, "Most Important Coronavirus Statistic."

"LONG-HELD BUT LITTLE DISCUSSED EUGENIC BELIEFS" Laura I. Appleman, "Pandemic Eugenics: Discrimination, Disability and Detention During COVID-19," *Loyola Law Review* 67, no. 2 (2021): 329.

"OFTEN OVERLOOKED" Joel Teitelbaum and Sara E. Wilensky, *Essentials of Health Policy and Law*, 3rd ed. (Sudbury, MA: Jones and Bartlett Learning, 2017), 22; on agencies' power, see also John McDermott, *Restoring Democracy to America* (University Park: Pennsylvania State University Press, 2010):187–89.

"HOW SKIMPY TRUMPCARE PLANS WILL BE" Ilene MacDonald, "Confirmation of CMS Chief Seema Verma: Industry Reaction," *Fierce Health Care*, March 14, 2017.

MEDICAID IS POPULAR Laura Katz Olson, *The Politics of Medicaid* (New York: Columbia University Press, 2010), 13.

SHE HAD SPENT ALMOST $6 MILLION Dan Diamond and Adam Cancryn, "Inspector General: Medicare Chief Broke Rules on Her Publicity Contracts," *Politico*, July 16, 2020.

THE INSPECTOR GENERAL WAS INVESTIGATING House Committee on Oversight and Reform, *Investigation of Administrator Seema Verma's Use of Private Communications Consultants* (Washington, DC: House Committee on Oversight and Reform, September 2020), 37.

"EVERYONE'S EYES SEEMED WIDER" John Okrent, *This Costly Season: A Crown of Sonnets* (Bristol: Arrowsmith, 2021), 11, 14.

SOCIAL SECURITY ACT . . . SECTION 1819 [AND] SECTION 1135 Sec. 1819 (42 U.S.C. 1395i–3), https://www.ssa.gov/OP_Home/ssact/title18/1819.htm; Sec. 1135. (42 U.S.C. 1320b–5), https://www.ssa.gov/OP_Home/ssact/title11/1135.htm.

CHANGING RULES OR REGULATIONS IS LEGITIMATE Office of the Federal Register, *Guide to the Rulemaking Process* (Washington, DC: Office of the Federal Register, 2011), https://www.federalregister.gov/uploads/2011/01/the_rulemaking_process.pdf.

TELEHEALTH Paige Winfield Cunningham, "The Health 202: The Trump Administration Is Pulling Medicare and Medicaid Levers to Combat Coronavirus," *Washington Post*, March 18, 2020.

ON THE OTHER HAND Lisa M. Koonin, Brooke Hoots, Clarisse A. Tsang, Zanie Leroy, Kevin Farris, Tilman Jolly, Peter Antall, Bridget McCabe, Cynthia B. R. Zelis, Ian Tong, and Aaron M. Harris, "Trends in the Use of Telehealth during the Emergence of the COVID-19 Pandemic—United States, January–March 2020," *Morbidity and Mortality Weekly Report* 69, no. 43 (October 30, 2020).

AN APPARENTLY INNOCUOUS PUBLIC DOCUMENT Seema Verma, "CMS Administrator Seema Verma's Remarks as Prepared for Delivery: Updates on Healthcare Facility Inspections in Light of COVID-19," *CMS.gov*, March 23, 2020.

INSPECTORS . . . SUPPOSEDLY MAKE UNSCHEDULED VISITS Tony Martins

Ajaero, "How to Become a State Inspector for Nursing Homes in 2022," *Profitable Venture*, accessed December 7, 2023, https://www.profitableventure.com/become-state-inspector-nursing-homes/.

IN PRACTICE . . . See the endnotes in Nina A. Kohn, "Nursing Homes, COVID-19, and the Consequences of Regulatory Failure," *Georgetown University Law School Online* 110 (2021): 8; see also Robert Gebeloff, Katie Thomas, and Jessica Silver-Greenberg, "How Nursing Homes' Worst Offenses Are Hidden from the Public," *New York Times*, December 9, 2021.

CUT HIS REQUEST 40 PERCENT Slavitt, *Preventable*, 84 and 188, citing a *Washington Post* article.

FIFTY GOVERNORS FIGHTING Teresa Murray, *Nursing Home Safety during Covid: Cases and Vaccines* (Denver, CO: US Public Interest Research Group Education Fund, March 2021).

FORMS OF SPEECH . . . "SET NORMS" Rae Langton, "Lies and Back-Door Lies," *Mind* 130, no. 517 (January 2021): 251–58.

"WHEN . . . INSPECTORS CAN'T ENTER" Verma, "Remarks as Prepared for Delivery."

NO MASK WAS VISIBLE "2020 CMS Quality Conference Day 2 Recap," QIO Program, March 7, 2020, video, minute 3, https://qioprogram.org/quality-conference-day-2-recap.

VERMA DECLINED TO APPEAR Congressman Lloyd Doggett explains in a C-SPAN video; see "House Ways and Means Subcommittee Hearing on COVID-19 and Nursing Homes," *C-SPAN*, June 25, 2020, 1:00 et seq., https://www.c-span.org/video/?473382-1/house-ways-means-subcommittee-hearing-covid-19-nursing-homes#.

"TO PROVIDE THE HEALTHCARE INDUSTRY *RELIEF* " "US Centers for Medicare and Medicaid Services Answers COVID-19 Questions on Hospital Industry Stakeholder Call," *Dentons.com*, March 23, 2020. This page describes a live Q and A session on March 16, 2020, but the listed link shows no transcript or recording.

INCENTIVE TO INVESTMENT FIRMS TO BUY Eleanor Laise, "As Pandemic Struck, a Private Equity Firm Went on a Nursing-Home Buying Spree," *Barron's*, August 6, 2020; Rebecca Tan and Rachel Chason, "An Investment Firm Snapped Up Nursing Homes during the Pandemic," *Washington Post*, December 21, 2020.

MARKET PERFORMANCE . . . WAS UP Andrew Cockburn, "Elder Abuse," *Harper's* (September 2020).

VERMA . . . SHARED THE NEOLIBERAL IDEOLOGICAL MISSION Jordyn Reiland, "Former CMS Chief Seema Verma Blasts Nursing Home Reform Proposals," *Skilled Nursing News*, March 14, 2022.

"ONLY ONE PIECE OF IT" David Hochman, "Four Months That Left 54,000 Dead from COVID in Long-Term Care: The Oral History of an American Tragedy," *AARP*, December 3, 2020: "February-March."

"PAY THE BILLS . . ." Paul Elstein, phone call and email exchange with author, "Talking about CMS," August 18, 2023.

TWO-FACED SPEECH Verma, "CMS Administrator Seema Verma's Remarks as Prepared for Delivery."

"*MINIMIZE THE IMPACT ON PROVIDER ACTIVITIES*" HHS, CMS, Center for Clinical Standards and Quality/ Quality, Safety and Oversight Group, "Prioritization of Survey Activities," memorandum to state survey agency directors from the quality, safety, and oversight group director, March 20, 2020, updated March 10, 2021, ref. QSO-20-20-All, https://www.cms.gov/files/document/qso-20-20-all.pdf, emphasis added. See also, from Wright: CMS/QSO, "On Suspension of Survey Activities to State Survey Agency Directors," memorandum to state survey agency directors from the quality, safety, and oversight group director, March 4, 2020, ref: QSO-20-12-All, https://www.cms.gov/files/document/qso-20-12-all.pdf.

CHECKLIST THAT FOLLOWED HHS, CMS, Quality, Safety, and Education Portal, "COVID-19 Focused Survey for Nursing Homes," survey, March 20, 2020: 3, https://qscp.cms.gov/data/274/COVID-19FocusedSurveyforNursingHomes.pdf.

"A SIGNIFICANTLY LESS COMPREHENSIVE MEASURE" "Rep. Neal Urges New CMS Administration to Take Bold Steps to Protect Medicare Beneficiaries in Nursing Facilities," *Targeted News Service*, February 26, 2021.

"RATINGS TEMPORARILY SUPPRESSED" HHS, CMS, *Design for* Nursing Home Compare *Five-Star Quality Rating System: Technical Users Guide* (Woodlawn, MD: CMS, July 2020), 2, https://www.hhs.gov/guidance/sites/default/files/hhs-guidance-documents/Five-Star%20Users_%20Guide%20July%202020-%20Updated%207-29-2020.pdf. The guidance was revised in 2021 and rescinded on March 30, 2023. See HHS, CMS, Center for Clinical Standards and Quality/Quality, Safety and Oversight Group, "RESCIND Revised COVID-19 Survey Activities, CARES Act Funding, Enhanced Enforcement for Infection Control Deficiencies, and Quality Improvement Activities in Nursing Homes," memorandum to state survey agency directors from the quality, safety, and oversight group director, June 1, 2020, revised January 4, 2021, rescinded March 30, 2023, ref. QSO-20-31-All, https://www.cms.gov/files/document/qso-20-31-all-revised.pdf. On how star ratings fail, see Tamara R. Konetzka, Kevin Yan, and Rachel M. Werner, "Two Decades of Nursing Home Compare: What Have We Learned?" *Medical Care Research and Review*, June 13, 2020.

PHYSICIANS AND PRACTITIONERS . . . COULD DELEGATE HHS, CMS, Center for Clinical Standards and Quality, Director of Quality, Safety, and Oversight Group, "Prioritization of Survey Activities," March 20, 2020, updated March 10, 2021: 3, 1, 14.

FEDERAL LAW REQUIRED National Consumer Voice for Quality Long-Term Care, "CMS Rescinds Emergency Waivers, Including of Training and Certification Requirements for Nurse Aides," *Voice* (e-newsletter), April 14, 2022.

FROM SIXTEEN HOURS TO ONE "Rep. Neal Urges New CMS Administration to Take Bold Steps."

FORTY-EIGHT STATES ASKED "Medicaid Emergency Authority Tracker: Approved State Actions to Address COVID-19," *Kaiser Family Foundation*, July 1, 2021.

THEY SHOULD NOT "HESITATE TO ASK" Verma, "CMS Administrator Seema Verma's Remarks as Prepared for Delivery."

ONLY A LITTLE OVER HALF OF NURSING HOMES HHS, CMS, Center for Clinical Standards and Quality/ Quality, Safety and Oversight Group, "RESCIND Revised COVID-19 Survey Activities, CARES Act Funding, Enhanced Enforcement for Infection Control Deficiencies, and Quality Improvement Activities in Nursing Homes," memorandum to state survey agency directors from the quality, safety, and oversight group director, June 1, 2020, revised January 4, 2021, rescinded March 30, 2023, ref. QSO-20-31-All, https://www.cms.gov/files/document/qso-20-31-all-rescinded.pdf.

THE STENCH SHE NOTICED Amanda James, "Witnesses Recount 'Dire Conditions' in Nursing Homes during Covid-19 in Congressional Hearing," *MedCity News*, September 23, 2022.

"DEGRADED PATIENT SAFETY" Lee A. Fleisher, Michelle Schreiber, Denise Cardo, and Arjun Srinivasan, "Health Care Safety during the Pandemic and Beyond — Building a System That Ensures Resilience," *New England Journal of Medicine* 386 (February 17, 2022): 609–11.

HUMAN RIGHTS WATCH Human Rights Watch, *US: Concerns of Neglect in Nursing Homes. Pandemic Exposes Need for Improvements in Staffing, Oversight, Accountability* (New York: Human Rights Watch, March 25, 2021).

HAD "REMOVED THE MINIMUM STANDARDS" HHS, CMS, Center for Clinical Standards and Quality/Quality, Safety and Oversight Group, "Update to COVID-19 Emergency Declaration Blanket Waivers for Specific Providers," memorandum to state survey agency directors from the quality, safety, and oversight group director, April 7, 2022, ref. QSO-22-15-NH & NLTC & LSC, https://www.cms.gov/files/document/qso -22-15-nh-nltc-lsc.pdf.

"THE ROLE OF REGULATORY REGIMES . . ." Joe Greener, "Performative Compliance and the State–Corporate Structuring of Neglect in a Residential Care Home for Older People," *Critical Criminology* 28 ((November 13, 2019): 651–68, emphasis added.

THE TESTIMONY OF A LAWYER "CMA Senior Policy Attorney Testifies before Congressional Committee," Center for Medicare Advocacy, June 25, 2020, https:// medicareadvocacy.org/cmas-toby-edelman-testifies-at-congressional-hearing-on -covid-in-nursing-homes/.

"OFTEN WORK OUT OF THE PUBLIC'S EYE" Teitelbaum and Wilensky, *Essentials*, 22.

"AREAS OF GREATEST NEED" Libby Cathey, "Trump Declares National Emergency Responding to Coronavirus: Here's What That Means," *ABC News*, March 13, 2020.

"POTENTIAL FINANCIAL PENALTIES OR SANCTIONS" Jacqueline LaPointe, "Documentation to Ease Medical Billing Issues Due to COVID-19," *RevCycle Intelligence*, March 24, 2020.

THE TRAILS WERE COLD Lauren J. Mapp, "Complaints Persisted at San Diego County Nursing Homes during Pandemic," *San Diego Union Tribune*, May 6, 2023.

CHAPTER THREE

"CLASSIFYING THE HORROR" Jacqueline Rose, "Pointing the Finger," *London Review of Books*, May 7, 2020: 3.

"MISSED THE WORST PART OF THE OUTBREAK" Danielle Ivory, quoted in David Hochman, "Four Months That Left 54,000 Dead from COVID in Long-Term Care: The Oral History of an American Tragedy," *AARP*, December 3, 2020.

SEVEN THOUSAND BY APRIL 3 Margaret Peacock and Erik L. Petersen, *A Deeper Sickness: Journal of America in the Pandemic* (Boston, MA: Beacon Press, 2023), 53, 58.

"MORE THAN 7,000 DEATHS IN NURSING HOMES" Danielle Ivory, quoted in Hochman, "Four Months."

BARELY VISIBLE IN FILM . . . Kathleen Woodward, "A Public Secret: Assisted Living, Caregivers, Globalization," *International Journal of Ageing and Later Life* 7, no. 2 (2012): 17–51.

BLACK OR LATINX RESIDENTS WERE LIKELIER TO SUFFER Amanda James, "Witnesses Recount 'Dire Conditions' in Nursing Homes during Covid-19 in Congressional Hearing," *MedCity News*, September 23, 2022.

UNDERSTAFFING HAD BEEN A CHRONIC ISSUE Government Accountability Office, *Infection Control Deficiencies Were Widespread and Persistent in Nursing Homes Prior to COVID-19 Pandemic*, report GAO-20–576R, (Washington, DC: GAO, May 20, 2020).

THE CONDITIONS OF THOSE WHO HAD BEEN NEGLECTED One story may suffice: Matt Sedensky and Bernard Condon, "Not Just COVID: Nursing Home Neglect Deaths Surge in Shadows," *AP News*, November 19, 2020.

"DEATH PITS" Betsy McCaughey is quoted in Farah Stockman, Matt Richtel, Danielle Ivory, and Mitch Smith, "'They're Death Pits': Virus Claims At Least 7,000 lives in US Nursing Homes," *New York Times*, April 17, 2020.

"HEROES WORK *HERE* TOO" Jasmine Travers, "Perspective Roundtable: Long-Term Care in the United States—Problems and Solutions," *New England Journal of Medicine*, May 19, 2022.

A "RATHER VAGUE DEFINITION" Medical University of South Carolina Health, "Frailty: A New Predictor of Outcome as We Age," *Healthy Aging Newsletter*, accessed December 8, 2023, https://muschealth.org/medical-services/geriatrics-and-aging/healthy-aging/frailty#.

"GOD'S WAITING ROOM" Mary Papenfuss, "Governor Ron DeSantis Calls Florida 'God's Waiting Room' for Retirees," *Huffington Post*, April 27, 2020.

"THAT MARVELOUS INDIFFERENCE" Simone Weil, "The Iliad, or the Poem of Force," trans. Mary McCarthy, *Politics* (November 1945), 326.

"SUPER-SURVIVORS" Alexis Shanes, "108-Year-Old New Jersey Woman Who Lived through Spanish Flu Survives Coronavirus," *USA Today*, May 14, 2020.

"FULLY ACCREDITED LONG-TERM HEALTH CARE FACILITY" Commonwealth of Massachusetts, "Veterans Home at Holyoke Residential Care," *Mass.gov*, accessed

February 5, 2024, https://www.mass.gov/info-details/veterans-home-in-holyoke -residential-care.

AN INDEPENDENT REPORT FOUND THE "MISTAKES" "UTTERLY BAFFLING" Hanna Krueger and Matt Stout, "Independent Report Slams Handling of Outbreak at Holyoke Soldiers' Home," *Boston Globe*, June 24, 2020.

DIED IN HIGHER PERCENTAGES CarePort, *Trends in Covid-19 Infection and Deaths Observed across 63,000 Nursing Home Residents* (Overland Park, KS: CarePort, 2020).

DEMENTISM Stephen Post, *The Moral Challenge of Alzheimer Disease: Ethical Issues from Diagnosis to Dying* (Baltimore: Johns Hopkins University Press, 2002), 29–32.

STATES THAT NEVER CARED ENOUGH Laura Katz Olson, *The Politics of Medicaid* (New York: Columbia University Press, 2010), 228.

"THE SMELL . . . OF THE ENTRENCHED RACKET" Andrew Wengraf, email to author, "Eldercide," January 11, 2021.

OWNED BY CORPORATE CHAINS Charles P. Sabatino and Charlene Harrington "Policy Change to Put the Home back into Nursing Homes," *ABA Law and Aging* (July–August 2021).

"BIASED TOWARD INSTITUTIONAL . . . CARE" Meg Coffin, letter to the editor, *Boston Globe*, July 12, 2021.

"WE COULD HAVE DONE BETTER" Elizabeth Dugan, quoted in Dasia Moore, "Virus Death Rate Still Higher Here Than in Similar Spots—but Why?" *Boston Globe*, October 14, 2020: A6.

"UGLY STEPCHILD" Edward Alan Miller, Elizabeth Simpson, Pamela Nadash, and Michael Gusmano, "Thrust into the Spotlight: COVID-19 Focuses Media Attention on Nursing Homes," *Journals of Gerontology: Series B* 76, no. 4 (March 14, 2021): gbaa103.

"SARS SCARED THE HELL OUT OF EVERYONE" *SARS in China: Prelude to Pandemic?*, ed. Arthur Kleinman and James L. Watson (Stanford, CA: Stanford University Press, 2006).

REPORTS FROM 2003 TO 2015 Aaron Blake, "The Trump Administration Just Changed Its Description of the National Stockpile to Jibe with Jared Kushner's Controversial Claim," *Washington Post*, April 3, 2020.

NOT ADEQUATELY REPLENISHED THE STOCKPILE Amy Sherman, "Trump Said the Obama Admin Left Him a Bare Stockpile. Wrong," *Politifact*, April 8, 2020, https://www.politifact.com/factchecks/2020/apr/08/donald-trump/trump-said -obama-admin-left-him-bare-stockpile-wro/.

TRUMP ADMINISTRATION HAD REDUCED THE AMOUNTS Jordan Rau, "Trump Administration Eases Penalties against Negligent Nursing Homes," CNN, January 3, 2018.

A MAXIMUM OF $22,000 Reed Abelson, "Nursing Homes May Face Steeper Safety Fines," California Advocates for Nursing Home Reform, *CANHR News*, July 28, 2021.

"UNDERMINE SAFETY" Rebecca Cokley and Valerie Novack, "The Trump Administration's Deregulation of Nursing Homes Leaves Seniors and Disabled at Higher Risk for COVID-19," *American Progress*, April 21, 2020.

"SHATTERING AND BULLETPROOF" STATISTICS Gretchen Morgenson and Joshua Rosner, *These Are the Plunderers: How Private Equity Runs—and Wrecks—America* (New York: Simon and Schuster, 2023), 189.

"INCREASE[D] THE SHORT-TERM PROBABILITY OF DEATH" Atul Gupta, Sabrina T. Howell, Constantine Yannelis, and Abhinav Gupta, "Does Private Equity Investment in Healthcare Benefit Patients? Evidence from Nursing Homes," NBER Working Paper no. 28474, (National Bureau of Economic Research, Cambridge, MA, February 2021). See also Robert Holly, "House Hearing Slams Private Equity's Troubling Expansion into Health Care," *Home Health Care News*, March 25, 2021.

FOR-PROFITS HAD AN AVERAGE OVERALL MORTALITY RATE CLOSE TO 20 PERCENT HHS, Office of the Inspector General, *More Than a Thousand Nursing Homes Reached Infection Rates of 75 Percent or More in the First Year of the COVID-19 Pandemic; Better Protections Are Needed for Future Emergencies*, OEI-02-20-00491 (Washington, DC: Office of the Inspector General, January 19, 2023).

"PERVASIVELY FAULTY AND MISLEADING COST REPORTS" Dave E. Kingsley, quoted in Richard Moore, "Are Nursing Homes Really in Tough Shape?" *Common-Wealth*, November 26, 2022.

MORE THAN ELEVEN THOUSAND NURSING HOMES . . . HAD SUCH BUSINESS DEALINGS Jordan Rau, "Neglect Unchecked: Care Suffers as More Nursing Homes Feed Money into Corporate Webs," *Kaiser Health News*, December 31, 2017.

"SLUMLORDS" Maureen Tkacik, "The Nursing Home Slumlord Manifesto," *American Prospect*, January 26, 2022. For analysis, see National Consumer Voice for Quality Long-Term Care, *Where Do the Billions of Dollars Go?* (Washington, DC: National Consumer Voice, April 6, 2023).

"RUSSIAN NESTING DOLL" Bill Pascrell Jr., "Private Equity's Growing Control of Health Care Endangers the Underserved," *USA Today*, April 8, 2021, https://www.northjersey.com/story/opinion/2021/04/08/private-equitys-control-long-term-care-endangers-underserved/7132417002/.

RESIDENTS WERE GOING HUNGRY Moe Tkacik, "Why Are America's Cash-Starved Nursing Homes Still Paying Their Rent?" *Medium*, March 30, 2021.

"CLEAN BILL OF HEALTH" Debbie Cenziper, Joel Jacobs, and Sean Mulcahy, "As Pandemic Raged and Thousands Died, Government Regulators Cleared Most Nursing Homes of Infection-Control Violations," *Washington Post*, October 29, 2020.

"THEY JUST ROLLED OVER" Charlene Harrington, quoted in Cenziper, Jacobs, and Mulcahy, "As Pandemic Raged."

"SENICIDE" David A. Swanson, "Senicide: The Lack of Containment Measures: Does It Constitute Senicide?" *Northwest Citizen*, May 7, 2020.

"CARNAGE" Julie Chang, "Months into Pandemic, Texas Reveals Ravages of COVID-19 Nursing Home Infections," *El Paso Times*, July 29, 2020. I prefer to give full names of residents—say their names! But the facility refused to reveal the name of Cindy's mother.

THIS SHIELD WAS "IMPERATIVE" Center for Medicare Advocacy, *Special Report: Nursing Home Industry Seeks Immunity during COVID Crisis; States Are Obliging* (Willimantic, CT: Center for Medicare Advocacy, May 14, 2020).

CORPORATE STATE CAPTURE The Center for Constitutional Rights website provides this definition and many instances. See "Corporate Capture," Center for Constitutional Rights, accessed December 8, 2023, https://ccrjustice.org/Corporate-Capture.

THE AUTHORS SENT A BEGGARS' LETTER National Association of Social Workers to Mitch McConnell and Charles Schumer, "NASW Opposes Granting Immunity to Nursing Homes," May 28, 2020, https://www.socialworkers.org/LinkClick.aspx ?fileticket=q2czO-x0_Bc%3D&portalid=0.

MEDICAID *CUTS* Lynn A. Blewett and Robert Hest, "Emergency Flexibility for States to Increase and Maintain Medicaid Eligibility for LTSS under COVID-19," *Journal of Aging and Social Policy* 32, nos. 4–5 (May 2020): 347.

"NEVER BE HELD ACCOUNTABLE" Samuel Brooks, Robyn Grant, and Michael F. Bonamarte, "States Move to Shield LTC Facilities from Civil Liability," ABA, Commission of Law and Aging, *Bifocal* 41, no. 6 (July–August 2020); Nina A. Kohn, "Nursing Homes, COVID-19, and the Consequences of Regulatory Failure," *Georgetown University Law School Online* 110 (2021).

DEATHS PER WEEK MORE THAN DOUBLED "What We're Reading," *American Journal of Managed Care*, November 9, 2020.

BROUGHT IN MOBILE HOMES Mark S. Lachs, "COVID-19 and Aging, a Tale of Two Pandemics," *Nature Aging* 1 (January 2021): 9.

DID NOT MEANINGFULLY IMPROVE THOSE CONDITIONS Brian E. McGarry, David C. Grabowski, and Michael L. Barnett, "Severe Staffing and Personal Protective Equipment Shortages," *Health Affairs* 39, no. 1 (August 2020).

WOUND "WENT DOWN TO THE BONE" Harold Brubaker, "After Cutting Staff at Darby Nursing Home, Former Manager Pleads No Contest to Recklessly Endangering Residents," *Philadelphia Inquirer*, June 2, 2021.

"THE ODDS OF SURVIVAL IS LOW" June M. McKoy, Anna Liggett, and Fernanda Heitor, "Are Nursing Home Residents Expendable?" *Hill*, April 24, 2020.

GUARDIAN HEADLINE Associated Press, "Coronavirus Outbreaks Like 'Wildfire' at US Nursing Homes under Lockdowns," *Guardian*, April 2, 2020.

A FIRE GOING THROUGH DRY GRASS Aditi Sangal, "Gov. Cuomo: Outbreak Is 'Like Watching a Fire Going through Dry Grass with a Strong Wind," CNN, April 13, 2020.

"WILDFIRE" Joseph G. Ouslander and David C. Grabowski, "COVID-19 in Nursing Homes: Calming the Perfect Storm," *Journal of the American Geriatric Society* 68, no. 10 (October 2020): 2153–62.

"CAUSES, VULNERABILITY, PREPAREDNESS . . ." Neil Smith, "There's No Such Thing as a Natural Disaster," *Social Science Research Council*, June 11, 2006. See also Margaret Morganroth Gullette, "Katrina and the Politics of Later Life," in *There Is No Such Thing as a Natural Disaster: Race, Class, and Hurricane Katrina*, ed. Gregory Squires and Chester Hartman (New York: Routledge, 2006), 103–19.

JUSTIFICATIONS "FACILITATE THE RELEASE OF GENUINE PREJUDICE" Kristen. P. Jones, Isaac E. Sabat, Eden B. King, Afra Ahmad, Tracy C. McCausland, and Tiffani Chen, "Isms and Schisms: A Meta-Analysis of the Prejudice-Discrimination Relationship across Racism, Sexism, and Ageism," *Journal of Organizational Behavior* 38 (2017): 1078.

"GET RID OF WHAT YOU CANNOT EFFECTUALLY SUCCOUR" Adam Phillips, *Promises, Promises: Essays on Psychoanalysis and Literature* (New York: Basic Books, 2001), 285.

RESENTMENT . . . FOUND ON TIKTOK UNDER THE #DEMENTIA TAG Abby Olhiser, "Dementia Content Gets Millions of Views on TikTok," *MIT Technology Review*, February 16, 2022, https://www.technologyreview.com/2022/02/16/1045322 /dementia-consent-tiktok-online-ethics/.

FANTASY OF EUTHANASIA Margaret Morganroth Gullette, "Euthanasia as a Caregiving Fantasy in the Era of the New Longevity," *Age Culture Humanities* (2014): 214.

DEATHS OF PEOPLE IN NURSING FACILITIES WERE UP 32 PERCENT David Grabowski, quoted in Ricardo Alonso-Zaldibar, "Nursing Home Deaths Up 32% in 2020 amid Pandemic," Associated Press, June 22, 2021. The report refers only to Medicare beneficiaries (including those dually eligible for both Medicare and Medicaid).

EXTRA DEATHS Amartya Sen, "More Than 100 Million Women Are Missing," *New York Review of Books*, December 20, 1990: 61–66.

THE MASSACHUSETTS ATTORNEY GENERAL INDICTED TWO ADMINISTRATORS Office of [MA] Attorney General Maura Healey, "AG Healey Announces Criminal Charges Against Superintendent and Former Medical Director," press release, *Mass.gov*, September 25, 2020, https://www.mass.gov/news/ag-healey-announces -criminal-charges-against-superintendent-and-former-medical-director-of-holyoke -soldiers-home-for-their-roles-in-deadly-covid-19-outbreak.

AMICUS BRIEF Disability Law Center, "Brief of Amicus Curiae in Support of Appellant, Commonwealth of Massachusetts v. David Clinton and Bennett Walsh," December 14, 2022: 15, 16, 18.

CHAPTER FOUR

"OLD PEOPLE'S LIVES APPEAR[ED] NOT TO MATTER" Thomas Scharf, "Reframing Ageing Covid-19 Webinar," University College Dublin, June 12, 2020, https:// framingageing.ucd.ie/podcasts/.

SERIOUS CHRONIC CONDITIONS Mary L. Adams, David L. Katz, and Joseph Grandpre, "Population-Based Estimates of Chronic Conditions Affecting Risk for Complications from Coronavirus Disease, United States," *Emerging Infectious Diseases* 26, no. 8 (August 2020): 1831–33.

THE CDC'S DATA INDICATED CDC, Jonathan M. Wortham, James T. Lee, Sandy Althomsons, et al., "Characteristics of Persons Who Died with COVID-19, United States, February 12–May 18, 2020," *Morbidity and Mortality Weekly Report* 69 (2020): 923–29, https://www.cdc.gov/mmwr/volumes/69/wr/mm6928e1.htm.

DYING A DECADE YOUNGER Age/race data from Tiffany Ford, Sarah Reber, and Richard V. Reeves, "Race Gaps in COVID-19 Deaths Are Even Bigger Than They Appear," *Brookings*, June 16, 2020.

"IT'S HARD TO REMEMBER A YEAR WHEN DEATH WAS SO IN YOUR FACE" Richard Harris, "Too Many Americans Still Can't Talk about Death, Even after 15 Months of Pandemic," *Boston Globe Magazine*, June 1, 2021.

80 PERCENT OF THE US DEAD WERE OVER THE AGE OF SIXTY-FIVE Kaiser Family Foundation, "8 in 10 People Who Have Died of COVID-19 Were Age 65 or Older," press release, July 24, 2020, https://www.kff.org/coronavirus-covid-19/press-release/8-in-10-people-who-have-died-of-covid-19-were-age-65-or-older-but-the-share-varies-by-state/.

"1 OF EVERY 100 OLDER AMERICANS HAS PERISHED" Julie Bosman, Amy Harmon, and Albert Sun, "As U.S. Nears 800,000 Virus Deaths, 1 of Every 100 Older Americans Has Perished," *New York Times*, December 14, 2021.

"PEOPLE WHOSE DISAPPEARANCE WOULDN'T DRAW ATTENTION" Mike Jay, "Lace the Air with LSD," *London Review of Books*, February 4, 2021: 18.

"[THE LABELS ARE] NOW APPLIED ROUTINELY" Chris Phillipson, email to author, "My Essay about 'Avoiding Bias and Tragedy in Triage' in *Tikkun* April 15," April 27, 2020.

"FOR EVERY 1,000 PEOPLE . . ." Smriti Mallapaty, "The Coronavirus Is Most Deadly If You Are Older and Male," *Nature*, August 28, 2020.

"RISK INCREASES WITH AGE" "Older Adults . . . Risk Increases with Age," CDC, updated February 26, 2021, https://www.cdc.gov/aging/covid19/index.html#:~:text=Older%20adults%20%28especially%20those%20aged%2050%20years%20and,COVID-19%20deaths%20occur%20in%20people%20older%20than%2065.

"BLACKOUT DRINKING" Rose Marie Ward, Benjamin C. Riordan, Jennifer E. Merrill, and Jacques Raubenheimer, "Describing the Impact of the COVID-19 Pandemic on Alcohol-Induced Blackout Tweets," *Drug and Alcohol Review* 40, no. 2 (2021–2022): 192–95.

REVELRY Florida Life, "Spring Break 2020 / Fort Lauderdale Beach / Video #001," March 3, 2020, YouTube video, 6:12, https://www.youtube.com/watch?v=1Z3xA3JqI1o.

HE DIDN'T THINK THE VIRUS WAS A "BIG DEAL" Jawontae Rodgers, quoted in Hillary Hoffower, "'We're Not Worried about It,'" *Business Insider*, March 19, 2020.

"WE'RE JUST OUT HERE HAVING A GOOD TIME" Brady Sluder, quoted in Lorraine King, "Coronavirus: Young Spring Break Party Animals Say 'If I Get Corona, I Get Corona,'" *Mirror*, March 19, 2020.

"SYMBOLIZE THE PAST" Sarah Falcus, email to author, ". . . for My Chapter on the Cult of Youth?" August 6, 2021.

ADS ON FOX NEWS Darryl Pinckney, "Georgia's Battle over the Ballot," *New York Review of Books*, November 24, 2022: 58–60.

"BECAUSE THE RECKLESSNESS OF ADOLESCENCE IS SUCH ELATION . . ."

Joyce Carol Oates, "To Marlon Brando in Hell," *Salmagundi Magazine* 190–91 (Spring–Summer 2016): 57.

"FEAR *FOR* THE OTHER" Sijin Yan and Patrick Slattery, "The Fearful Ethical Subject: On the Fear for the Other, Moral Education, and Levinas in the Pandemic," *Studies in Philosophy and Education* 40 (2021): 81–92.

AGEISM AS A BUFFER Lauren E. Popham, Shelia M Kennison, and Kristopher I. Bradley, "Ageism and Risk-Taking in Young Adults: Evidence for a Link Between Death Anxiety and Ageism," *Death Studies* 35, no. 8 (2011): 751–63.

FORBADE HIS SON "New York Dad Refuses to Allow His College Kid Son, 21, Home . . . ," *Daily Mail* (UK), March 8, 2020, https://www.dailymail.co.uk/news/article-8163907/New-York-dad-locks-son-family-home-21-year-old-returns-spring-break-partying.html.

"ASSESSING ONE ANOTHER" Louise Erdrich, *The Sentence* (New York: Harper Perennial, 2021), 209.

CELLPHONE DATA HELPED RESEARCHERS PROVE Daniel Mangrum and Paul Kniekap, "College Student Travel Contributed to Local COVID-19 Spread," *Journal of Urban Economics*, June 18, 2020.

A DESPAIRING LAUGH Lawrence Wright, *The Plague Year: America in the Time of COVID* (New York: Knopf, 2021), 195.

AGEIST ALGORITHMS Kevin Collier, "Twitter's Racist Algorithm Is Also Ageist, Ableist and Islamaphobic, Researchers Find," *NBC News*, August 9, 2021.

"REASSURING MESSAGES WERE DEFINITELY NOT INTENDED FOR ME" Sonia Kruks, "Alterity and Intersectionality: Reflections on Old Age," *Hypatia* 37, no. 1 (Winter 2022): 196–209, at 197.

"IT WAS ALL OF A SUDDEN" Chip Conley, quoted in Katherine Ellison, "With the Novel Coronavirus, Suddenly at 60 We're Now 'Old,'" *Washington Post*, June 22, 2020.

"ELDERLY" IS A LABEL JOURNALISTS SHOULD AVOID Kristen Senz, "6 Tips for Improving News Coverage of Older People," *Journalist's Resource*, Harvard Kennedy School, November 15, 2022, https://journalistsresource.org/home/6-tips-for-improving-news-coverage-of-older-people/.

"AGEISM MAY BE THE FIRST MAJOR TYPE OF DISCRIMINATION" Julie O. Allen, email to author, "Social Class and Ageism," November 17, 2022.

"THE IMAGE OF OLDER PEOPLE" Marta, age 62, quoted in Stefan Hopf, Kieran Walsh, Eilionóir Flynn, and Nena Georgantzi, "The Relationship between Ageism and Well-Being as Mediated through COVID-19-Related Experiences and Discourses," *International Journal of Environmental Research and Public Health* 18, no.19 (October 2021): 10490, https://doi.org/10.3390/ijerph181910490.

CRITICS, INCLUDING ME, HAVE DISSECTED IT Margaret Morganroth Gullette, "From Adorable Baby Bulge to "#BoomerRemover," *Age, Culture, Humanities* 6 (September 2022).

AARP SURVEYS SHOWED Kimberly Palmer, "10 Things You Should Know about

Age Discrimination," *AARP*, updated September 1, 2022, https://www.aarp.org/work/age-discrimination/facts-in-the-workplace/.

LOST THE CHANCE TO SAVE Yimeng Yin, Anqi Chen, and Alicia H. Munnell, "The National Retirement Risk Index: Version 2.0," *Center for Retirement Research at Boston College*, May 9, 2023.

APPEARED ON FOX NEWS *Tucker Carlson Tonight*, episode dated March 23, 2020, written by Tucker Carlson, aired on Fox News.

"CLEAR THEMES OF POPULATION CLEANSING" Brad Meisner, "Are You OK, Boomer? Intensification of Ageism and Intergenerational Tensions on Social Media amid COVID-19," *Leisure Sciences* 43, nos. 1–2 (June 24, 2020): 56–61.

CULLING OF THE LEAST FIT "Great Barrington Declaration," accessed February 5, 2024, https://gbdeclaration.org/.

JOHN SNOW MEMORANDUM "John Snow Memorandum," accessed February 5, 2024, https://www.johnsnowmemo.com/john-snow-memo.html; see also "Official Endorsements," John Snow Memorandum, accessed February 5, 2024, https://www.johnsnowmemo.com/endorsements.html.

"THEIR RHETORIC INVALIDATES PUBLIC HEALTH POLICY" Stephen L. Archer, "5 Failings of the Great Barrington Declaration's Dangerous Plan for COVID-19 Natural Herd Immunity," *Conversation*, November 2, 2020.

"SACRIFICE THE WEAK" Bronwen Lichtenstein, "From 'Coffin Dodger' to 'Boomer Remover': Outbreaks of Ageism in Three Countries with Divergent Approaches to Coronavirus," *Journals of Gerontology: Social Sciences* 76, no. 4 (2021): e210.

"I REMEMBER SO VIVIDLY THE REST OF US BEING TOLD" Lisa Iezzoni, interviewed in Holly J. Humphrey, "Addressing Ableism in Health Professions Learning Environments," January 10, 2022, episode 8, *Vital Voices* (Josiah Macy Jr. Foundation podcast), MP3 audio, 22:49, transcript available at https://macyfoundation.org/assets/img/podcast-transcripts/episode-8_vital-voices_iezzoni_transcript_1.pdf.

ROAD SIGNS Richard P. Gale, Christopher P. Gale, T. A. Roper, and Graham P. Mulley, "Depiction of Elderly and Disabled People on Road Traffic Signs: International Comparison," *BMJ* 327, no. 7429 (December 20, 2003): 1456–57, https://www.ncbi.nlm.nih.gov/pmc/articles/PMC300805/.

OLDER READERS WROTE TO AARP Postings to the AARP website, March 24 and March 30, 2020, quoted in Lichtenstein, "From 'Coffin Dodger,'" e209.

"DEATHS OF SUCH PEOPLE COULD NOT BE PREVENTED" Age Platform Europe, quoted in Linda Naughton, Miguel Padeiro, and Paula Santana, "The Twin Faces of Ageism, Glorification and Abjection: A Content Analysis of Age Advocacy in the Midst of the COVID-19 Pandemic," *Journal of Aging Studies* 57 (June 2021): 14.

CHAPTER FIVE

"ELDER ABUSE" S. Duke Han and Laura Mosqueda, "Elder Abuse in the COVID-19 Era," letter in the *Journal of the American Geriatrics Society* 68, no. 7 (April 27, 2020).

"AS MUCH AS 84 PERCENT" E-Shien Chang and Becca R. Levy, "High Prevalence of Elder Abuse during the COVID-19 Pandemic: Risk and Resilience Factors," *American Journal of Geriatric Psychiatry* 29, no. 11 (November 2021): 1152–59.

FEDERAL TRADE COMMISSION AND THE AMERICAN BAR ASSOCIATION . . . ISSUED RESPECTIVE WARNINGS For the FTC warning, see Colleen Tressler, "Consumer Alert: Scammers Follow the Headlines," Federal Trade Commission Consumer Advice, February 10, 2020, https://consumer.ftc.gov/consumer-alerts/2020/02/coronavirus-scammers-follow-headlines; the American Bar Association warning is cited in Han and Mosqueda, "Elder Abuse," n3.

IRS HAD TO REMIND NURSING FACILITIES Anonymous, "IRS Lists 'Dirty Dozen' Tax Scams for 2020 with Focus on COVID-19," *Journal of Taxation* 133, no. 3 (September 2020): 33.

"VITAL TASKS" Congress of the United States Representative Mike Levin and ten others to Seema Verma, "Nursing Home Medical Director Registry Letter," *PALTC*, May 26, 2020.

"CHEMICAL RESTRAINTS" Katie Thomas, Robert Gebeloff, and Jessica Silver-Greenberg, "Phony Diagnoses Hide High Rates of Drugging at Nursing Homes," *New York Times*, updated September 16, 2021.

WORLD HEALTH ORGANIZATION "Elder Abuse," World Health Organization, June 15, 2021.

SOME RESIDENTS STARVED Mary-Therese Connelly, in a Woodrow Wilson Center interview entitled "Protecting the Elderly," October 2, 2013, YouTube video, 28:30, https://www.youtube.com/watch?v=I_1jVHwY58s.

DIRECTORS "IN NAME ONLY" Levin et al. to Verma, "Nursing Home Medical Director Registry Letter."

BARRED BY LOCKDOWNS FROM VISITING Emily Paulin, "Have a Nursing Home Complaint?" AARP, May 1, 2020, https://www.aarp.org/caregiving/health/info-2020/long-term-care-complaints-ombudsman.html. The Elder Justice Act of 2010, including its essential Ombudsman program, was more adequately supported later, in 2021.

REPORTS TO ADULT PROTECTIVE SERVICES ACTUALLY DECREASED Lena K. Makaroun, Scott Beach, Tony Rosen, and Ann-Marie Rosland, "Changes in Elder Abuse Risk Factors Reported by Caregivers of Older Adults during the COVID-19 Pandemic," letter to the editor, *Journal of the American Geriatrics Society*, December 21, 2020.

"THE EPICENTER IN DEATHS WAS NURSING HOMES" David Hochman, "Four Months That Left 54,000 Dead from COVID in Long-Term Care: The Oral History of an American Tragedy," *AARP*, December 3, 2020.

A BRANDEIS UNIVERSITY THESIS Kacy Jordan Ninteau, "Palliative Care in Nursing Homes during the COVID-19 Public Health Emergency" (BS thesis, Brandeis University, 2021), 20, https://doi.org/10.48617/etd.560.

"OUR CULTURAL FEAR AND SOCIETAL REVULSION" Christopher E. Laxton, David A. Nace, and Arif Nazir, "Special Article: Solving the COVID-19 Crisis in Post-Acute and Long-Term Care," *JAMDA* 21 (2020): 886.

FEARED HAVING TO "SELECT" FURTHER Denise Chow and Emmanuelle Saliba, "Italy Has a World Class Health System. The Coronavirus Has Pushed It to the Breaking Point," *NBC News*, March 18, 2020, https://www.nbcnews.com/health/health-news/italy-has-world-class-health-system-coronavirus-has-pushed-it-n1162786.

OATH OF GENEVA World Medical Association, "WMA Declaration of Geneva," July 9, 2018, https://www.wma.net/policies-post/wma-declaration-of-geneva/.

"VIRAL UNDERCLASS" *The Viral Underclass* is the title of a book by Steven Thrasher (New York: Celadon, 2022).

RUSHED TO CREATE TRIAGE GUIDELINES Wayne Martin, "Ethics of Triage: Philosophy in the Time of COVID-19," University of Essex webinar, April 29, 2020, https://www.essex.ac.uk/events/2020/04/29/the-ethics-of-triage.

UNIVERSITY OF PITTSBURGH University of Pittsburgh Department of Critical Care Medicine, "Allocation of Scarce Critical Care Resources during a Public Health Emergency," policy declaration, March 23, 2020: 6, https://bioethics.pitt.edu/sites/default/files/Univ%20Pittsburgh%20-%20Allocation%20of%20Scarce%20Critical%20Care%20Resources%20During%20a%20Public%20Health%20Emergency.pdf.

"GUT-WRENCHING" Liz Kowalczyk, "Who Gets a Ventilator? New Gut-Wrenching State Guidelines Issued on Rationing Equipment," *Boston Globe*, April 7, 2020.

THE MASSACHUSETTS GUIDELINE Commonwealth of Massachusetts, Department of Public Health, *Crisis Standards of Care: Planning Guidance for the COVID-19 Pandemic* (Boston, MA: Department of Public Health, April 7, 2020; revised April 20, 2020), 4, 11; on age priorities, see 21.

"SCHEMES USING POINT SCALES" Michelle D. Holmes, "Re-Opening America," *Vox Populi*, May 16, 2020.

"OTHER FACTORS THAT TAKE AGE INTO ACCOUNT" "Statement on Discriminatory Denial of Care to Older Adults," Justice in Aging, April 4, 2020. See also Thomas A. Bledsoe, Janet A. Jokela, Noel N. Deep, and Lois Snyder Sulmasy, "Universal Do-Not-Resuscitate Orders, Social Worth, and Life-Years: Opposing Discriminatory Approaches to the Allocation of Resources during the COVID-19 Pandemic and Other Health System Catastrophes," *Annals of Internal Medicine*, August 4, 2020.

"I THINK IT WOULD BE BIZARRE" Lachlan Forrow, email to author, "MA Crisis Standard of Care Document—A Query," August 2, 2022.

"WORST OFF" Ezekiel J. Emanuel, Govind Persad, Ross Upshur, Beatriz Thome, Michael Parker, Aaron Glickman, Cathy Zhang, Connor Boyle, Maxwell Smith, and James P. Phillips, "Fair Allocation of Scarce Medical Resources in the Time of Covid-19," *New England Journal of Medicine*, March 23, 2020, emphasis added, https://www.nejm.org/doi/full/10.1056/NEJMsb2005114.

PITTSBURGH GUIDELINE University of Pittsburgh, Department of Critical Care Medicine, "Allocation of Scarce Critical Care Resources during a Public Health Emergency," 6, 8, emphasis added.

CMS HAD BANNED QALY Andrés J. Gallegos to Charles Schumer, Nancy Pelosi, and Steny Hoyer, "NCD Letter to Congress Recommending QALY Ban in Build

Back Better Act," National Council on Disability, November 12, 2021, https://ncd.gov/publications/2021/ncd-letter-qaly-ban.

FEARS OF RATIONING LED THE OFFICE OF CIVIL RIGHTS TO ISSUE A STATE-MENT Sheri Fink, "U.S. Civil Rights Office Rejects Rationing Medical Care Based on Disability, Age," *New York Times*, March 28, 2020.

ADVOCATED A LOTTERY Holmes, "Re-Opening America."

"THE FIRST THING YOU HAVE TO COMMIT TO" Arthur Caplan, interviewed in James Hamblin, "No Shirt. No Shoes. No Shot. No Service," April 1, 2020, *Social Distance* (*Atlantic* podcast), MP3 audio, 40:28, https://www.theatlantic.com/health/archive/2021/04/no-shirt-no-shoes-no-shots-no-service/618487/.

"VIRTUALLY NO CHANCE OF SURVIVAL" Alex Wigglesworth, Rong-Gong Lin II, Soumya Karlamangla, and Luke Money, "Ambulance Crews Told Not to Transport Patients Who Have Little Chance of Survival," *Los Angeles Times*, January 4, 2021.

"WOULD YOU WANT TO GO TO THE ICU?" Celina Carter, Shan Mohammed, Ross Upshur, and Pia Kontos, "How the *More Life* Discourse Constrains End-of-Life Conversations in the Primary Care of Medically Frail Older Adults: A Critical Ethnography," *SSM—Qualitative Research in Health* 2 (December 2022): 12, 11.

NOT MEANT TO BE "A MEDICAL PROFESSIONAL'S ASSESSMENT" Valerie Gut-mann Koch and Susie A. Han, "Denying Ventilators to Covid-19 Patients with Prior DNR Orders is Unethical," *Hastings Center*, April 21, 2020.

DNR DOES NOT MEAN "DO NOT TREAT" Patricia A. Kelly, Kathy A. Baker, Karen M. Hodges, Ellen Y. Vuong, Joyce C. Lee, and Suzy W. Lockwood, "Original Research: Nurses' Perspectives on Caring for Patients with Do-Not-Resuscitate Orders," *American Journal of Nursing* 121, no. 1 (January 2021): 26–36.

WHAT THEY WOULD *NOT* DO FOR YOU Jacqueline K. Yuen, M. Carrington Reid, and Michael D. Fetters, "Hospital Do-Not-Resuscitate Orders: Why They Have Failed and How to Fix Them," *Journal of General Internal Medicine* 26, no. 7 (July 2011): 791–97.

"DYING, NOT RECOVERING" Betsy McCaughey, "Do Not Sign a DNR before You Read This," *Investor's Business Daily*, March 28, 2018.

MANY DOCTORS ARE ALSO IGNORANT Anthony C. Breu and Shoshana J. Her-zig, "Differentiating DNI from DNR: Combating Code Status Conflation," *Journal of Hospital Medicine* 9, no. 10 (October 2014): 669–70.

"MY DAD COULD HAVE BEEN SAVED" Mark Randlett, quoted in Shawne K. Wickham, "23 COVID-19 Deaths in NH, Each One a Family Tragedy," *Union Leader*, April 14, 2020.

EIGHTY-EIGHT PERCENT OF PHYSICIANS SAY THEY WOULD CHOOSE A DNR Tracie White, "Study: Doctors Would Choose Less Aggressive End-of-Life Care for Themselves," *Scope*, May 28, 2014.

BARBARA REICH Barbara Reich, *Intimations of Mortality: Medical Decision-Making at the End of Life* (New York: Cambridge University Press, 2022), 47.

PATIENTS ARE CHARACTERIZED AS "GOOD" Carter et al., "How the *More Life* Discourse Constrains," 8.

IGNORANCE OF GERIATRIC MEDICINE See Julia Mastroianni, "'Real People Won't Die': Rhetoric around Who Is at Risk of Coronavirus Infection Sparks Debate over Ageism, Ableism," *National Post*, March 3, 2020.

SUPPLY OF STUDENTS STUDYING GERIATRICS Aldis H. Petriceks, John C. Olivas, and Sakti Srivastava, "Trends in Geriatrics Graduate Medical Education Programs and Positions, 2001 to 2018," *Gerontology and Geriatric Medicine*, May 18, 2018.

"DESPAIR AT THE FUTILITY OF CARE" Louise Aronson, *Elderhood: Redefining Aging, Transforming Medicine, Reimagining Life* (New York: Bloomsbury, 2019), 343 and 429n.

"THEIR OWN FUTURE DECLINE" Ben Lerner, *10:04: A Novel* (New York: Farrar, Straus and Giroux, 2014), 6.

DOCTORS. . . IGNORED THEM Judith Graham, "Seniors Decry Age Bias, Say They Feel Devalued When Interacting with Health Care Providers," *Kaiser Health Network*, October 17, 2021.

"INSTANTLY OVERWHELMED" Mark S. Lachs, "COVID-19 and Aging: a Tale of Two Pandemics," *Nature Aging* 1 (January 14, 2021): 9, emphasis added.

"THERE WAS SUBSTANTIAL OPPORTUNITY" Michelle J. Berning, Emily Palmer, Timothy Tsai, Susan L. Mitchell, and Sarah D. Berry, "An Advance Care Planning Long-Term Care Initiative in Response to COVID-19," *Journal of the American Geriatric Society* 69, no. 4 (April 2021): 861–67, at 861.

$13.02 AN HOUR Daniel Moore, "How to Spend $400 billion on Home Care?" *Pittsburgh Post Gazette*, July 18, 2021.

DO NOT HOSPITALIZE ORDERS INCREASED Ping Ye, Liam Fry, and Jane Dimmitt Champion, "Changes in Advance Care Planning for Nursing Home Residents During the COVID-19 Pandemic," *JAMDA* 22 (2021): 209–14.

PATIENTS ADMITTED TO CALIFORNIA HOSPITALS Derek K. Richardson, Dana Zive, Mohamud Daya, and Craig D. Newgard, "The Impact of Early Do Not Resuscitate (DNR) Orders on Patient Care and Outcomes Following Resuscitation from Out of Hospital Cardiac Arrest," *Resuscitation*, September 3, 2012.

"SOME EXISTING AND PROPOSED GUIDELINES" Koch and Han, "Denying Ventilators."

"A PATIENT WHO WOULD NOT HAVE SURVIVED" Jeffrey P. Bishop, Kyle B. Brothers, Joshua E. Perry, and Ayesha Ahmad, "Reviving the Conversation around CPR/DNR," *American Journal of Bioethics* 10, no. 1 (January 2010): 66.

DOCTORS ACROSS HIS HOSPITAL "WERE IMPLORING US" Joseph J. Fins, "Resuscitating Patient Rights during the Pandemic: COVID-19 and the Risk of Resurgent Paternalism," *Cambridge Quarterly of Healthcare Ethics* 30, no. 2 (April 2021): 215–21.

"A PUBLIC HEALTH MANIFESTO" Rainbow Push Coalition and National Medical Association, "Joint Statement on the Response to the Coronavirus/COVID-19 Pandemic: A Public Health Manifesto," April 15, 2020, https://www.nmanet.org

/news/503170/Joint-Statement-on-the-Response-to-the-CoronavirusCOVID-19 -Pandemic.htm.

SAID THEY WOULD FORGO AGGRESSIVE TREATMENTS Anthony Breu, email to author, "Confusing DNR and DNI — Implications for the COVID Era of 2020?" July 25, 2020.

"MANY FAMILY MEMBERS ARE MAKING THE DIFFICULT CHOICE" Ariana Eunjung Cha, "Hospitals Consider Universal Do-Not-Resuscitate Orders for Coronavirus Patients," *Washington Post*, March 3, 2020.

DR. JOSEPH FINS . . . HAD FELT "A QUEASINESS" Fins, "Resuscitating Patient Rights."

"COLLECT AND REPORT ALL INVOLUNTARY DNR ORDERS" Rainbow Push Coalition and National Medical Association, "Joint Statement."

"WHEN THE PATIENT'S WISHES ARE NOT KNOWN" "Do Not Attempt Resuscitation Orders in the Out-of-Hospital Setting," American College of Emergency Physicians policy resource and education paper, October 2003, https://www.acep.org/life -as-a-physician/ethics--legal/ethics/dnar-orders-in-the-out-of-hospital-setting.

"THEY'RE NOT GIVING PEOPLE A SECOND CHANCE" Oren Barzilay, quoted in Danielle Wallace and Nick Givens, "New York State Rescinds DNR Orders for Cardiac Patients amid Coronavirus Crisis," *Fox News*, April 22, 2020.

"WE NEVER COMPLIED" Oren Barzilay, telephone interview with author, September 9, 2021.

"THIS GUIDANCE" Wallace and Givens, "New York State Rescinds DNR Order."

BLANKET DNACPR . . . NOTICES Clare Dyer, "Some Care Home Residents May Have Died because of Blanket DNR Orders, Says Regulator," *British Medical Journal*, December 3, 2020.

"THROWING HERSELF OFF A BRIDGE" Lucy Jeal, quoted in Deborah Mahmoudieh, "Britain's Throw Away People," *Medium*, January 12, 2021.

"SOME FORM OF TRIAGE" John Lanchester, "As the Lock Rattles," *London Review of Books*, December 16, 2021: 14; data from George Arbuthnott and Jonathan Calvert, *Failures of State: The Inside Story of Britain's Battle with Coronavirus* (London: Harper Collins, 2021).

SUFFICIENTLY PROVED For one example, see Aikaterini Gkoufa, Eleni Maneta, Georgios N. Ntoumas, Vasiliki E. Georgakopoulou, Athina Mantelou, Stelios Kokkoris, and Christina Routsi, "Elderly Adults with COVID-19 Admitted to Intensive Care Unit: A Narrative Review," *World Journal of Critical Care Medicine* 10, no. 5 (September 9, 2021): 278–89.

"WHEN OLDER PEOPLE DIE" Connelly, "Protecting the Elderly."

CASH COW Dylan Scott, "Private Equity Ownership Is Killing People at Nursing Homes," *Vox*, February 22, 2021; this article goes only through 2017 data.

"ELDERLY PEOPLE WHO I ADORE" Quoted in Sarah Lamb, "On Vulnerability, Resilience, and Age: Older Americans Reflect on the Pandemic," *Anthropology and Aging* 41, no. 2 (2020): 177–86.

"WALKING THEM TO THEIR DEATH" Katie Lannan, "Report Details 'Utterly Baffling' Decisions at Holyoke Soldiers' Home," *New England Public Media*, June 24, 2020.

"ISOLATED INCIDENTS OF IRRATIONALITY" Jennifer J. Yeager, introduction, in Sue E. Meiner and Jennifer J. Yeager, *Gerontologic Nursing* (New York: Elsevier Health Sciences, 2018), 40.

"MISSED COVID-19 DIAGNOSES" Tucker Doherty, "Summer Wave of Dementia Deaths Adds Thousands to Pandemic's Deadly Toll," *Politico*, September 16, 2020.

NO COVID-19-RELATED DEATHS IN THE TEN MONTHS OF 2020 Caroline Pearson, David Rein, Mairin Mancino, Lindsey Schapiro, and Claudia Gorman, *Final Report: The Impact of COVID-19 on Seniors Housing* (Chicago: National Opinion Research Center (NORC) at the University of Chicago, June 3, 2021): 3, https://info.nic .org/hubfs/Outreach/2021_NORC/20210601%20NIC%20Final%20Report%20and %20Executive%20Summary%20FINAL.pdf.

"THE TEMPLATE FOR A NEW NORMAL THAT WE MIGHT COME TO REGRET" Fins, "Resuscitating Patient Rights."

CHAPTER SIX

"LOVE SONG TO THE CARE INDUSTRY" Jack Thorne, quoted in K. J. Yossman, "Acorn TV Unveils New 'Help' Trailer Starring 'Killing Eve's' Jodie Comer as COVID-Hit Care Nurse," *Variety*, January 10, 2022.

"'WE'D RATHER JUST NOT BE INCONVENIENCED'" Tara Swanigan, quoted in Ariana Eunjung Cha and Dan Keating, "Covid Becomes Plague of Elderly," *Washington Post*, November 30, 2022.

140 TIMES AS LIKELY Centers for Disease Control and Infection (CDC), "Risk for COVID-19 Infection, Hospitalization, and Death by Age Group," *CDC.gov*, updated May 30, 2023, https://archive.cdc.gov/#/details?url=https://www.cdc.gov /coronavirus/2019-ncov/covid-data/investigations-discovery/hospitalization-death -by-age.html.

"WHEN I SAY 'THIS'" John Okrent, *This Costly Season: A Crown of Sonnets* (Bristol: Arrowsmith, 2021), 14.

GREY'S ANATOMY Valentina Possenti and Debora Serra, "Narrating the COVID-19 Pandemic by Medical Drama: The Case of Grey's Anatomy," *Academia Letters*, December 21, 2021: 5.

"CRASHED" CNNWire, "Silent Hypoxia," CNN, May 8, 2020.

"SELF-DEFENSIVE PROCESS OF PSYCHOLOGICAL DISTANCING" Anthony Terracciano, Yannick Stephan, Damaris Aschwanden, Ji Hyn Lee, Amanda A. Sesker, Jason E. Strickhouser, Martina Luchetti, and Angelina R. Sutin, "Changes in Subjective Age during COVID-19," *Gerontologist* 61, no. 1 (January 2021): 13–22, https://doi.org /10.1093/geront/gnaa104.

REMINDED OF THEIR OWN DEATH, [COLLEGE STUDENTS] Andy Martens, Jeff Greenberg, Jeff Schimel, and Mark J. Landau, "Ageism and Death: Effects of Mortality

Salience and Perceived Similarity to Elders on Reactions to Elderly People," *Personality and Social Psychology Bulletin* 30, no. 12 (December 2004): 1532, https://journals.sagepub.com/doi/abs/10.1177/0146167204271185.

THEY REPORTED FEELING *YOUNGER* Terracciano et al., "Changes in Subjective Age."

"SOCIAL STIGMA IN THE CONTEXT OF A HEALTH OUTBREAK" United Nations Department of Economic and Social Affairs (UN DESA), *Issue Brief: Older Persons and COVID-19* (New York: UN DESA, April 2020), https://www.un.org/development/desa/ageing/wp-content/uploads/sites/24/2020/04/POLICY-BRIEF-ON-COVID19-AND-OLDER-PERSONS.pdf.

"LIKE A DOOR IN A HORROR MOVIE" Okrent, *This Costly Season*, 37.

REPORTED THE SHAME Margaret Morganroth Gullette, *Ending Ageism, or How Not to Shoot Old People* (New Brunswick, NY: Rutgers University Press, 2017), chapter 7, "Induction into the Hall of Shame and the Way Out."

SECOND SIGHT W. E. B. DuBois, *The Souls of Black Folk: Essays and Sketches* (Chicago: A. C. McClurg, 1903), 1, 3; Laura Mulvey, "Visual Pleasure and Narrative Cinema," *Screen* 16, no. 4 (1975): 6–18.

"SUPERFLUOUS" Laurie Carter Noble, letter to the editor, *Boston Globe Magazine*, September 24, 2022.

THE RUN OF RISING LONGEVITY DROPPED A FULL 1.5 YEARS Nazrul Islam, Dmitri A. Jdanov, Vladimir M. Shkolnikov, Kamlesh Khunti, Ichiro Kawachi, Martin White, Sarah Lewington, and Ben Lacey, "Effects of Covid-19 Pandemic on Life Expectancy and Premature Mortality in 2020: Time Series Analysis in 37 Countries," *British Medical Journal* 375 (November 2021): 1–14.

REGISTER OF SHAME Andre M. Perry, Carl Romer, and Anthony Barr, "Why Is Life Expectancy So Low in Black Neighborhoods?" *Brookings Institute*, December 20, 2021.

LIFE EXPECTANCY CONTINUED TO DROP Akilah Johnson and Sabrina Malhi, "U.S. Life Expectancy Down for Second-Straight Year, Fueled by Covid-19," *Washington Post*, August 31, 2022.

THAT TOTAL WAS INADEQUATE Neil A. Halpern and Kay See Tan, "United States Resource Availability for COVID-19," *Society of Critical Care Medicine* (blog), March 2020, https://sccm.org/blog/march-2020/united-states-resource-availability-for-covid-19.

"FIRST COME, FIRST SERVED" Robert D. Truog, "Ventilator Allocation Protocols: Sophisticated Bioethics for an Unworkable Strategy," *Hastings Center Report* 51, no. 5 (September 16, 2021): 56–57.

"AN UNJUST ALLOCATION OF RESOURCES" Commonwealth of Massachusetts, Department of Public Health, *Crisis Standards of Care: Planning Guidance for the COVID-19 Pandemic* (Boston, MA: Department of Public Health, revised April 20, 2020), 11, 23.

DAWN KELLY TOLD THE DOCTORS The *New York Times* and CNN versions of Kelly's story have details other accounts lack. See Jan Benzel, "51 Days on a Ventilator:

How 'Miracle Larry' Survived," *New York Times*, July 17, 2020; and Alicia Lee, "After 128 Days in a Hospital—51 on a Ventilator—Covid-19 Survivor 'Miracle Larry' Is Finally Home," CNN, July 23, 2020.

IN KELLY'S CASE Debbie Humphrey, "Seniors Can Survive COVID-19 with Help, Hope and Support," *Home Helpers*, July 23, 2020. Kelly also appeared on *CBS This Morning*, "'Miracle Larry' Kelly Leaves Hospital after 128 Days Battling Coronavirus, 51 Days on Ventilator," reported by Tara Narula, aired July 24, 2020, on CBS, https://www.cbsnews.com/video/miracle-larry-kelly-leaves-hospital-after-128-days-battling-coronavirus-51-days-on-ventilator/#x.

"THESE PATIENTS MAY EVENTUALLY RECOVER" Greer Waldrop, Seyed A. Safavynia, Megan E. Barra, Sachin Agarwal, David A. Berlin, Amelia K. Boehme, Daniel Brodie, Jacky M. Choi, Kevin Doyle, Joseph J. Fins, Wolfgang Ganglberger, Katherine Hoffman, Aaron .M Mittel, David Roh, Shibani S. Mukerji, Caroline Der Nigoghossian, Soojin Park, Edward J. Schenck, John Salazar-Schicchi, Qi Shen, Evan Sholle, Angela G. Velazquez, Maria C. Walline, M. Brandon Westover, Emery N. Brown, Jonathan Victor, Brian L. Edlow, Nicholas D. Schiff, and Jan Claassen, "Prolonged Unconsciousness Is Common in COVID-19 and Associated with Hypoxemia," *Annals of Neurology* 91, no. 6 (March 7, 2022): 740–55.

"OLDEST ELDERLY" DID WELL Wei Yu, Arlene S. Ash, Norman G. Levinsky, Mark A. Moskowitz, "Intensive Care Unit Use and Mortality in the Elderly," *Journal of General Internal Medicine* 15, no. 2 (February 2000): 97–102.

"ALL MEDICINE WANTS" Jelaluddin Rumi, "Cry Out in Your Weakness," in *The Essential Rumi*, trans. Coleman Barks (Edison, NJ: Castle Books, 1997), 156.

SUCCESS IN MEDICINE REQUIRES NOT SUPERIOR INTELLIGENCE BUT "CHARACTER" Atul Gawande, *Better: A Surgeon's Notes on Performance* (New York: Metropolitan, 2007), 9.

"WHOLE PERSON CARE" Archie S. Golden, "A Definition of Primary Care for Educational Purposes," in *The Art of Teaching Primary Care*, ed. Archie S. Golden, Denis G. Carlson, and Jan L. Hagen (New York: Springer: 1982), 6.

"DOCTORS HAVE BECOME PEOPLE" Laura Kolbe, "The Moment. The Physician as Patient: Medicine after COVID-19," *Yale Review* (Summer 2022): 6.

WHEN MANUALS AND CURRICULA CHANGE See Christopher C. Colenda, Charles F. Reynolds, William B. Applegate, Philip D. Sloane, Sheryl Zimmerman, Anne B. Newman, Suzanne Meeks, and Joseph G. Ouslander, "COVID -19 Pandemic and Ageism: A Call for Humanitarian Care," *Journal of the American Geriatrics Society*, July 14, 2020.

"AN OLDER PHYSICIAN WHO HAS SHARED EXPERIENCES" Jane Mansbridge, email to author, "How Physicians 'Represent' Their Patients," August 25 and 26, 2022.

"COMMUNICATIVE DISTRUST" Liz Mineo, "Jane Mansbridge Talks about Her 'Jagged Trajectory' to Becoming One of the World's Leading Scholars of Democratic Theory," *Harvard Gazette*, September 20, 2020.

"BASED ON THE ALTERNATIVES TO TRUST" Bradford H. Gray, "Trust and

Trustworthy Care in the Managed Care Era," *Health Affairs* 16, no. 1 (January–February 1997): 34–49.

"I WILL NEVER . . . ABANDON YOU" Abraham Verghese, "A Doctor's Touch," *TEDGlobal*, July 2011, video, 18:16, at 18:00, https://www.ted.com/talks/abraham _verghese_a_doctor_s_touch.

"TRYING TO ISOLATE AND IDENTIFY" George Orwell, "Notes on Nationalism," in *The Collected Essays, Journalism, and Letters of George Orwell Vol. III (1943–1945)*, ed. Sonia Orwell and Ian Angus (New York: Harcourt Brace Jovanovich, 1968), 10.

CHAPTER SEVEN

"BETTER THAN YOU THINK" Pew Research Center, *Growing Old in America: Expectations vs. Reality* (Washington, DC: Pew Research Center, June 29, 2009), https://www.pewresearch.org/social-trends/2009/06/29/growing-old-in-america -expectations-vs-reality/.

BRISKLY SUMMARIZED FOR ME Peter Whitehouse, email to author, "Your POV on 'Dementism,'" July 6, 2021.

THAT GLORIOUS FAKE FACT BECAME CONVENTIONAL WISDOM Margaret Morganroth Gullette, "History of Longevity Discourses," in *Encyclopedia of Gerontology and Population Aging*, eds. Danan Gu and Matthew E. Dupre (New York: Springer, 2019), 2407–12.

FEARED OUR TENACIOUS LIFE SPANS Margaret Morganroth Gullette, "Why We Fear Aging More Than We Should," *Next Avenue*, April 13, 2012.

SIX TIMES HIGHER Reuben Ng, "Societal Age Stereotypes in the U.S. and U.K. from a Media Database of 1.1 Billion Words," *International Journal of Environmental Research and Public Health* 18, no. 16 (2021): 8822.

"THE LARGEST SINGLE NEWS STORY" John Baron, quoted in Heather Hanlon, Judy Farnsworth, and Judy Murray, "Ageing in American Comic Strips: 1972–1992," *Ageing and Society* 17 (May 1997): 299.

FOOLISH GENERATIONAL WARNS Margaret Morganroth Gullette, "The 'Xers' versus 'the Boomers': A Contrived War," in Gullette, *Aged by Culture* (Chicago: University of Chicago Press, 2004), 42–60; and Dan Bouk, "Generation Crisis: How Population Research Defined the Baby Boomers," *Modern American History* 1, no. 3 (November 2, 2018).

"VOODOO DEMOGRAPHY" See Ellen Gee, "Voodoo Demography, Population Ageing, and Canadian Social Policy," in *The Overselling of Population Ageing: Apocalyptic Demography, Intergenerational Challenges and Social Policy*, ed. Ellen Gee and Gloria Gutman (New York: Oxford University Press, 2000), 5–35.

"EXAGGERATION OF THE SIZE OF THE RESOURCES" Jason L. Powell and John Martyn Chamberlain, *Social Welfare, Aging, and Social Theory* (Lanham, MD: Lexington Books, 2012), 43.

"TRIBUTARY NEGLIGENCE" Paul Goldberg, *The Château* (New York: Picador,

2018), quoted in Cathleen Schine, "Comic Noir," *New York Review of Books*, August 16, 2018: 54.

"A MERCY" Louise Penny, *The Madness of Crowds* (New York: Minotaur Books, 2021), 70.

"WE REALLY DO SPEND TOO MUCH" Joshua Rothman, "Thinking It Through," *New Yorker*, August 23, 2021: 28.

A US CORRELATIONAL STUDY Betül Kanık, Özden Melis Uluğ, Nevin Solak, and Maria Chayinska, "'Let the Strongest Survive': Ageism and Social Darwinism as Barriers to Supporting Policies to Benefit Older Individuals," *Journal of Social Issues* 78 (2022): 804, https://doi.org/10.1111/josi.12553.

EMANUEL AND HIS COAUTHOR ALAN WERTHEIMER Ezekiel Emanuel and Alan Wertheimer, "Who Should Get Influenza Vaccine When Not All Can?" *Science* 312 (May 12, 2006): 854–55.

EZEKIEL EMANUEL Ezekiel Emanuel, Govind Persad, Ross Upshur, Beatriz Thome, Michael Parker, Aaron Glickman, Cathy Zhang, Connor Boyle, Maxwell Smith, and James P. Phillips, "Fair Allocation of Scarce Medical Resources in the Time of Covid-19," *New England Journal of Medicine*, March 23, 2020.

"FURIOUS CRITICISM" See Christopher S. Wareham, "Between Hoping to Die and Longing to Live Longer," *History of Philosophy and the Life Sciences* 43, no. 40 (2021): 2.

"THE COMING DEATH SHORTAGE" Charles C. Mann, "The Coming Death Shortage," *Atlantic Monthly* (May 2005).

"OUR DUTY MAY BE" Daniel Callahan, "On Dying after Your Time," *New York Times*, December 1, 2013.

"WICKEDNESS" James Baldwin, *Notes of a Native Son* (Beacon Press, 1955), 43.

THE COSTLIEST TO TREAT WERE MIDLIFE MEN Christopher Hogan, June R. Lunney, Jon Gabel, and Joanne Lynn, "Medicare Beneficiaries' Costs of Care in the Last Year of Life," *Health Affairs* 20, no. 4 (July–August 2001): 188–95, at 191.

"NOT AN ABERRATION, BUT INSTEAD A REFLECTION" Laura I. Appleman, "Pandemic Eugenics: Discrimination, Disability and Detention During COVID-19," *Loyola Law Review* 67, no. 2 (2021).

NAZI TEXTBOOKS Examples can be found in Kurt-Ingo Flessau, *Schule der Diktatur: Lehrpläne und Schulbücher des Nationalsozialismus* (Frankfurt / Main: Fischer, 1984/2018), 201, translated for me by Rüdiger Kunow. Robert Proctor, *Racial Hygiene* (Cambridge, MA: Harvard University Press, 1988), 184, provides similar examples.

"DEPENDENCY RATIOS" Grayson K. Vincent and Victoria A. Velkoff, *The Next Four Decades: The Older Population in the United States, 2010 to 2050*, report no. P25-1138 (Washington, DC: US Census Bureau, Department of Commerce, May 2010).

"TEXTUALITY AS THE SITE OF LIFE AND DEATH" Stuart Hall, "Cultural Studies and Its Theoretical Legacies," in Hall, *Essential Essays*, vol. 1 (Durham, NC: Duke University Press, 2019), 83.

"BEGINS TO CIRCULATE IN THE CAPILLARIES" Rüdiger Kunow, *Material Bodies: Biology and Culture in the United States*, American Studies vol. 286 (Heidelberg:

Universitätsverlag Winter, 2018), 181–82. Kunow attributes the body metaphor to Scott Lash.

"HUMANIZATION AND DEHUMANIZATION OCCUR CEASELESSLY" Judith Butler, *Precarious Life: The Powers of Mourning and Violence* (New York: Verso, 2004), 141.

"OFFICIOUSLY TO KEEP ALIVE" Arthur Hugh Clough, "The Latest Decalogue," 1862, https://allpoetry.com/The-Latest-Decalogue.

A BRILLIANT PLAY CALLED CRACKED Collective Disruption, *Cracked: New Light on Dementia*, written by Julia Gray, produced by the Partnerships in Dementia Care Alliance, premiered in 2017 in Ontario, Canada. A donation of $100 provides a download of the play; see https://crackedondementia.ca/donate. The teaching tool, which includes clips, is free; see https://crackedondementia.ca/dementia-in-new-light/.

A CLIP SHOWING PEOPLE IN WHEELCHAIRS PBS Wisconsin, "Director's Cut—A Scene from 'Penelope: A Theatrical Odyssey,'" June 20, 2014, YouTube video, 1:44, https://www.youtube.com/watch?v=NNJw26U6_Ug. See also Anne Basting, Maureen Towey, and Ellie Rose, *The Penelope Project: An Arts-Based Odyssey to Change Elder Care* (Iowa City: University of Iowa Press, 2016).

KIRKWOOD'S ACCLAIMED PLAY Lucy Kirkwood, *The Children* (New York: Dramatists' Play Service, Inc., 2018), https://dramatists.com/previews/5667.pdf.

"LIFE-ALTERING DECISION" Stage Buddy [unsigned], *Theater Review*, December 27, 2019.

"ONCE-VITAL PARTY PEOPLE" Jim Burke, "*The Children* Shakes Up the Centaur with a Very English Apocalypse," special to *Montreal Gazette*, November 13, 2018, emphasis added.

"WHAT TODAY'S ELDERS OWE THE YOUNG" "Announcing Aurora's 28th Season: 2019/2020," Aurora Theatre Company, 2019, https://www.auroratheatre.org/1920season, emphasis added.

"WHO'S SELFISH NOW?" Jesse. Green, "Review: In 'The Children,' the Waters Rise and a Reckoning Comes Due," *New York Times*, December 12, 2017, emphasis added.

"SELFISH" "The Children Post-Show Talk: Q and A with Lucy Kirkwood," Royal Court Theatre, 2017, https://royalcourttheatre.com/whats-on/the-children/#extras.

"KAMIKAZE HEARTS" Katy Waldman ("Let There Be Darkness," *New Yorker*, September 27, 2021) quotes Joy Williams in her review of *Harrow* (New York: Knopf, 2021).

"THE INTERGENERATIONAL UNFAIRNESS NARRATIVE" Anne Karpf, "Don't Let Prejudice against Older People Contaminate the Climate Movement," *Guardian*, January 18, 2020.

"GENERATIONAL CONFLICT WILL BE PROMINENT" Jesse Ballenger, email to author, "Your Point of View," July 22, 2021.

"CRISIS OF AGING" Núria Casado-Gual, "Staging the 'Crisis of Aging': Old Age as the New Apocalypse in *The Children* and *Escaped Alone*," in *Understanding the Discourse of Aging: A Multifaceted Perspective*, ed. Vicent Salvador and Agnese Samprieto (Newcastle upon Tyne: Cambridge Scholars, 2021), 233–58.

A 2017 REPORT Daniel R. Levinson to Seema Verma, "SUBJECT: Early Alert: The

Centers for Medicare & Medicaid Services Has Inadequate Procedures to Ensure That Incidents of Potential Abuse or Neglect at Skilled Nursing Facilities Are Identified and Reported in Accordance with Applicable Requirements (A-01-17-00504)," memorandum, HHS, Office of the Inspector General, August 24, 2017, https://oig.hhs.gov/oas/reports/region1/11700504.pdf.

UNDERSTAFFING IS PERMITTED "What's Needed for Transformational Nursing Home Reform to Improve Quality and Oversight," statement, Dignity Alliance Massachusetts, July 2023, https://dignityalliancema.org/wp-content/uploads/2023/07/Dignity-Alliance-Whats-Needed-for-Transformational-Reform.pdf. Their recommendations are based on Kaiser Health News analysis of payroll records.

"WHY ARE WE SO QUICK TO ALWAYS PROTECT THEM?" Sarah Waddle, quoted in "Critics Say Indiana COVID-19 Law Allows Nursing Home Neglect," *AP News*, May 8, 2021.

"SUBSEQUENTLY CITED FOR CAUSING SERIOUS HARM" Clark Kaufman, "Five Iowa Nursing Homes Have Spent Years on Federal List of the Nation's Worst Care Facilities," Iowa Public Radio, June 7, 2021, https://www.iowapublicradio.org/health/2021-06-07/five-iowa-nursing-homes-have-spent-years-on-federal-list-of-the-nations-worst-care-facilities. Kaufman's data comes from Jordan Rau, "Poor Patient Care at Many Nursing Homes Despite Stricter Oversight," *New York Times*, July 5, 2017, https://www.nytimes.com/2017/07/05/health/failing-nursing-homes-oversight.html.

TAKE OVER AT LEAST THE WORST Margaret Morganroth Gullette, "Everyone in a Nursing Home Deserves a Single Room," *Boston Globe*, March 15, 2023.

"A HUGE THREAT TO THE U.S. BUDGET HAS RECEDED" Margot Sanger-Katz, Alicia Parlapiano, and Josh Katz, "A Huge Threat to the U.S. Budget Has Receded. And No One Is Sure Why," *New York Times*, September 5, 2023.

OFFICIALLY FAVORED WITH THE FIRST VACCINE Jennifer Tolbert, Jennifer Kates, and Josh Michaud, "The COVID-19 Vaccine Priority Line Continues to Change as States Make Further Updates," *Kaiser Family Foundation*, January 21, 2021, https://www.kff.org/policy-watch/the-covid-19-vaccine-priority-line-continues-to-change-as-states-make-further-updates/.

RANKED BY THE NUMBER OF COVID-19 DEATHS PER HUNDRED THOUSAND Mississippi was the worst in this ranking, but as noted, states do not all count the same way. See "Death Rates from COVID-19 in the United States as of October 24, 2022, by State," *Statista*, October 24, 2022. https://www.statista.com/statistics/1109011/coronavirus-covid19-death-rates-us-by-state/.

"BOOMERS GOT THE VAX" "Boomers Got the Vax," *Saturday Night Live*, aired March 28, 2021, on NBC, https://www.youtube.com/watch?v=2hekDuCBxCc.

ONLY 30 PERCENT OF THOSE OVER FIFTY WHO LOST JOBS WERE RE-EMPLOYED Laura Putre, "Age Discrimination and 'The Great Shedding,'" *Industry Week*, November 23, 2022.

"FAR FROM HAVING FLATTENED THE CURVE ON THE VIRUS OF AGEISM"

Susan Flory, "Ageism and the Virus," April 17, 2020, episode 54, *The Big Middle* (podcast), MP3 audio, 51:48, https://susanflory.com/margaret-morganroth-gullette-2/.

CHAPTER EIGHT

"SNUGGED INTO LIFE" Richard Ford, *The Lay of the Land* (New York: Knopf, 2006), 75, 76.

THE FIRST BIAS SOME FORTUNATE WHITES EXPERIENCE Julie Ober Allen, Erica Solway, Matthias Kirch, Dianne Singer, Jeffrey T. Kullgren, Valerie Moïse, and Preeti N. Malani, "Experiences of Everyday Ageism and the Health of Older US Adults," *JAMA Network Open* 5, no. 6 (June 15, 2022): 9.

95 PERCENT OF THE PARTICIPANTS ... HELD NEGATIVE VIEWS Becca Levy, "Eradication of Ageism Requires Addressing the Enemy Within," *Gerontologist* 41, no. 5 (2001): 578–79.

THE RISK OF BAD PHYSICAL AND MENTAL HEALTH OUTCOMES See Becca R. Levy, Martin D. Slade, E-Shien Chang, Sneha Kannoth, and Shi-Yi Wang, "Ageism Amplifies Cost and Prevalence of Health Conditions," *Gerontologist* 60, no. 1 (February 2020): 174–81.

AS AARP SURVEYS SHOWED Joe Kita, "Workplace Discrimination Still Flourishes in America," *AARP*, December 30, 2019.

THE AVERAGE PERSON RESENTED HARSH BIRTHDAY CARDS Margaret Morganroth Gullette, "Are Old People Still Human? On Ageist Humor," *Palgrave Handbook of Literature and Age*, ed. Valerie Lipscomb and Aagje Swinnen (New York: Palgrave Macmillan, forthcoming 2024).

"SUBJECT TO PERSONAL CONTROL" Toni Calasanti, "A Feminist Confronts Ageism," *Journal of Aging Studies* 22, no. 2 (April 2008): 152–57.

"MOST AMERICANS HAVE YET TO PUT THEIR CONCERNS" Ashton Applewhite, *This Chair Rocks* (Networked Books, n.d.), 14.

"AGE-ISM MIGHT PARALLEL OR REPLACE RACISM AS THE GREAT ISSUE" Robert Butler, quoted in Andrew W. Achenbaum, "A History of Ageism Since 1969," *Generations* 39, no. 3 (Fall 2015): 10–16.

"BEST TO DO IT SOMEWHERE ELSE" Nicole Hollander, *Tales of Graceful Aging from the Planet Denial* (New York: Broadway Books, 2007).

"THE CHRONOLOGICAL AND BIOLOGICAL DIMENSIONS OF AGING" Corinne T. Field, "Anti-Feminism, Anti-Blackness, and Anti-Oldness: The Intersectional Aesthetics of Aging in the Nineteenth-Century United States," *Signs* 47, no. 4 (Summer 2022).

"ERAS WHERE FOOTWEAR DEFORMS LESS" Marguerite Yourcenar, *Mémoires d'Hadrien* (Paris: Plon, 1951), 333. My translation.

"*A COLLECTION OF DISEASES*" Colin Farrelly, "Rethinking the Definition of Aging," *Boston Globe*, July 7, 2008, quoting Dr. David Sinclair of Harvard Medical School, http://colinfarrelly.blogspot.com/2008/07/boston-globe-article-on-aging.html.

"BYPASSED GERONTOLOGY" Stephen Katz, "Five Eye-Openers in My Life of Critical Gerontology," *International Journal of Ageing and Later Life* 10, no. 1 (2015): 25.

I WISHFULLY NAMED THE POTENTIAL FIELD "AGE STUDIES" Margaret Morganroth Gullette, "Creativity, Aging, Gender: A Study of Their Intersections, 1910–1935," in *Aging and Gender in Literature: Studies in Creativity*, ed. Anne M. Wyatt-Brown and Janice Rossen (Charlottesville: University Press of Virginia, 1993), 19–48; see also Gullette, "What Is Age Studies?" in *Aged by Culture* (Chicago: University of Chicago Press, 2004), 101–19; Stephen Katz, "What Is Age Studies?" *Age, Culture, Humanities* 1 (January 2014): 17–23.

"ALTERNATIVE . . . CONDITIONS OF AGING" Stephen Katz, "Critical Gerontological Theory: Intellectual Fieldwork and the Nomadic Life of Ideas," in *The Need for Theory: Critical Approaches to Social Gerontology*, ed. Simon Biggs, Ariela Lowenstein, and Jon Hendricks (Amityville, NY: Baywood, 2003), 15–32, at 25.

"WHAT EXACTLY HAS *AGE* GOT TO DO WITH IT?" Margaret Morganroth Gullette, "What Exactly Has Age Got to Do With It? My Life in Critical Age Studies," *Journal of Aging Studies* 22, no. 2 (2008): 109–14. I wrote this autobiographical essay at the journal's request.

"WHAT ROUGH TERRITORY" Leni Marshall, *Age Becomes Us: Bodies and Gender in Time*, SUNY Series in Feminist Criticism and Theory (Albany, NY: SUNY Press, 2015), 14.

"SCORES OF RESEARCHERS" Erdman Palmore, "Ageism Comes of Age," *Journals of Gerontology: Series B* 70, no. 6 (November 2015): 873–75.

"AN ESSENTIAL ELEMENT OF ALL ENDEAVOR" Kate de Medeiros, "Confronting Ageism: Perspectives from Age Studies and the Social Sciences," *Gerontologist* 59, no. 4 (August 2019): 799–800, at 800, emphasis added.

ANY UNIFIED CALL MAY BE RESISTED AS "OVER-ORGANIZATION" Karl Mannheim, "The Sociological Problem of Generations," in Mannheim, *Essays on the Sociology of Knowledge: Collected Works*, vol. 5 (New York: Routledge, 1998), 163–93, at 164.

WHY ANTI-AGEIST WORK "HAD NOT PACKED A BIGGER WALLOP" Erdman Palmore, "Three Decades of Research on Ageism, *Generations* 29, no. 3 (September 2005): 87–90. See also Erdman Palmore, "The Future of Ageism," in *The Encyclopedia of Ageism*, ed. Erdman B. Palmore, Laurence Branch, and Diana K. Harris (New York: Routledge, 2013), 155–58.

"THE SENSE OF THE CONCRETE HISTORICAL INSTANCE" Stuart Hall, "Two Paradigms," in Hall, *Essential Essays*, vol. 1 (Durham, NC: Duke University Press, 2019), 67.

ERDMAN PALMORE['S] . . . RESPONSE Erdman Palmore, emails to author, "Why 'Ageism' Hasn't Packed a Bigger Wallop," August 28, 2018.

LESS EFFECTIVE AS CULTURAL CRITIQUE Rüdiger Kunow, *Material Bodies: Biology and Culture in the United States*, American Studies vol. 286 (Heidelberg: Universitätsverlag Winter, 2018).

"CONTEMPORARY OBSESSION" Sarah Lamb, ed., *Successful Aging as a Contem-*

porary Obsession: Global Perspectives (New Brunswick, NJ: Rutgers University Press, 2017).

THE SUMMATION OF TWO HUMANISTIC AGE CRITICS James Chappell and Sari Edelstein, "No One Is Too Old to Be President," *Washington Post*, April 28, 2019.

RISK [TO] BELOVED GOVERNMENT PROGRAMS Michael C. Kearl, Christa Moore, and J. Scott Osberg, "The Political Implications of the 'New Ageism,'" *International Journal of Aging and Human Development* 15, no. 3 (October 1982): 181–82, https://doi.org/10.2190/63BC-UE77-33J6-XY0P.

PROBLEMS INHERENT IN THE CONTINUING USE OF THE TERM *AGING* Margaret Morganroth Gullette, "Against 'Aging': How to Talk about Growing Older," *Theory, Culture and Society* (blog), December 21, 2017, https://www.theoryculturesociety.org/blog/margaret-morganroth-gullette-aging-talk-growing-older.

THE PROFESSION'S AVOIDANCE OF REAL SOCIAL CONDITIONS Stephen Katz, email to author, "Re: Why Did 'Ageism' Not Matter in Gerontology until Very Recently?" September 9, 2020.

"RECLAIMING OLD AGE AS A VALUABLE STATUS" Toni Calasanti, email to author, "Why Did Anti-Ageism (before Covid-19 Era) Have So Little Clout?" September 17, 2020.

"THE TARGET IS CONSTANTLY SHIFTING" Alan Walker, email to author, "Fighting Ageism," April 15, 2019.

FEW MAINSTREAM JOURNALISTS CONCENTRATED ON AGE ISSUES Paul Kleyman, email to author, "My Latest Uplift: Better Care and Good Grief!" March 14, 2022.

"LEADS INEXORABLY TO ARGUMENTS IN FAVOUR OF EUTHANASIA" Alan Walker, "The New Ageism," *Political Quarterly* 83, no. 4 (October–December 2012): 812–19, at 813, 814. On the globalized duty to die, see also Margaret Morganroth Gullette, "The 'Christine Lagarde Memo': For Your Eyes Only," *Monthly Review* online, October 9, 2018.

"AGEISM IS OFTEN HARD TO PROVE" Erdman Palmore, email to author, "Why 'Ageism' Hasn't Packed a Bigger Wallop," August 14, 2018.

ONLY IN 2019 WAS THE TERM *RACISM* DECISIVELY ADDED TO THE *AP STYLEBOOK* Janine Jackson, "Calling Racism by Its Real Name," *FAIR*, April 5, 2019.

"REPLACEMENT BIASES" This tern means that ageism has revived or replaced some other earlier prejudice; for example, although one may have overcome homophobia toward young adults, one may find sexually active, older gays or lesbians disgusting. See Margaret Morganroth Gullette, *Ending Ageism, or How Not to Shoot Old People* (New Brunswick, NJ: Rutgers University Press, 2017).

"A HOMOLOGOUS RELATIONSHIP WITH ALL OLDER PEOPLE AS ALLIES" Stephen Katz, email to author, "Re: Why Did 'Ageism' Not Matter in Gerontology until Very Recently?" September 9, 2020.

"ALMOST NEVER HAVE ACTUAL 'ELDERS'" Harry Moody, email to author, "On Anti-Ageism, Why It Doesn't Pack a Bigger Wallop," March 16, 2019.

"MAYBE IF THE FIELD WERE WOMAN-DOMINATED" Margaret Cruikshank, email to author, "Re: On the Belatedness of 'Ageism' Discourse," April 23, 2019.

"THE BODILY VARIABILITIES WE TODAY CATEGORIZE AS 'DISABILITIES'"
Joel Michael Reynolds and Anna Landre, "Ableism and Ageism: Insights from Disability Studies for Aging Studies," in *Critical Humanities and Ageing*, ed. Kate de Medeiros, Marlene Goldman, and Thomas Cole (London: Routledge, 2022), 118–29.

"LITTLE DISCUSSION BETWEEN THESE FIELDS" Joel Michael Reynolds, "The Extended Body: On Aging, Disability, and Well-Being," *Hastings Center Report*, October 11, 2018.

WOMEN'S SALARIES Jenee Wilde, "AAUP Report Shows Challenges Faced by Women in Academia," *Center for the Study of Women and Society*, January 11, 2021.

"THE PLACE FROM WHICH YOU TAKE YOUR ORDERS" Athol Fugard, interviewed in Lloyd Richards, "Athol Fugard, The Art of Theater No. 8," *Paris Review* 111 (Summer 1989).

"WITHOUT CHANGING THEIR MARGINAL STATUS" Margaret Cruikshank, *Learning to Be Old: Gender, Culture, and Aging* (Plymouth, UK: Rowman and Littlefield, 2013), 121.

"MUCH OF GERONTOLOGY IS ABOUT CHANGING THE INDIVIDUAL" Martha Holstein, "Looking Forward to Seeing You—and Hearing You," emails to author, April 23–24, 2019.

"WITHOUT MUCH REGARD FOR LARGER THEORETICAL CONSIDERATIONS" Larry Polivka, "Gerontology for the 21st Century," *Gerontologist* 46, no. 4 (August 2006): 558–63, at 558.

TIKKUN CONTEMPLATED *Tikkun* published an article by Ruth Ray Karpen (which was also a review of my book *Ending Ageism*) under the title "Anti-Ageism: The Next Big Social Movement," December 7, 2017.

"FOURTH AGEISM" . . . EXPLAINED AND PROMOTED Chris Gilleard and Paul Higgs, "An Enveloping Shadow? The Role of the Nursing Home in the Social Imaginary of the Fourth Age," in *Care Home Stories: Aging, Disability, and Long-Term Residential Care*, ed. Sally Chivers and Ulla Kriebernegg (Bielefeld: Transcript Verlag, 2017), 229–46.

REQUIRED ALL HER NEW EMPLOYEES Pedtke also wrote a book, *What Living as a Resident Can Teach Long-Term Care Staff* (Baltimore: Health Professions Press, 2018). Hear Pedtke delivering a Gray Panthers NYC webinar of the same title, February 1, 2024, https://www.youtube.com/watch?v=DKcDaiFyTUY.

GREEN HOUSES . . . THAT DID SO WELL Rob Waters, "The Big Idea behind a New Model of Small Nursing Homes," *Health Affairs* 40, no. 3 (March 2021), https://doi.org/10.1377/hlthaff.2021.00081; see also Green House Project, "The Shahbazim: In Their Own Words," 2010, Vimeo video, 4:21, https://vimeo.com/5807912.

"HANGS, POISED AND READY" Simone Weil, 'The Iliad, or the Poem of Force," trans. Mary McCarthy, *Politics* (November 1945), 326.

"HOW LITTLE WE'VE BEEN ABLE TO CHANGE ANYTHING" Stuart Hall, "Cultural Studies and Its Theoretical Legacies," in Hall, *Essential Essays*, vol. 1, 83.

"INTERNAL DESIRE" TO SUBDUE ONE'S OWN SENSE OF PRIORITY Judith Butler, *Precarious Life: The Powers of Mourning and Violence* (New York: Verso, 2004), 137.

"MORE STRONGLY THAN OTHER OPPRESSED GROUPS" Sonia Kruks, "Alterity and Intersectionality: Reflections on Old Age," *Hypatia* 37, no. 1 (Winter 2022): 196–209, at 204.

"YOUNG PEOPLE NEED TO FIGHT THE FIGHT" Liat Ayalon, email to author, "Re: Good Review of *Ending Ageism* and Liat Ayalon's *Ageism* Collection in *The Gerontologist*," April 20, 2019.

CHAPTER NINE

"A LOT OF FRIENDS THAT USED TO COME EVERY WEEK" Ms. Marquez referred to seven hundred high school students in a program developed by Columbia University Teachers College to train students for jobs as Certified Nursing Assistants by having them get to know people in nursing homes.

A STUDY OF THE HEALTH STATUS OF COVID SURVIVORS Michael Levere, Patricia Rowan, and Andrea Wysocki, "The Adverse Effects of the COVID-19 Pandemic on Nursing Home Resident Well-Being," *JAMDA* 22, no. 5 (May 1, 2021): 948–54.

I ASKED MY INTERN . . . TO SELECT ONLY THE ARTICLES THAT QUOTED RESIDENTS We omitted residents of assisted living or other LTC communities; the government is not responsible for private places. I asked Vishni Samaraweera to read articles from databases like Lexis-Uni and Newsstream on dates early in the pandemic (March–April), during the second surge, and at random dates during the rest of the year and early in 2021.

"I CONSULTED SOME EXPERTS" Eleanor Feldman Barbera, "The World According to Dr. El," *McKnights.com*, November 3, 2020.

"ADULT CHILDREN DON'T WANT TO UPSET THE STAFF" Whitney Bryen, phone interview with author, March 24, 2021.

"WHEELING A MILE IN ANOTHER PERSON'S WHEELCHAIR" Marilyn R. Gugliucci and Audrey Weiner, "Learning by Living: Life-Altering Medical Education through Nursing Home-Based Experiential Learning," *Gerontology and Geriatrics Education* 34, no. 1 (2013): 60–77.

"I AM IMMUNE-COMPROMISED, STAY AWAY" Quoted in Laura Crimaldi, "COVID-19 Sweeps through State Prisons," *Boston Globe*, December 25, 2020: B1, B3.

LOST MORE THAN 2,100 DAILY AND WEEKLY LOCAL NEWSPAPERS Renee Loth, "Saving Democracy's Frontlines—Local Newspapers," *Boston Globe*, December 17, 2021.

"REFRESHED ON AN ONGOING BASIS" Paul Kleyman, email to author, "Paul Kleyman on the Media Sources on Age," July 14–15, 2021.

"THE RISE OF THE INTERNET HAS MEANT BLOGS AND PODCASTS" Paul Kleyman, email to author, "Paul Kleyman on the Media Sources on Age," July 14–15, 2021.

HAWKINS'S RESEARCH CONCLUDED B. Denise Hawkins, "Black-Owned Nursing Homes Continue Little-Known Legacy, Fill Needs Unmet by Troubled Industry," National Association of Black Journalists, *Black News and Views*, October 30,

2023, https://blacknewsandviews.com/black-owned-nursing-homes-continue-little-known-legacy-fill-needs-unmet-by-troubled-industry/.

DERRICK Z. JACKSON . . . EXPOSED THAT DISREGARD Derrick Jackson, "Environmental Justice? Unjust Coverage of the Flint Water Crisis," Shorenstein Center, July 11, 2017.

"THOSE [WHOM REPORTERS] SEE AS HAVING SUFFICIENT RIGHT TO OPINE" Derrick Z. Jackson, phone interview with author, July 30, 2021.

"EVERYONE LIVING IN A NURSING HOME ISN'T COGNITIVELY COMPROMISED" Judith E. Graham, email to author, "Excellent Article about Medical Ageism," October 22, 2021.

"KITBAG" Tom Kitwood, quoted in Nader Shabahangi, Geoffrey Faustman, Julie N. Tahi, and Patrick Fox, "Some Observations on the Social Consequences of Forgetfulness and Alzheimer's Disease: A Call for Attitudinal Expansion," *Journal of Aging, Humanities, and the Arts* 3 (2009): 1–15, at 5.

"FEATURES OF 'TOTAL' INSTITUTIONS" Jari Pierhonen and Ilkka Pietila, "Patient, Resident, or Person: Recognition and the Continuity of Self in Long-Term Care for Older People," *Journal of Aging Studies* 35 (December 2015): 95–103.

"DRAW ON THEIR FULL RESOURCES" Paul Johnson, quoted in Michael Mangan, *Staging Ageing: Theatre, Performance and the Narrative of Decline* (Bristol: Intellect, 2013), 37.

"I GOT THERAPY" Emily Hopkins, quoted in Naseem S. Miller, "How They Did It: *Indianapolis Star* Reporters Uncover How Billions in Nursing Home Medicaid Dollars Were Diverted to County Hospitals," *Journalist's Resource*, March 30, 2021.

"SKIN FLAKES ALL OVER THE MATTRESS" Kianna Gardner, "History of Deficiencies Documented at COVID-Infected Whitefish Care Center," *Daily Inter Lake*, September 13, 2020.

REBECCA WEST The first quotation is from West's biography *St. Augustine*; the second is from her fictional story "Parthenope." Both can be found in Rebecca West, *Rebecca West: A Celebration* (New York: Penguin, 1979), 201, 491.

"THOSE WHO GAIN REPRESENTATION" Judith Butler, *Precarious Life: The Powers of Mourning and Violence* (New York: Verso, 2004), 141.

ALTARUM FOUND THOSE RESIDENTS Liz Seegert, "COVID-19 Is Taking a Huge Emotional Toll on Nursing Home Residents," *PBS.org*, October 20, 2020.

THE "FIRST KNOWN POLL OF ITS KIND" Liz Seegert "I'm Very Lonely and Depressed—Many Nursing Home Residents Say They Feel Like They Are in Prison," *Marketwatch*, October 12, 2020.

"ESSENTIAL AND UNTOLD STORIES" Julie Golia, email to author, "Re: How to Access Pandemic Diaries of People Residing in Long-Term Care Facilities," December 23, 2020. Golia was director of the New York Public Library's Pandemic Diaries program.

NO AUDIO DIARIES FROM RESIDENTS Julie Golia, emails to author, "Re: Endnote on Pandemic Diaries of People Residing in Long-Term Care Facilities: The Pandemic Diary Collection, NYPL," May 9, 2022.

CULTURE-CHANGE MOVEMENT A. N. Rahman and J. F. Shnelle, "The Nursing Home Culture-Change Movement: Recent Past, Present, and Future Directions for Research," *Gerontologist* 48, no. 2 (April 2008): 142–48.

CHAPTER TEN

NO ACKNOWLEDGMENT OF LOST PEERS Anne Montgomery, Sarah Slocum, and Christine Stanik, *Experiences of Nursing Home Residents during the Pandemic*, special report (Ann Arbor, MI: Altarum, October 2020), 15, https://www.ipfcc.org/resources /Nursing-Home-Resident-Survey_Altarum-Special-Report.pdf.

"BEREAVEMENT IS THIS FEELING OF PROFOUND LOSS" Toni Miles, quoted in Jeannette Galvanek, "Bereavement Researcher: We Must Do Better for the Grief-Stricken," *CareWise Solutions* (blog), February 15, 2020, https://carewisesolutions .com/bereavement/.

"AN INCALCULABLE LOSS" "U.S. Deaths Near 100,000, An Incalculable Loss," *New York Times*, May 24, 2020.

"I GUARANTEE YOU" Chris Kocher, "Healing Hearts—Moving Forward from COVID-19 Loss," Gray Panthers webinar, Transformation Tuesday, December 14, 2021, organized by Jack Kupferman, https://www.youtube.com/watch?v=USfd -FKEHg4&t=28s.

"WEIGHT BEGINNING TO LIFT FROM MY SHOULDERS" Suzanne Brennan Firstenberg, "What the 700,000 Flags I Put on the National Mall Really Mean," opin-ion column, *Washington Post*, October 1, 2021.

FRONTLINE MEDICAL PERSONNEL FIRST, SURVIVING RESIDENTS SECOND Jennifer Tolbert, Jennifer Kates, and Josh Michaud, "The COVID-19 Vaccine Priority Line Continues to Change as States Make Further Updates," *Kaiser Family Foundation*, January 21, 2021, https://www.kff.org/policy-watch/the-covid-19-vaccine-priority -line-continues-to-change-as-states-make-further-updates/.

VETERANS ADMINISTRATION HAD ISSUED A MANDATE Eric Katz, "Some Agencies Are Keeping a Vaccine Mandate in Place and Enforcing It," *Government Executive*, January 31, 2022, https://www.govexec.com/workforce/2022/01/some -agencies-are-keeping-vaccine-mandate-place-and-enforcing-it/361384/.

SUPREME COURT CAUSED PART OF THE DELAY Aaron Gould Sheinin, "Su-preme Court Blocks Biden Vaccine Mandate for Businesses," *Web MD*, January 13, 2022.

"WHO IS CARING FOR THEM?" Dorothy Weitzman, "Nursing Home Residents Continue to Be Overlooked," letter to the editor, *Boston Globe*, March 10, 2022.

UNDERUSE OF . . . PAXLOVID PARTICULARLY IN NURSING HOMES The JAMA study is cited and linked, and Barnett and McGarry are interviewed, in Christopher Rowland, "Paxlovid Is Underused at Nursing Homes, Study Says," *Washington Post*, July 14, 2023.

"INATTENTIVE TO THE ELDERS' PLIGHT" Liz Kowalczyk and Robert Weisman, "A Home to Die In," *Boston Globe*, September 27, 2020.

UNMOURNABLE I borrow the term from Teju Cole, "Unmournable Bodies," *New Yorker*, January 9, 2015, and from the title of Tsitsi Dangarembga's novel, *This Mournable Body* (New York: Faber and Faber, 2018). Judith Butler has offered a related term, *ungrievable*.

THEATER OF WAR Theater of War Productions, "Homelessness: The Oedipus at Colonus Project," accessed February 10, 2024, https://theaterofwar.com/projects/the -oedipus-at-colonus-project.

"NEVER AGAIN" Diana I. Popescu and Tanja Schult, "Introduction," *Holocaust Studies: A Journal of Culture and History* 26, no. 2 (2020).

AWARDED EACH FAMILY OF SURVIVORS ON AVERAGE $445,000 Tracy Tulley, "Families of Veterans Who Died of Covid Win $53 Million Legal Settlement," *New York Times*, January 7, 2022.

"YOU HAVE NO IDEA" Karen Tei Yamashita, *Letters to Memory* (Minneapolis: Coffee House Press, 2017), 35, 95.

"BROAD PUBLIC SUPPORT WAS NEVER GOING TO DEVELOP" Grant Ujifusa, interviewed in Justin McDonnell, "Interview: Japanese American Grant Ujifusa Defied Odds in Face of Historic U.S. Error," *Asia Society* (blog), June 17, 2013.

FORMALLY ACKNOWLEDGED "Patriotism and Prejudice: Japanese Americans and World War II," *National Park Service*, accessed February 10, 2024, https://www .nps.gov/articles/patriotism-prejudice-japanese-americans.htm.

UJIFUSA . . . TOLD ME Grant Ujifusa, telephone interviews with author, March 12 and 13, 2021.

THAT VISION WAS NOT REALIZED The Manzanar National Historic Site in California, by contrast, was created to honor the internees alone; it is located on the former site of one of the concentration camps.

A HISTORY PRODUCED BY THE EQUAL JUSTICE INITIATIVE Equal Justice Initiative, *Lynching in America: Confronting the Legacy of Racial Terror (Third Edition)* (Montgomery, AL: Equal Justice Initiative, 2017), Key Findings #5.

"AFRICAN AMERICAN VICTIMS OF RACIAL TERROR LYNCHING" Equal Justice Initiative, *Lynching in America: Confronting the Legacy of Racial Terror County Data Supplement* (Montgomery, AL: Equal Justice Initiative, updated February 2020).

I INTERVIEWED SIA SANNEH Sia Sanneh, telephone interview with author, January 6, 2022.

"BLOOD IN THAT SOIL" Bryan Stevenson, quoted in "Blood in the Soil: How Equal Justice Initiative Confronts our History of Racial Violence," *Emerson Collective*, December 2016.

A SHOP AT THE MUSEUM SELLS AN ARTIST'S IMAGE "Soil Collection Print," Equal Justice Initiative online shop, accessed December 16, 2023, https://shop.eji.org /products/soilcollectionprint.

A REMORSEFUL DEATHBED CRY Susan Righi, "Remembering: The Equal Justice Initiative," *Center for Community Solutions*, November 23, 2020.

"THE REPORT OF 2015 GOT SO MUCH PUBLICITY" Sanneh, telephone interview with author, January 6, 2022.

ENCOUNTERED OUTRIGHT HOSTILITY Sam Levin, "Lynching Memorial Leaves Some Quietly Seething: 'Let Sleeping Dogs Lie,'" *Guardian*, April 28, 2018.

SANNEH CONFIRMED Sanneh, telephone interview with author, January 6, 2022.

"FORCED TO ACKNOWLEDGE" "The Visitor's Corner with Sia Sanneh and Bryan Stevenson of the Equal Justice Initiative," *Modern American History*, September 3, 2018.

"EVASIVE MEMORY" Lawrence L. Langer, "The Afterdeath of the Holocaust," MS of a talk Professor Langer gave at the opening of a new museum in Bergen-Belsen. Sent privately as a Word document. See also Langer, "The Afterdeath of the Holocaust," in *The Afterdeath of the Holocaust: The Holocaust and its Contexts* (Cham: Palgrave Macmillan, 2021), https://doi.org/10.1007/978-3-030-66139-7_1; and Langer, *Using and Abusing the Holocaust* (Bloomington: Indiana University Press, 2006).

"FOR THAT HE PAID WITH HIS LIFE" Kristin Urquisa, quoted in Nicole Narea, "Watch: A Covid-19 Victim's Daughter Delivered a Moving Account of Her Father's Death—and a Searing Critique of Trump," *Vox*, August 17, 2020.

"A SMALL DIGITAL SCREEN" Ariel Dorfman, "Chile: Now More Than Ever," *New York Review of Books*, August 16, 2018: 55.

"NOT SO ALONE" Dorfman, "Chile: Now More Than Ever," 55.

"LOGICAL FULFILLMENT" E. J. Emanuel and D. J. Skorton, "Mandating COVID-19 Vaccinations for Health Care Workers," *Annals of Internal Medicine*, July 30, 2021.

EPILOGUE

"AND MORAL DEBTS NEED TO BE PAID" Shennette Garrett-Scott, "What Price Wholeness?" *New York Review of Books*, February 11, 2021: 20.

SOCRATES SAYS Plato, *Republic*, book 1, trans. Benjamin Jowett, https://www.gutenberg.org/files/55201/55201-h/55201-h.htm.

ROSE EXPLAINED WHAT HAPPENED NEXT Emails to author, "Cheering News Today," January 31, 2021, and "Quote from [Vera]," February 2 and 3, 2021.

"WHEN EXPENSIVE RISKS TRANSPIRE" Ben Veghte, email to author, "Term: 'Defined Contributory Benefit Sponsored by the Government,'" January 14, 2022.

MIDDLE-CLASS PEOPLE . . . SPEND DOWN THEIR ASSETS E. Kathleen Adams, Mark R. Meiners, and Brian O. Burwell, "Asset Spend-Down in Nursing Homes: Methods and Insights," *Medical Care* 31, no. 1 (1993): 1–23.

"LONGEST STEP I EVER TOOK" Mrs. Smith, quoted in Patricia Worth Simmons, *Yesterday's Children* (Nashville, TN: Aurora Publishers, 1972), 46.

"AFTER THREE DECADES WITH *NO GROWTH*" Ben Veghte, "Sen. Sanders' Bold Plan to Expand Social Security," *Huffpost*, updated December 6, 2017, now available at https://register.cnbc-newsletter.com/entry/sen-sanders-bold-plan-to_b_6879582 /amp. See also Yimeng Yin, Anqi Chen, and Alicia H. Munnell, "The National Retirement Risk Index: Version 2.0," *Center for Retirement Research at Boston College*, May 9, 2023.

"INEFFECTIVE, INEFFICIENT, INEQUITABLE . . ." David C. Grabowski, Marilyn Rantz, and Jasmine L. Travers, "Report: U.S. Nursing Home Care Is Ineffective, Inefficient, Inequitable, Fragmented, and Unsustainable," *STAT News,* April 6, 2022.

"THE WORST ASPECTS OF THE PRIVATIZATION" Laura Katz Olson, *The Politics of Medicaid* (New York: Columbia University Press, 2010), 8.

"FAILURE BY ALL STANDARDS" Trudy Lieberman, "The Long-Term Care Insurance Market Is a Disaster. Can Washington State Offer a Better Path Forward?" *Center for Health Journalism,* March 21, 2022.

COMPREHENSIVE REFORM Rachel M. Werner, R. Tamara Konetzka, David C. Grabowski, and David G. Stevenson, "Reforming Nursing Home Financing, Payment, and Oversight," *New England Journal of Medicine* 386 (May 19, 2022): 1869–71.

LEADINGAGE . . . DARED TELL Katie Smith Sloan to Charles Grassley and Ron Wyden, December 6, 2019: 1–4, https://www.leadingage.org/sites/default/files /Grassley-Wyden%2012-6.pdf.

"YOU COULD FILL A LIBRARY" Ron Wyden, "Wyden Statement at Finance Committee Hearing on the Impacts of COVID-19 on Nursing Homes," March 17, 2021: 1, https://www.finance.senate.gov/imo/media/doc/031721%20Wyden%20nursing %20homes%20hearing%20opener.pdf.

POLICY CHANGE . . . WAS LONG OVERDUE Werner, Konetzka, Grabowski, and Stevenson, "Reforming Nursing Home Financing, Payment, and Oversight."

[BIDEN'S] SECOND STATE OF THE UNION ADDRESS Joseph Biden, "State of the Union Address," March 1, 2022, https://www.whitehouse.gov/state-of-the-union -2022/; see also White House, "Fact Sheet: Protecting Seniors and People with Disabilities by Improving Safety and Quality of Care in the Nation's Nursing Homes," February 28, 2022, https://www.presidency.ucsb.edu/documents/fact-sheet-protecting -seniors-and-people-with-disabilities-improving-safety-and-quality.

FEWER THAN 0.5 PERCENT OF [FACILITIES] Amanda Seitz, "Failing US Nursing Homes to Face Tougher Federal Penalties," *Seattle Times,* October 21, 2022, https://www.seattletimes.com/seattle-news/health/failing-nursing-homes-to-face -tougher-penalties/.

CLYBURN'S SELECT SUBCOMMITTEE ON THE CORONAVIRUS CRISIS US House Select Subcommittee on the Coronavirus Crisis, *Preparing for and Preventing the Next Public Health Emergency: Lessons Learned from the Coronavirus Crisis* (Washington, DC: Select Subcommittee on the Coronavirus Crisis, December 2022).

THESE ARE THE HARD FACTS Zhe Li and Joseph Dalaker, *Poverty among the Population Aged 65 and Older,* report R45791 (Washington, DC: Congressional Research Service, April 14, 2021).

A FULL HALF . . . WILL BE UNABLE TO AFFORD THE BASICS Joanne Lynn, "100 Days for Biden et al. to Change the Course of Elderhood," *Generations Today,* January–February 2021, https://generations.asaging.org/100-days-biden-change -course-elderhood.

MORE THAN 260,000 ARE STILL ENROLLED "About Us," Federal Long Term

Care Insurance Program, accessed December 17, 2023, https://www.ltcfeds.com /about.

WA CARES FUND WA Cares is located in the Department of Social and Health Services.

"DEFINED CONTRIBUTORY INSURANCE PROGRAM" Veghte, email to author, "Term: 'Defined Contributory Benefit Sponsored by the Government,'" January 14, 2022.

GENWORTH COST OF CARE "Calculate the Cost of Care in Your Area," *Genworth*, November 2021, https://www.genworth.com /aging-and-you /finances /cost-of-care .html.

"LO AND BEHOLD . . ." Elaine Waxman, quoted in Helena Bottemiller Evich, "Could Covid-19 End Hunger in America?" *Politico*, September 9, 2021.

"GLARING INABILITY" Olson, *Politics of Medicaid*, 228.

BILL HENNING TOLD ME Bill Henning, email to author, "RE: Ageism Presentation," October 13, 2022.

"A DIGNITY THAT COMES WITH AGING IN THE HOME" Mike Batista, quoted in Tom Lutey, "Montanans See Senior Care Benefits in Democrat Spending Plan," *Billings Gazette*, December 21, 2021.

THE NUMBER . . . IN THE FACILITIES WAS DOWN TO THIRTY-ONE THOUSAND Dignity Alliance Massachusetts, "Fact Sheet: Massachusetts Nursing Homes," April 2022, https://dignityalliancema.org/wp-content /uploads/2022/04/Fact-U -0422-1-Nursing-Home-Fact-Sheet1.pdf.

LAWSUIT . . . THAT SOUGHT TO COMPEL "ADA Class Action Seeks to Compel Massachusetts to Stop Unnecessary Institutionalization of People with Disabilities," Center for Public Representation, October 11, 2022, https://www.centerforpublicrep .org /news /ada-class-action-seeks-to-compel-massachusetts-to-stop-unnecessary -institutionalization-of-people-with-disabilities/. The suit was brought under the Baker administration, as *Simmons v. Baker*.

OCCUPANCY . . . WENT DOWN FROM 81 PERCENT BEFORE COVID TO 68 PERCENT David C. Grabowski, "Studying the Nursing Home Workforce: Lessons and Opportunities," with comments from Charlene Harrington, Advancing Workforce Analysis and Research for Dementia (AWARD) Network inaugural research webinar, University of California-San Francisco, December 7, 2022, https://www.youtube .com /watch?v=aZTwYyD7PpU&list=PLPdSQGGMt89fUixYqDZDYyG1Jw1ja8hFo &index=2.

88 PERCENT OF PEOPLE OVER SIXTY-FIVE WOULD PREFER TO [AGE AT HOME] "Long-Term Care in America: Americans Want to Age at Home," AP-NORC Center for Public Affairs, May 3, 2021.

"DIE UNDER BRIDGES" Lamont McClure, quoted in Jeff Ward, "Northampton County Puts Together Scenarios for Gracedale under Potential Federal, State Rule Changes," *Lehigh Valley Regional News*, June 2, 2022.

"AN INCREDIBLE ASSET" David Gifford, quoted in Susan Mitchell, Shawn Bloom,

David Gifford, David Grabowski, and Jasmine Travers, "Perspective Roundtable: Long-Term Care in the United States—Problems and Solutions," *New England Journal of Medicine* 386 (May 19, 2022): 6.

"THE BEST OPPORTUNITY WHEN BUYING AN ASSET" Josh Jandris, quoted in Amy Stulick, "Buyers Have 'Voracious Appetite' for Skilled Nursing Facilities," *Skilled Nursing News*, May 24, 2021.

END UP HOMELESS Aaron Bolton, "Homelessness among Older People Is on the Rise, Driven by Inflation and the Housing Crunch," *Kaiser Health News*, November 10, 2022, https://tinyurl.com/2c3sdvtd.

AN ILLEGAL "TAKING" Maureen Tkacik, "The Nursing Home Slumlord Manifesto," *American Prospect*, January 26, 2022, https://prospect.org/health/nursing-home-slumlord-manifesto/.

"CONFLATING THEIR [BUSINESS] NEEDS Olson, *Politics of Medicaid*, 6.

CONSERVATIVES . . . "DESTROY" . . . SAFETY NETS James Crotty, "The Great Austerity War: What Caused the US Deficit Crisis and Who Should Pay to Fix It?" *Cambridge Journal of Economics* 36, no. 1 (January 2012): 79.

STATE CAPTURE APPEARS PERMANENT Martha Patterson-Cohen, email to author, "Comment on SAGE Article," September 29, 2022.

ARGUMENTS . . . FOR SAFETY [AND] PRIVACY Sharon Silow-Carroll, Deborah Peartree, Susan Tuck, and Anh Pham, "Fundamental Nursing Home Reform: Evidence on Single-Resident Rooms to Improve Personal Experience and Public Health," *Health Management Associates*, March 2021.

"TWO MINUTES NOT BEING ABLE TO BREATHE" Health Care Financing Administration, 4.7.3.1: Sources Used to Identify a Deficient Practice—II. Resident Interviews," in *Report to Congress: Appropriateness of Minimum Nurse Staffing Ratios in Nursing Homes* (Washington, DC: HCFA, draft July 20, 2000), 25. Staff also described the harms they necessarily inflict when they are short-staffed; see *Report to Congress*, 27–31.

A TWENTY-MINUTE INCREASE IN CARE Based on nursing facilities with confirmed cases. See Yue Li, Helena Temkin-Greener, Gao Shan, and Xueya Cai, "COVID-19 Infections and Deaths among Connecticut Nursing Home Residents: Facility Correlates," *Journal of the American Geriatrics Society* 68 (2020): 1899–1906.

"ONE THING EVERYONE AGREES ON" Tamara R. Konetzka, "A National Tragedy: COVID-19 in the Nation's Nursing Homes," a virtual hearing before the United States Senate Finance Committee, March 17, 2021.

"GOALS, PREFERENCES AND VALUES" CMS, "Person-Centered Care," *CMS. gov*, accessed February 8, 2024, https://www.cms.gov/priorities/innovation/key-concepts/person-centered-care.

MASSACHUSETTS . . . ASKED TO BE KEPT ON THE LOWER STANDARD Rachana Pradhan, "End of COVID Emergency Will Usher In Changes across the U.S. Health System," *Kaiser Health News*, March 22, 2023.

MASSACHUSETTS ALSO RATES BADLY Long Term Care Community Coalition, *Broken Promises* (New York: LTCC, 2021), 13, figure 6.

FEDERAL FUNDING HAS BEEN STAGNANT Noble Brigham, "Idaho Nursing Homes Haven't Had Full Inspections in Years. How Did This Happen?" *Idaho Statesman*, August 15, 2023.

MASSACHUSETTS . . . IN THE BOTTOM 10 PERCENT OF STATES IN . . . RESOLVING COMPLAINTS Office of the Inspector General, *States Continued to Fall Short in Meeting Required Timeframes for Investigating Nursing Home Complaints: 2016–2018*, report OEI-01-19-00421 (Washington, DC, OIG, September 2020), 6.

A PATCHWORK OF AGENCIES Liz Kowalczyk and Robert Weisman, "A Home to Die In," *Boston Globe*, September 27, 2020.

THIRTY-TWO HOMES HAVEN'T HAD A RECERTIFICATION SURVEY SINCE 2019 Kerry Kavanaugh and Marina Villeneuve, "Mass Fails to Conduct Full Inspections of Some Nursing Homes for Years, 25 Investigates Finds," *Boston25 News*, June 8, 2023.

KRISTA RUFFINI . . . ESTIMATES Krista Ruffini, "Better Workplace Conditions for Long-Term Eldercare Staff Are Key to Promoting Resident Safety amid the Coronavirus Pandemic," *Equitable Growth*, June 4, 2020.

"1 IN 5 OF ALL THE PEOPLE LIVING IN SENIOR CARE SITES" Robert Weisman, "'You Are My Sunshine': For Nursing Homes, COVID-19 Vaccinations Bring Hope amid an Uncertain Future," *Boston Globe*, March 20, 2021.

ALMOST A THIRD OF STATE FACILITIES ADMITTED SPENDING LESS THAN REQUIRED MassHealth, *DCC-Q Report: July 1, 2021–June 30, 2022* (Boston, MA: MassHealth, December 8, 2022), 1, unadjusted column.

MASSACHUSETTS ADVOCATES FOR NURSING HOME REFORM See https://manhr.org/, accessed December 17, 2023.

"WE ARE FAILING" Gray Panthers NYC, "Town Hall Featuring the Honorable Ron Kim," October 25, 2022, YouTube video, 1:02:47, https://www.youtube.com/watch?v=wD_lY485Nho.

ACCORDING TO DICK MOORE Richard T. Moore, "Are Nursing Homes Really in Tough Shape?" *CommonWealth Magazine*, November 26, 2022.

"NO NURSING HOME SHALL REASSIGN" See 193rd General Court of the Commonwealth of Massachusetts, *Acts of 2023*, "An Act Making Appropriations for the Fiscal Year 2024," chapter 28, line item 4000–0601, https://malegislature.gov/Laws/SessionLaws/Acts/2023/Chapter28.

ACCORDING TO THE OFFICE OF CAMPAIGN AND POLITICAL FINANCE Joe Dwinell, "Charlie Baker Defends Nursing Homes, Calls Toll of Coronavirus 'Tremendous Tragedy,'" *Boston Herald*, May 13, 2020.

THE BIDEN WHITE HOUSE BOLDLY ACKNOWLEDGED White House Briefing Room, "Fact Sheet: Biden-Harris Administration Takes Steps to Crack Down on Nursing Homes that Endanger Resident Safety," September 1, 2023, https://www.whitehouse.gov/briefing-room/statements-releases/2023/09/01/fact-sheet-biden-harris-administration-takes-steps-to-crack-down-on-nursing-homes-that-endanger-resident-safety/.

"PUBLICLY KNOWN FACT TO POLITICAL CONSEQUENCE" James Butler, "The World According to Dom," *London Review of Books*, May 28, 2021.

CONGRESS HAS NEVER SET A NATIONAL STAFFING FLOOR Mary Beth Musumeci, Emma Childress, and Belle Harris, "State Actions to Address Nursing Home Staffing during COVID-19," *Kaiser Family Foundation*, May 16, 2022.

CONGRESSIONAL COMMISSION Abt Associates Inc., *Appropriateness of Minimum Nurse Staffing Ratios in Nursing Homes*, report to Congress, phase II final, vol. 1 (Cambridge, MA: Abt Associates, December 2001).

IN 2021, ONLY 6 PERCENT OF US NURSING HOMES ACHIEVED 4.1 HOURS PER PERSON Victoria Bailey, "Minimum Staffing Requirements Could Cost Nursing Homes $10B Annually," *RevCycle Intelligence*, July 20, 2022.

"INSUFFICIENT STAFFING" . . . ACCOUNTED FOR JUST 1 PERCENT OF CITATIONS Jayme Fraser and Nick Penzenstadler with Jeff Kelly Lowenstein, "Many Nursing Homes Are Poorly Staffed. How Do They Get Away with It?" *US News*, December 2, 2022.

"ENDING THE ABUSE TODAY" President Joe Biden, "President Biden: Nursing Homes Are Putting Residents at Risk. We're Ending the Abuse Today," *USA Today*, September 1, 2023.

"HUNDREDS OF THOUSANDS OF VULNERABLE RESIDENTS . . . COULD BE FORCED OUT" Bailey, "Minimum Staffing Requirements."

POSITION OF DIGNITY ALLIANCE MASSACHUSETTS Paul J. Lanzikos "Medicare and Medicaid Programs: Minimum Staffing Standards for Long-Term Care Facilities and Medicaid Institutional Payment Transparency Reporting—Comments Submitted by Dignity Alliance Massachusetts," November 6, 2023, CMS-2023-0144-0001, https://dignityalliancema.org/wp-content/uploads/2023/11/Dignity-Alliance-Official-Comments-on-Nurse-Staffing-Regulatons_2023-10.30.pdf.

THE RULE HAD BEEN ADJUSTED *UP* White House, "Fact Sheet: Vice President Harris Announces Historic Advancements in Long-Term Care to Support the Care Economy," April 22, 2024, https://www.whitehouse.gov/briefing-room/statements-releases/2024/04/22/fact-sheet-vice-president-harris-announces-historic-advancements-in-long-term-care-to-support-the-care-economy/

"DANGEROUSLY INADEQUATE" Nina A. Kohn, Charlene Harrington, and Lori Smetanka, "Biden's Nursing Home Staffing Proposal Is Dangerously Inadequate," *Hill*, September 22, 2023.

NEARLY THREE-QUARTERS . . . FELL BELOW Dignity Alliance Massachusetts, *What's Needed for Transformational Nursing Home Reform to Improve Quality and Oversight* (Boston: Dignity Alliance Massachusetts, July 2023), n7.

A READABLE MAP SHOWS YOUR STATE'S MINIMUM STAFFING LEVEL See Fraser, Penzenstadler, and Lowenstein, "Many Nursing Homes Are Poorly Staffed."

"SAD CEMETERIES" Translated and adapted by the author from Marguerite Yourcenar, *Mémoires d'Hadrien* (Paris: Plon, 1951), 228.

"INSTITUTIONAL FAILURE TO ACT" Christopher L. Brown, "Later, Not Now," *London Review of Books*, July 15, 2021: 25.

"LET THIS BOOK ERASE THAT DOUBT" Erdrich, *Night Watchman*, 451.

THE BIG QUESTION Grabowski, Rantz, and Travers, "Report: U.S. Nursing Home Care Is Ineffective."

"TINKERING WITH SMALL WAYS TO MAKE INCREMENTAL IMPROVEMENTS" Tamara Konetzka, "Improving the Fate of Nursing Homes during the COVID-19 Pandemic: The Need for Policy," *American Journal of Public Health* 111, no. 4 (April 2021): 632–34.

KILLS PEOPLE Elizabeth Warren, "Opening Remarks by Senator Warren as Prepared for Delivery," April 3, 2024; https://www.warren.senate.gov/newsroom/press-releases/icymi-warrens-opening-remarks-at-senate-hearing-in-boston-steward-health-care-is-a-clear-cut-case-of-private-equity-exploiting-for-profit-health-care. The Markey quotation comes from a televised hearing. Ed Markey, "Senate Field Hearing in Boston, MA, 'When Health Care Becomes Wealth Care,'" April 3, 2024, https://www.youtube.com/watch?v=AL3R6n_-4uA.

"LET THIS BOOK GIVE YOU HEART" Erdrich, *Night Watchman*, 451.

DIGNITY ALLIANCE MASSACHUSETTS WROTE UP A 2025 BUDGET Dignity Alliance Massachusetts, *The Dignity Budget Overview*, fact sheet, November 17, 2023, https://dignityalliancema.org/wp-content/uploads/2023/11/The-Dignity-Budget-Overview.pdf.

APPENDIX

ELIZABETH WHITE Elizabeth M. White, "Underreporting of Early Nursing Home COVID-19 Cases and Deaths in Federal Data," *JAMA Network Open* 4, no. 9 (September 9, 2021): e2123696.

ADDS 40,000 This data comes from only thirty-nine states reporting as of May 28, 2020: see Jerry H. Gurwitz and Alice Bonner, "Nursing Homes, the Pandemic, and Caring Enough," *Journal of General Internal Medicine* 35, no. 9 (September 2020): 2752–54 n1, using Kaiser Family Foundation (KFF) data, https://doi.org/10.1007%2Fs11606-020-06022-7.

AARP NURSING HOME DASHBOARD "AARP Nursing Home COVID-19 Dashboard," AARP Public Policy Institute, updated December 14, 2023, https://www.aarp.org/ppi/issues/caregiving/info-2020/nursing-home-covid-dashboard.html?cmp=RDRCT-350d888f-20201013; scroll down to "Comparability to Other Data Sources."

OBSCURE COMMON OWNERSHIP Kimberly Marselas, "Breaking: Congressional Study Eviscerates For-Profit Nursing Homes," *McKnight's Long Term Care News*, September 21, 2022, https://www.mcknights.com/news/breaking-congressional-study-eviscerates-for-profit-nursing-homes/. See also House Select Subcommittee on the Coronavirus Crisis, *Preparing for and Preventing the Next Public Health Emergency: Lessons Learned from the Coronavirus Crisis. Final Report* (Washington, DC: Select Subcommittee on the Coronavirus Crisis, December 2022), 51.

RAISED SERIOUS QUESTIONS Kay Lazar, "Is Massachusetts Undercounting COVID-19 Deaths in Nursing Homes?" *Boston Globe*, April 23, 2021.

ALSO REPORTED BY GBH NEWS Barbara Anthony and Mary Z. Connaughton, "COVID-19: How the Baker Administration Ill Serves Those in Elder Care," *GBH*, February 11, 2022, https://www.wgbh.org/news/commentary/2022-02-11/covid-19-how-the-baker-administration-ill-serves-those-in-elder-care.

NO WAY TO DETERMINE ACTUAL COVID DEATHS EVEN APPROXIMATELY An expert in reading Chapter 93 data told me, "DPH is still including the huge file by facility, but has eliminated cumulative totals at the end of column A, just past line 700ish. . . . There's a note in column C that says 'Facility has had resident deaths, no deaths reported yesterday.'" In the Chapter 93 archive, for the first date, July 1, 2020, one can download the spreadsheet. See Massachusetts Department of Public Health, "Archive of Chapter 93 COVID-19 Data (2020-2022)," *Mass.gov*, https://www.mass.gov/info-details/archive-of-chapter-93-covid-19-data-2020-2022.

"NEW YORK . . . REPORTS LTC DEATHS ONLY WHEN Whet Moser and Conor Kelly, "Introducing the Long-Term Care COVID Tracker," *Atlantic* online, September 1, 2020, https://covidtracking.com/analysis-updates/long-term-care.

INDEX

DNR = Do Not Resuscitate (order)
NH = nursing facility ("home") operating under the Centers for Medicare and Medicaid Services (CMS) and the states; excludes assisted living, rest homes, and continuing-care retirement communities (CCRCs)

justice for residents
bills to reform NHs, 142, 230, 243, 264, 277, 280
legal suits, 89, 230, 241
a monument, 243–44, 251–56
public health reform, 255
recognizing the Eldercide, 7, 25, 252, 254
recognizing equal right to live, 7–8, 25, 37, 88, 123, 125, 151, 173, 178, 243–44, 247, 256
remembering them, 236, 254
restoring the social embrace, 173, 181, 208, 230, 243, 247, 282
unlearning bias, 23, 243–44
See also monuments; nursing facilities: reformers

kindness, 183, 205

language, 169, 170
lack of language for writing residents' experiences, 214
need for residents' stories and archive, 229–31, 254–55
textuality constructs: decline over life course, 100, 111, 128, 180; dependency, 9; doomed-to-die narrative, 64, 91–92, 116, 215, 252; duty-to-die argument, 166–67, 170–75, 180–81, 183, 255; generational difference, 107, 163, 178, 181, 201; horror of COVID in NHs, 77, 91–92, 94; sense of futility of medical care, 92, 116
See also narrative(s)
Latinx, 98, 205
NH residents, 79
law, 63, 67, 73, 74, 135, 248
DNR and last wishes, 129, 151
Eldercide as violation of, 35
in relation to NH industry, 89–90, 284
in relation to residents, 7, 28, 34, 70, 190, 230, 236, 267
LGBTQ+, 11, 65
longevity, 102, 110, 131
drops with COVID deaths, 149–50

treated as a costly problem, 163–64
treated as a US success, 149, 161
"treatments," 166
long-term care (LTC) insurance, 282
CLASS (Community Living Assistance Services and Supports) Act, 265
need for, 159, 207, 260, 263, 265–66
in Washington State, 265–66

marriage, 11, 12
masculinity and aging, 19, 56, 104, 105, 106, 190
mask wearing, import of, 34, 36, 109, 141, 147, 252
anti-mask Trump, 55–56, 105
media and age, before COVID, 220–21
ageism in, 201–2
a billion uses of the term "aging," 162, 171
coverage of age issues, 171–72, 181–82, 200, 221–22
publishing "aging America" theme, 163
media in the COVID Era
capturing the NH story, 29, 77–78, 99, 123, 215, 223, 239, 285
counting the dead, 77–78, 184, 227, 286
overlooking the voices of NH residents, 217–28
publishing the "doomed-to-die" narrative, 59–60, 91–92
vicarious vulnerability of journalists, 225
See also social media
Medicaid, as NH program, 14, 35, 73, 84, 119, 222, 278
fraud, 164, 225, 271
low funding per day vs. Medicare, 33–34, 47, 126
pauperizes residents, 207, 259–60
stigma of needing "welfare," 69, 226, 259–60
vulnerable to cost cutting, 64, 90, 267
medical advances in COVID Era
cohorting, 34